Hematology

Guest Editor

JOANNE B. MESSICK, VMD, PhD

VETERINARY CLINICS OF NORTH AMERICA: SMALL ANIMAL PRACTICE

www.vetsmall.theclinics.com

January 2012 • Volume 42 • Number 1

SAUNDERS an imprint of ELSEVIER, Inc.

W.B. SAUNDERS COMPANY
A Division of Elsevier Inc.

1600 John F. Kennedy Blvd. • Suite 1800 • Philadelphia, PA 19103-2899

http://www.vetsmall.theclinics.com

VETERINARY CLINICS OF NORTH AMERICA: SMALL ANIMAL PRACTICE Volume 42, Number 1
January 2012 ISSN 0195-5616, ISBN-13: 978-1-4557-3956-1

Editor: John Vassallo; j.vassallo@elsevier.com
Developmental Editor: Teia Stone

Veterinary Clinics of North America: Small Animal Practice (ISSN 0195-5616) is published bimonthly (For Post Office use only: volume 42 issue 1 of 6) by Elsevier Inc., 360 Park Avenue South, New York, NY 10010-1710. Months of issue are January, March, May, July, September, and November. Business and Editorial Offices: 1600 John F. Kennedy Blvd., Ste. 1800, Philadelphia, PA 19103-2899. Customer Service Office: 3251 Riverport Lane, Maryland Heights, MO 63043. Periodicals postage paid at New York, NY and additional mailing offices. Subscription prices are $283.00 per year (domestic individuals), $455.00 per year (domestic institutions), $138.00 per year (domestic students/residents), $375.00 per year (Canadian individuals), $559.00 per year (Canadian institutions), $416.00 per year (international individuals), $559.00 per year (international institutions), and $201.00 per year (international and Canadian students/residents). To receive student/resident rate, orders must be accompanied by name of affiliated institution, date of term, and the signature of program/residency coordinator on institution letterhead. Orders will be billed at individual rate until proof of status is received. Foreign air speed delivery is included in all Clinics subscription prices. All prices are subject to change without notice. **POSTMASTER:** Send address changes to Veterinary Clinics of North America: Small Animal Practice, Elsevier Health Sciences Division, Subscription Customer Service, 3251 Riverport Lane, Maryland Heights, MO 63043. Customer Service (orders, claims, online, change of address): Elsevier Periodicals Customer Service, Elsevier Health Sciences Division, Subscription Customer Service, 3251 Riverport Lane, Maryland Heights, MO 63043. Tel: 1-800-654-2452 (U.S. and Canada); 314-447-8871 (outside U.S. andCanada). Fax: 314-447-8029. E-mail: journalscustomerservice-usa@elsevier.com (for print support); journalsonlinesupport-usa@elsevier.com (for online support).

Reprints. For copies of 100 or more of articles in this publication, please contact the Commercial Reprints Department, Elsevier Inc., 360 Park Avenue South, New York, NY 10010-1710. Tel.: 212-633-3812; Fax: 212-462-1935; E-mail: reprints@elsevier.com.

Veterinary Clinics of North America: Small Animal Practice is also published in Japanese by Inter Zoo Publishing Co., Ltd., Aoyama Crystal-Bldg 5F, 3-5-12 Kitaaoyama, Minato-ku, Tokyo 107-0061, Japan.

Veterinary Clinics of North America: Small Animal Practice is covered in Current Contents/Agriculture, Biology and Environmental Sciences, Science Citation Index, ASCA, MEDLINE/PubMed (Index Medicus), Excerpta Medica, and BIOSIS.

Printed in the United States of America.

Contributors

GUEST EDITOR

JOANNE B. MESSICK, VMD, PhD
Diplomate, American College of Veterinary Pathologists; Associate Professor,
Department of Comparative Pathobiology, Purdue University, School of Veterinary
Medicine, West Lafayette, Indiana

AUTHORS

ANNE C. AVERY, VMD, PhD
Associate Professor and Director, Clinical Immunology Laboratory, Department of
Microbiology, Immunology and Pathology, College of Veterinary Medicine and
Biomedical Sciences, Colorado State University, Fort Collins, Colorado

ANNE M. BARGER, DVM, MS
Diplomate, American College of Veterinary Pathologists; Clinical Associate Professor,
Department of Pathobiology, College of Veterinary Medicine, University of Illinois,
Urbana, Illinois

MARY K. BOUDREAUX, DVM, PhD
Professor, Department of Pathobiology, Auburn University College of Veterinary
Medicine, Auburn, Alabama

MICHAEL O. CHILDRESS, DVM, MS
Diplomate, American College of Veterinary Internal Medicine (Oncology); Assistant
Professor of Comparative Oncology, Department of Veterinary Clinical Sciences, Purdue
University School of Veterinary Medicine, West Lafayette, Indiana

PETE W. CHRISTOPHERSON, DVM, PhD
Diplomate, American College of Veterinary Pathologists; Assistant Professor,
Department of Pathobiology, Auburn University College of Veterinary Medicine, Auburn,
Alabama

BENTE FLATLAND, DVM
Diplomate, American College of Veterinary Internal Medicine; Diplomate, American
College of Veterinary Pathologists; Assistant Professor of Clinical Pathology,
Department of Biomedical and Diagnostic Sciences, College of Veterinary Medicine,
University of Tennessee, Knoxville, Tennessee

MICHAEL M. FRY, DVM, MS
Diplomate, American College of Veterinary Pathologists (Clinical Pathology), Associate
Professor, Department of Biomedical and Diagnostic Sciences, College of Veterinary
Medicine, University of Tennessee, Knoxville, Tennessee

LUCA GIORI, DVM
Resident, Clinical Pathology, Department of Veterinary Pathology, Hygiene and Health,
Università degli Studi di Milano, Milano, Italy

CAROLYN N. GRIMES, DVM
Resident, Clinical Pathology, Department of Biomedical and Diagnostic Sciences,
College of Veterinary Medicine, University of Tennessee, Knoxville, Tennessee

JOHN W. HARVEY, DVM, PhD
Diplomate, American College of Veterinary Pathologists; Professor of Clinical Pathology
and Executive Associate Dean, College of Veterinary Medicine, University of Florida,
Gainesville, Florida

SHANNON JONES HOSTETTER, DVM, PhD
Diplomate, American College of Veterinary Pathologists; Assistant Professor,
Department of Veterinary Pathology, College of Veterinary Medicine, Iowa State
University, Ames, Iowa

JOANNE B. MESSICK, VMD, PhD
Diplomate, American College of Veterinary Pathologists; Associate Professor,
Department of Comparative Pathobiology, Purdue University, School of Veterinary
Medicine, West Lafayette, Indiana

JENNIFER L. OWEN, DVM, PhD
Clinical Pathology Resident, Department of Physiological Sciences, University of Florida
College of Veterinary Medicine, Gainesville, Florida

ROSE E. RASKIN, DVM, PhD
Diplomate, American College of Veterinary Pathologists; Department of Comparative
Pathobiology, Purdue University, School of Veterinary Medicine, West Lafayette, Indiana

AMY N. SCHNELLE, DVM
Veterinary Resident in Clinical Pathology, Department of Pathobiology, College of
Veterinary Medicine, University of Illinois, Urbana, Illinois

ELIZABETH A. SPANGLER, DVM, PhD
Diplomate, American College of Veterinary Internal Medicine; Diplomate, American
College of Veterinary Pathologists; Associate Professor, Department of Pathobiology,
Auburn University College of Veterinary Medicine, Auburn, Alabama

TRACY STOKOL, BVSc, PhD
Diplomate, American College of Veterinary Pathologists (Clinical Pathology); Associate
Professor, Department of Population Medicine and Diagnostic Sciences, College of
Veterinary Medicine, Cornell University, Ithaca, New York

LINDA M. VAP, MT, DVM
Diplomate, American College of Veterinary Pathologists; Instructor, Department of
Microbiology, Immunology, and Pathology, College of Veterinary Medicine and
Biomedical Sciences, Colorado State University, Fort Collins, Colorado

K. JANE WARDROP, DVM, MS
Diplomate, American College of Veterinary Pathologists; Department of Veterinary
Clinical Sciences, College of Veterinary Medicine, Washington State University, Pullman,
Washington

ELIZABETH G. WELLES, DVM, PhD
Diplomate, American College of Veterinary Pathologists; Professor, Department of
Pathobiology, Auburn University, Auburn, Alabama

MELINDA J. WILKERSON, DVM, MS, PhD
Associate Professor, Diagnostic Medicine/Pathobiology, Director of Clinical Immunology
and Flow Cytometry Laboratory, College of Veterinary Medicine, Kansas State
University, Manhattan, Kansas

Contents

> The decision to purchase an in-office hematology instrument is typically
> based on the desire to have immediate access to complete blood count
> (CBC) data for disease diagnosis and follow-up and perhaps add to the
> financial bottom line of your practice. The decision regarding which
> in-office hematology instrument to purchase requires comparison of
> available instruments, how they function and knowledge of their strengths
> and limitations, what analytes they report, their ease of use, and their initial
> and continued costs. Other considerations include instrument space
> requirements, ability to interact with your existing data management
> system, the methods used by analyzers, and data accuracy.

> This chapter provides recommendations for minimizing preanalytical,
> analytical, and postanalytical error during hematology testing of mam-
> mals. These recommendations are not intended to be all-inclusive;
> rather, they provide a minimum standard for hematology quality assur-
> ance and the maintenance and use of hematology point-of-care ana-
> lyzers. Written with the private practice setting in mind, the recommen-
> dations are also applicable to hematology in academic veterinary
> medical centers. Outlined are considerations for choosing a hematol-
> ogy instrument, nonstatistical quality assurance procedures important
> to hematology, and considerations for analyzing quality control mate-
> rials. A commitment to quality, including ongoing continuing education
> and training of veterinarians and veterinary technicians, is required to
> yield reliable results.

> Complete bone marrow evaluation should include a complete blood
> count (CBC), bone marrow cytologic biopsy, and bone marrow histo-
> logic biopsy. The CBC provides excellent quantitative and morphologic
> information. This information is complemented by the marrow cytology.
> When the cellularity of a bone marrow aspirate is low, it is difficult to

determine if this finding is due to "real" pathology or hemodilution of the sample. Histologic biopsy gives the best quantitative information regarding overall marrow cellularity. Methodical assessment should be made. Neglecting one or two parts of the evaluation often leaves unanswered questions; these three tests should be performed at the same time.

Coombs' Testing and Its Diagnostic Significance in Dogs and Cats   43

K. Jane Wardrop

The Coombs' test can detect both immunoglobulin and complement on the surface of red blood cells (RBCs), and as such can be of value as an aid in the diagnosis of immune-mediated hemolytic anemia (IMHA). Techniques that may improve sensitivity include use of monovalent reagents, increased dilutions of antiglobulin to avoid a prozone effect, and testing at 4°C. These techniques are not without controversy; positive tests should always be interpreted in the presence of other clinical and hematologic evidence for IMHA. Alternate techniques, such as flow cytometry, can improve detection of RBC-bound immunoglobulin but require a flow cytometer and further laboratory standardization.

Principles and Applications of Flow Cytometry and Cell Sorting in Companion Animal Medicine   53

Melinda J. Wilkerson

Flow cytometry measures multiple characteristics of single cells using light scatter properties and fluorescence properties of fluorescent probes with specificity to cellular constituents. The use in the veterinary clinical laborary has become more routine in veterinary diagnostic laboratories and institutions and reference laboratories. Common applications in small animal medicine includes quantitation of erythrocytes and leukocytes in automated hemology instruments, detection of antibodies to erythrocytes and platelets, immunophenotyping of leukocytes and lymphocytes in immunodeficiency syndromes or leukemias and lymphomas. DNA content analysis has not gained routine acceptance. Other applications including cell sorting and multiplexing are potential assays of the future.

Hemolytic Anemia in Dogs and Cats Due to Erythrocyte Enzyme Deficiencies   73

Jennifer L. Owen and John W. Harvey

The pathogenesis, laboratory diagnosis, and clinical implications of erythrocyte enzyme deficiencies in small animals are reviewed. Deficiencies of enzymes involved in erythrocyte metabolism can have significant effects on erythrocyte function and survival, resulting in hemolytic anemia. Animals with pyruvate kinase or phosphofructokinase deficiencies have shortened erythrocyte life spans and regenerative anemias, although the clinical presentations are very different. Understanding erythrocyte enzyme deficiencies and the tests needed to diagnose them is important in the differential diagnoses of anemia in small animals. Although enzymopathies are rare causes of anemia, the ability to identify deficient animals allows for the possibility of eliminating these undesirable traits in future breeding.

dyscrasias. These hematologic alterations may be hallmark features of certain malignancies and thus may serve as biomarkers of response to treatment or remission status, may complicate the therapeutic approach to the underlying tumor, and may have prognostic relevance. The etiopathogenesis, clinical significance, and tumor types most frequently associated with each of these abnormalities will be discussed. Where appropriate, a comparative review of similar hematologic findings in human cancer patients will be reviewed.

Neutrophil Function in Small Animals

Shannon Jones Hostetter

Neutrophils are motile phagocytes traditionally recognized for their role in innate immunity, representing the initial effector cell to eliminate bacterial and fungal pathogens. New evidence has highlighted their importance in numerous other processes, including the promotion and resolution of inflammation, amplification of adaptive immunity, and coagulation. Neutrophils are able to phagocytose and kill microbes, and create extracellular traps to ensnare and eradicate extracellular pathogens. Many of their diverse functions are linked to preformed proteins and effector molecules stored in granules. The importance of neutrophil function for animal health is emphasized through the discussion of inherited disorders of neutrophil function.

Evaluation and Clinical Application of Platelet Function Testing in Small Animal Practice

Pete W. Christopherson, Elizabeth A. Spangler, and Mary K. Boudreaux

Tests that evaluate many aspects of platelet function have been applied in both human and veterinary medicine to monitor treatment with platelet function inhibitors and detect platelet function abnormalities. Interspecies variation in the response to various platelet agonists is an important consideration when methods developed for people are applied in other species. Many of these assays are not available in standard veterinary practice. Advanced platelet function testing for veterinary patients is offered at select academic institutions. Discussion with a specialist is recommended when considering the use of these tests, and their relative strengths and limitations should be considered in interpretation of test results.

Laboratory Diagnosis of Disseminated Intravascular Coagulation in Dogs and Cats: The Past, the Present, and the Future

Tracy Stokol

The hemostatic system is an intricate co-operative network of proteins and cells that produces then dissolves fibrin clots. Disruptions in the balance between stimulatory and inhibitory forces that drive clotting and fibrinolysis cause hemorrhagic or thrombotic disorders, the most severe of which is disseminated intravascular coagulation (DIC). DIC is a secondary complication of infections, inflammation and neoplasia. It contributes to morbidity and mortality through systemic microvascular thrombosis. Since clinical signs and imaging techniques are insensitive to thrombosis, laboratory testing is essential for DIC detection. Early diagnosis and mitigation can potentially improve survival and decrease hospitalization costs of affected animals.

THE CLINICS ARE NOW AVAILABLE ONLINE!

Access your subscription at:
www.theclinics.com

Preface

Hematology

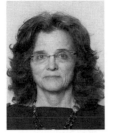

Joanne B. Messick, VMD, PhD
Guest Editor

As the standard of care changes in veterinary medicine, as novel technologies and treatment options develop, we are challenged to keep pace and understand the many advances. This is particularly true of veterinary hematology and is the impetus for this edition. We begin our hematology issue of *Veterinary Clinics of North America: Small Animal Practice* with a discussion of the newest and most widely used in-clinic hematology analyzers. These bench top systems are often smaller versions of large capacity laboratory analyzers providing blood cell counts with red cell indices and either a five- or a three-part white cell differential. Equally important is the inclusion of a complementary article that provides information and suggestions for using these systems and for providing reliable hematology results. These two articles as well as those related to Coombs' testing, understanding the causes and consequences of neutropenia, and diagnosis and monitoring disseminated intravascular coagulation provide an overview as well as information about more recent studies and advances related to these topics. Major hematologic abnormalities that may be identified in small animal cancer patients, including increases or decreases in the numbers of circulating blood cells, coagulopathies, and plasma protein dyscrasias, are also reviewed. There is clearly a need for future studies addressing the risk and clinical significance of these, and perhaps other, hematologic abnormalities to determine whether therapeutic intervention to correct them may improve patient outcome. Advances in molecular diagnostic techniques are not only changing the way in which we diagnose hematologic malignancies but are also providing us with new tools for making prognostic and treatment decisions in canine and feline malignancies. The principles and limitation of these procedures are an essential part of discussions in this article. While platelet and neutrophil function assays and testing for erythrocyte enzyme deficiencies are not readily available in standard veterinary practice, they are offered at select academic institutions. In separate articles, the importance of these assays is emphasized through a discussion of several inherited disorders. By identifying deficient animals, it may be possible to eliminate these undesirable traits in future breeding. Finally, we glimpse into the future, looking at the promising

Vet Clin Small Anim 42 (2012) xi–xii
doi:10.1016/j.cvsm.2011.11.002
0195-5616/12/$ – see front matter

diagnostic and therapeutic implications of hepcidin for veterinary species. This article also provides a review of the role of this hormone in physiologic homeostasis and pathologic processes.

I am greatly indebted to and thank all the authors for their outstanding contributions! It is my hope that we have included articles that will serve to increase the reader's knowledge of veterinary hematology while being of interest to a broad audience that includes the student, practitioner, specialist, and academic.

Joanne B. Messick, VMD, PhD
Department of Comparative Pathobiology
Purdue University
School of Veterinary Medicine
725 Harrison Street
West Lafayette, IN 47907, USA

E-mail address:
jmessic@purdue.edu

Automated In-Clinic Hematology Instruments for Small Animal Practitioners: What is Available, What Can They Really Do, and How Do I Make a Choice?

Elizabeth G. Welles, DVM, PhD

KEYWORDS

- Hematology • CBC • In-clinic hematology analyzers

WHAT IS AVAILABLE?

Instruments with 3 different methods of cell counting, or a combination of methods, are available and reasonably priced for purchase by individual or small groups of practitioners. These methods are quantitative buffy coat analysis, impedance analysis, and flow-cytometric analysis.

Quantitative Buffy Coat Analysis

An instrument based on quantitative buffy coat (QBC) analysis was the first in-clinic instrument available to veterinary practitioners; unfortunately, it is the least automated, provides the least number of analytes, and is the least accurate. The QBC Vet AutoRead is made by IDEXX Laboratories (Westbrook, ME, USA). This instrument is only semiautomated; it requires several manual steps, which are potential sources for the introduction of human errors. To perform counts and classify cell types, a person must draw blood into a specific tube by use of a dedicated pipetter, cap the tube, place a plastic float into the tube after mixing blood with a dye on the tube's interior, and properly load the tubes in a dedicated centrifuge. The principle of cell counting by the QBC is that after high-speed centrifugation of whole anticoagulated blood in a tube slightly longer and fatter than a typical microhematocrit tube, cells settle out in

---

The author has nothing to disclose.
Department of Pathobiology, Auburn University, 171 Greene Hall, Auburn, AL 36849-5519, USA
E-mail address: welleeg@auburn.edu

Vet Clin Small Anim 42 (2012) 1–9
doi:10.1016/j.cvsm.2011.09.003
0195-5616/12/$ – see front matter © 2012 Elsevier Inc. All rights reserved.

layers based on their density. This process is called differential centrifugation.[1,2] In order of greatest (bottom of the tube) to lowest (top of the tube) density, the cells layer in this order: erythrocytes, granulocytes, monocytes and lymphocytes, platelets, and then plasma. Leukocytes and platelets together constitute the buffy coat, which should never be used via direct visualization to estimate a total white count or platelet count. With QBC analysis, a small cylindrical plastic float with similar density as the buffy coat is placed in the tube prior to centrifugation. The float migrates to the area of the buffy coat during centrifugation and by displacement of cell-containing fluid around the float the buffy coat is expanded such that the length of each layer can be used to quantify the numbers of cells. A dye, acridine orange, coats the inside of each tube and binds to DNA, RNA, and lipoproteins in cells, which facilitates cell layer measurement via fluorescence with exposure to ultraviolet light. The automated reader of the samples determines changes in cell types by abrupt changes in fluorescence (slope) and produces a printout with analyte information in three different formats: as numbers (such as hematocrit, total white blood cells, WBC/μL, etc), as bars on an "idiot chart" that designate low, normal or high, and as a graph called a buffy coat analysis. The QBC does not provide a complete differential. Rather, the lymphocytes are grouped with monocytes and eosinophils are grouped with neutrophils (as granulocytes). In canine samples, eosinophil counts will be displayed separately from neutrophils if the eosinophils are a significant population within the leukocytes.

The QBC analyzer requires little or no maintenance. There is a calibration rod (painted metal rod) that should be run daily, but there are no real control materials available that can be run to allow the practitioner sufficient confidence that the results provided by the instrument are as accurate as possible. The sample run time is approximately 7 minutes (centrifugation and tube scanning/analysis). Evaluation of peripheral blood smears for cell morphology and verification of generated data should still be part of the routine CBC analysis.

Impedance Technology

Impedance technology–based instruments are the most numerous. These instruments are real workhorses with high reliability and dependability, fast sample cycle time, and high accuracy. They are relatively inexpensive to operate and have moderate in-house repair capabilities if you are willing to learn. Several instruments are available from different manufacturers including, but not limited to, Vet Scan ®HM II and HM V (Abaxis North America, Union City, CA, USA), scil Vet abc, scil Vet abc Plus, and scil Vet Focus 5 hematology analyzers (scil Animal Care Company, Gurnee, IL, USA), CBC-Diff and HemaTrue (Heska Corporation, Loveland, CO, USA), and Hemavet 950, Hemavet 950LV, Hemavet 950FS, and Hemavet 1700 (Drew Scientific Inc, Oxford, CT, USA). Each instrument has its own somewhat different bells and whistles, but essentially they are quite similar. These instruments can count and size cells. The principle of cell counting[1] is that cells proceed in single-cell fashion after dilution through a small aperture on either side of which are electrodes and between which a small electrical current flows. The cells moving through the aperture change the electrical impedance between electrodes and produce a voltage pulse that can be measured. Cells are enumerated by the numbers of generated voltage pulses within a designated time frame and cell size is proportional to the degree of voltage change. Leukocytes are enumerated after a solution is added to lyse erythrocytes. Differentiation of leukocyte types and platelets from erythrocytes is based on size as determined by magnitude of the change in voltage. Some manufacturer differences involve use of various lysing agents to which different cells show varying degrees of susceptibility to lyse, which helps distinguish cell types, while others use patented flow technology and software (Drew Scientific Inc has Focused Flow[R] technology)[3] for cell separation and categorization.

Impedance type counters use small volumes of anticoagulated blood (12 to 125 μL) and most have means of analyzing very small (12 to 25 μL) samples (micro-sample system for Heska instruments and predilution setting with Abaxis) when only very small sample volume is available, either because the patient is extremely small (such as mice, kittens, puppies), is very anemic, is dehydrated, or is uncooperative. Any size blood tube or syringe containing anticoagulant can be used.

Impedance type counters typically require minimal maintenance. The instruments automatically self-clean at specified intervals—6, 12, or 24 hours—which varies by instrument. Some require that a blank be used to test the background counts in the fluidics systems (Abaxis). The sample run times are short, typically between 1 and 3 minutes. The instruments have variable capacity for data storage. Liquid external control samples are available from manufacturers and should be used on a regular basis; daily prior to any patient samples are analyzed is best.

Flow Cytometric Analysis

The principle of flow-cytometry[1,2] is that micro-droplets of diluent containing single cells pass into a chamber through which a laser beam of light is shined. The absorption and scatter of the light after striking each cell are measured as forward angle scatter or side angle scatter. The diameter of each cell is determined by how long it takes to traverse the beam of light. Forward angle scatter (low) is used to count and size cells. Forward angle scatter (high) assesses the complexity of each cell and wide angle (right angle) scatter is affected by nuclear and internal cytoplasmic structures (granularity) and is used to differentiate leukocyte types and platelets from erythrocytes.

The LaserCyte made by IDEXX Laboratories is a flow-cytometry–based instrument. It is fully automated, which includes closed tube sampling to avoid sample contamination or spillage and within-instrument sample mixing (all instrument sample handling occurs beneath a cover and is not visualized by the user). For each sample the instrument uses individual tubes of reagent that contain tiny beads (qualiBeads[R]) that serve as internal controls in each sample run and across runs to assess that there has been correct pipetting and laser performance; however, there are no external control materials available for use as quality control samples. The instrument requires no daily maintenance owing to use of the qualiBeads[R], but the beads are not cells and cannot replace the use of external liquid controls. The instrument cycle time is quite long; results are provided in approximately 8 to 10 minutes and then the instrument continues cleaning itself for 5 to 7 additional minutes. And there are very limited to no means of performing any in-house troubleshooting.

The ProCyte Dx by IDEXX Laboratories utilizes a combination of flow-cytometric, optical fluorescence, and impedance analysis to count and differentiate cells.[2] Impedance technology is used to analyze erythrocytes, flow-cytometry and fluorescence are used to count leukocytes and perform leukocyte differential counts, and optical fluorescence is used to perform reticulocyte and platelet counts. The optical fluorescence analysis of cells eliminates interference between large erythrocytes and clumped platelets and provides additional specificity for analysis of leukocytes. External liquid quality controls are available.

As with the LaserCyte, the ProCyte Dx requires no sample preparation after proper collection of blood into specialized EDTA-containing tubes and seven or eight inversions to ensure proper mixing of blood with anticoagulant. There is closed tube sampling and on-board sample mixing. Sample cycle time is 2 minutes for the ProCyte Dx.

The IDEXX LaserCyte and ProCyte Dx use special blood tubes called IDEXX VetCollect[R] tubes. These tubes contain EDTA and are the size of a typical 5-mL sample draw tube, but they are intended to hold only 0.5 to 1.5 mL of whole blood. Although each instrument requires a small sample (95 or 30 μL for LaserCyte or ProCyte Dx, respectively), the instrument automated sampling system will not function properly if less than 0.5 mL or more than 1.5 mL of blood is present in the tubes.

WHAT CAN IN-CLINIC HEMATOLOGY INSTRUMENTS REALLY DO?

The IDEXX QBC provides the least CBC analytes (**Table 1**) and has the least accuracy of the various instruments based on results from several studies.[4,5] The instrument is semiautomated with several manual steps, which allow introduction of human error. The hematocrit from the QBC is quite accurate because it is basically a spun hematocrit (or packed cell volume [PCV]). The platelet count is provided as the number of platelets per microliter, but it is really a plateletcrit that has been converted to a platelet count. For dogs with macrothrombocytopenia,[6] this method of platelet enumeration (plateletcrit) appears to be more accurate than counts from instruments with other methodologies. The QBC method of platelet counting theoretically should be more accurate for cats and samples with clumped platelets[7,8]; however, this has not been found.[4] Feline platelets are often large and may have size overlap with their erythrocytes.[8] Impedance and, to a lesser extent, flow-cytometric instruments often count larger platelets and clumps of platelets as erythrocytes.[9] Platelet clumping is another problem often encountered in cats owing to the reactive nature of their platelets and because feline patients are often difficult to collect blood from with first-time, clean venipuncture. The inclusion of some platelets as erythrocytes has an almost imperceptible effect on red blood cells (RBCs) because there are only thousands of platelets and there are millions of erythrocytes. However, the patients are often reported to have thrombocytopenia. One should never believe a cat is thrombocytopenic based on instrument-derived values until a blood smear has been evaluated and platelet numbers have been estimated. With the ×100 (oil) objective, there should be an averaged minimum of 8 to 10 platelets per field; this is approximately 150,000 to 200,000 platelets/μL [formula: estimated platelet count/μL = average platelets per 100 (oil) objective field × 15,000 to 20,000].[10] Dogs with macrothrombocytopenia[11] (nearly all Cavalier King Charles Spaniels and a few individuals in several other breeds) have low numbers of platelets (30,000 to 100,000/μL often) that have large volume (12 to 34 fL or larger) such that the "platelet mass," which is typically normal (no bleeding tendency), is better represented by the plateletcrit.[6] Other measured analytes from the IDEXX QBC are less accurate than their counterparts as measured on impedance of flow-cytometric instruments.[5]

The main differences between the available analytes (see **Table 1**) from impedance-based and flow-cytometric/flow plus impedance–based instruments fall into 3 areas: nucleated RBC (nRBC) inclusion in the WBC, leukocyte differential, and reticulocyte determination results. Impedance-based instruments add lysing agents for erythrocyte removal prior to enumeration of leukocytes; however, the lysing agents actually lyse all cells. The nuclei of cells from which the cytoplasm is stripped are counted and sized; therefore, the nuclei of nRBCs are included as WBCs. This occasionally can lead to erroneous diagnoses when numerous nRBCs are in circulation such as in strongly regenerative anemias, in situations of vascular injury (sepsis or heat stroke), or in neoplastic or dysplastic conditions (erythroleukemia or

Table 1
Analytes included in CBC results from various in-clinic hematology instruments

Analyte	IDEXX QBC[2]	Vet Scan HMII[17] Vet Scan HMV	Heska CBC-Diff[18] Heska HemaTrue	Hemavet 950[3,c] Hemavet 1700[c]	scil Vet abc[19] scil Vet abc Plus scil Vet Focus 5[d]	IDEXX LaserCyte[2] IDEXX ProCyte[e]
RBC		X	X	X	X	X
HGB	X	X	X	X	X	X
HCT	X	X	X	X	X	X
MCV		X	X	X	X	X
MCH		X	X	X	X	X
MCHC	X	X	X	X	X	X
RDW		X	X	X		X
Reticulocytes, %	X					X
Absolute reticulocyte count						X
PLT	X	X	X	X	X	X
MPV		X	X	X		X
PDW						X
PCT						X
WBC	X	X	X	X	X	X
Neutros, %	X[a]	X	X	X	X	X
Lymphs, %		X	X	X	X	X
Monos, %		X	X	X	X	X
Lymph + mono, %	X					
Eos, %	X[a]	X[b]		X	Flagged if >5%	X
Baso, %		X[b]		X		X
Neutros, n	X[a]	X	X	X	X	X
Lymphs, n		X	X	X	X	X
Monos, n		X	X	X	X	X
Lymph + mono, n	X					
Eos, n	X[a]	X[b]		X	If >5%	X
Baso, n		X[b]		X		X

Abbreviations: HCT, hematocrit; HGB, hemoglobin; MCH, mean corpuscular hemoglobin; MCHC, mean corpuscular hemoglobin concentration; MCV, mean corpuscular volume; MPV, mean platelet volume; PCT, plateletcrit; PDW, platelet distribution width; PLT, platelets; RDW, red cell distribution width.

[a] Eosinophils cannot be differentiated from neutrophils in cats or horses.[2]

[b] Leukocyte 5-part differential available on HMV[16] for dogs, cats, and horses. Leukocyte 3-part differential available on HMV for mice, rabbits, rats, ferrets, pigs, cattle, and monkeys (research). Vet Scan HMII provides a 3-part leukocyte differential only on all validated species.

[c] Hemavet 950[3] offers CBC analysis on dogs, cats, calves, cattle, ferrets, foals, goats, Guinea pigs, horses, pigs, sheep, and rabbits. Hemavet 1700 has additional species including camel, deer, elephants, llamas, monkeys, mice, rats, and pre-diluted rats and mice.

[d] scil Vet Focus 5[18] appears to be identical to Hemavet 950 from Drew Scientific Inc.[3]

[e] IDEXX LaserCyte and ProCyte Dx[2] provide a 5-part differential on dogs, cats, horses, cattle, and ferrets. The 24 listed analytes are not available depending on species, such as retic percent and nRBC values are not available for horses.

Information obtained from manufacturer websites: IDEXX.com, Abaxis.com, Heska.com, Drew-scientific.com, and scil.com.

myelodysplastic syndrome-erythroid dominant). A 5-part leukocyte differential is available on dogs, cats, and horses on the Vet Scan HMV and on dogs, cats, horses, cattle, and ferrets on the IDEXX LaserCyte and ProCyte Dx.[2] The leukocyte differential is the weakest part of the CBC on all semiautomated and fully automated instruments, regardless of the manufacturers' claims.[5,6,12–16] A 5-part differential (neutrophils, lymphocytes, monocytes, eosinophils, and basophils) should provide the practitioner more information than does a 3-part differential (neutrophils, lymphocytes, and monocytes), but the cell types other than the most numerous type of cells (typically neutrophils) have questionable accuracy[12,15,16] and none of the instruments identify band neutrophils. Thus examination of cell morphology on a blood smear is essential for validation of data from these instruments as well as for identification of nucleated erythrocytes, neutrophilic left shifts (band neutrophils or earlier precursor cells), toxic changes in neutrophils, and lymphocyte and other leukocyte abnormalities and for the detection of low numbers of circulating blast-type cells or mast cells. Additionally, erythrocyte morphologic evaluation from blood smears is extremely beneficial in the pursuit of a cause of anemia. Flow cytometry–based instruments provide reticulocyte enumeration, which is quite helpful in determination of presence of regeneration in anemia, especially in dogs and cats. Results of reticulocyte analysis on a LaserCyte instrument showed only moderate accuracy compared with results from an Advia 120 (Siemens Healthcare Diagnostics, Deerfield, IL, USA; multispecies software), an instrument often considered a "gold standard" in diagnostic hematology. Reticulo-cytes were underreported in patients shown to have reticulocytes from Advia 120 data, and in those where they were reported, they were enumerated at lower values.[16]

HOW DO I DECIDE WHICH HEMATOLOGY INSTRUMENT IS BEST FOR ME AND MY PRACTICE?

There are numerous considerations that need to be made in the selection of the most suitable in-office hematology instrument for any particular practice (**Table 2**). How much space is available in which the instrument must fit? Does the instrument need to be near a sink for reagent disposal or in a cooler section of the building owing to sensitivity to heat or on a surface with no vibration such as avoidance of placement near a centrifuge? Some obvious considerations involve money issues. How much is the initial financial outlay to purchase the instrument? What are the costs of reagents, controls, and disposables? What is the warranty on the instrument and the cost of a service or repair contract after the warranty period? What is provided in the service or repair contract; for what exactly are you paying? I would suggest that you always have a service or repair contract because once you get accustomed to having an in-office hematology instrument you will not want to be without one. Can the instrument interface with other in-office instruments in your practice, such as a clinical chemistry or blood gas/electrolyte instrument? Is report storage in the instrument important to you? How important is the ability of the instrument to analyze blood from multiple different species? How important is the speed with which results are provided by the instrument? How important is it that the instrument has the capability to function with very small sample volume?

Some less obvious questions also must be considered. How is the in-office hematology instrument going to be used? Who will run the samples and control materials on the instrument? Does the manufacturer provide control reagents and what is their cost? Can data from control samples be stored and tracked for quality control assessment? (In the future in order to pass hospital inspections, clinics that use in-house hematology instruments and other analyzers may be required to show quality control records—that is, not just that appropriate controls are being run, but

Table 2
Selected characteristics of the various in-office hematology instruments

Parameter	IDEXX QBC	Vet Scan HMII Vet Scan HMV	Heska CBC-Diff Heska HemaTrue	Hemavet 950 Hemavet 1700	scil Vet abc scil Vet abc Plus scil Vet Focus 5	IDEXX LaserCyte IDEXX ProCyte
Sample size	~200 μL	50 μL	125 μL	20 μL	12 μL	95 μL LaserCyte 30 μL ProCyte
Microsample mode and amount	Not available	Automated calculations for 1:5 dilution for high values and small volume samples	20 μL True 20 sampling	Not needed, sample volume required very small	Not needed, sample volume required very small	Not available, sample volume required for ProCyte very small
Minimum blood in tube required	~500 μL	~100 μL ~20 μL for dilution	~200 μL ~20 μL for microsampling	~50 μL	~25 μL	0.5 mL (500 μL)
Sample run time	7 minutes	2–3 minutes	57 sec CBC-Diff 55 sec HemaTrue	2 min	1–1.5 min	Results in ~10 min, total time ~15 min for LaserCyte ~2 min ProCyte
Maintenance	Calibration rod daily	Self-cleaning daily Blank for fluidics every 12 hours	Self-cleaning daily	Self-cleaning daily	Self-cleaning daily	No daily maintenance for LaserCyte Cleaning for ProCyte touch button
Data storage	Not available	1000-2000 reports	Large volume	50 reports	300 reports	Large volume
Interaction with data management systems	IDEXX VetLab data management system	VetScan VS2 Analyzer and data management system	Heska data management system	Yes	Yes	IDEXX VetLab data management system

Information obtained from manufacturer websites: IDEXX.com, Abaxis.com, Heska.com, Drew-scientific.com, and scil.com.

that if there are problems, corrective actions are being taken.) And, finally, who will be in charge of the instrument care, maintenance, and record keeping?

My suggestions for how an in-office automated hematology instrument would be used are the following. (1) Use the hematology instrument to do CBCs on well patients prior to elective surgery, for obtainment of baseline data on geriatric well patients, or on minimally ill patients prior to needed surgery (such as cystotomy, subcutaneous mass removal, drain placement in abscesses, clean and repair trauma-induced wounds, etc). If the values from all analytes are within their reference intervals, then a blood smear may not have to be evaluated. You will miss a few inflammatory leukograms where the total leukocyte and neutrophil counts are within reference limits (no band neutrophils or earlier precursor cells are identified by any instrument), a few eosinophilias (if the instrument performs only a 3-part differential or even if a 5-part differential is provided, the differential data are questionable), some lymphoma/leukemia cases where the total numbers of leukocytes and the differentials are within reference limits, and a few other types of hematologic abnormalities. (2) Perform CBCs on ill patients, and if they have ANY values outside the reference intervals, then a blood smear should be evaluated by you, your technician, or sent to a laboratory where blood smears are evaluated on a daily basis. (3) Perform CBCs on patients for evaluation of disease progression or response to treatment. Compare and contrast the findings with previous data. These patients may or may not need to have blood smears evaluated dependant on the disorder being treated. Regardless of the desire of many busy practitioners that the in-office hematology instrument do a truly COMPLETE CBC, all hematology analyzers have limitations—cell morphologic changes cannot be assessed by any instrument. A pair of trained human eyes still must evaluate a well-made blood smear! Your decision to have an in-office hematology analyzer likely includes the desire to have more immediate diagnostic data towards disease identification, determination of health status of a patient, and evaluation of patient disease response to treatment. Additionally, the performance of diagnostic testing can offer a means of revenue generation once the initial investment has been recovered. These instruments, with proper care and maintenance, typically far outlast recovery of investment costs even if the CBC is priced fairly low. Remember to factor-in the cost of control materials into your prices; it is all part of providing accurate and reliable data for your clients.

Who will run the hematology instrument needs to be determined. The instruments last a lot longer if only a limited number of individuals have access to them. These individuals need to be trained, which is often a service provided by the instrument manufacturer, and then these individuals gain considerable insight into the nuances of their instrument based on daily use. The care of the instrument is paramount to its longevity. Most of these in-office hematology instruments are fairly rugged, some are virtual workhorses, but all will have longer life if proper care is provided. Cleanliness is next to godliness is aptly applied to these situations.

SUMMARY

To have an in-clinic hematology instrument in your practice and how it is used are decisions that precede the purchase of an instrument. Advantages and limitations of the various instruments should be considered. Initial purchase cost, reagent/disposable costs, costs of training personnel in the use and care of the instrument, and service/repair contract costs need to be considered.

Once the decision is made to have an in-office hematology instrument in your practice you should benefit from having nearly immediate CBC data results that enable you to provide better quality medicine, more rapid clinical decisions, more closely monitor patients for complications of disease or response to treatment. It should also generate revenue and allow some of your staff members to expand and develop their technical skills as they learn the nuances of a new diagnostic tool and how to provide you with the most accurate CBC information. In the final assessment, the addition of an in-office hematology instrument should improve the quality and efficiency of the medical care you provide patients and generate additional practice income.

REFERENCES

1. Rebar AH, MacWilliams PS, Feldman BF, et al. IDEXX Laboratories Guide to Hematology in dogs and cats. Jackson (WY): Teton NewMedia; 2002. p. 22–8.
2. IDEXX Laboratories. Website. http://www.IDEXX.com.
3. Drew Scientific, Inc. Website. http://www.Drew-scientific.com.
4. Papasouliotis K, Cue S, Graham M, et al. Analysis of feline, canine and equine hemograms using the QBC VetAutoread. Vet Clin Pathol 1999;28:109–15.
5. Bienzle D, Stanton JB, Embry JM, et al. Evaluation of an in-house centrifugal hematology analyzer for use in veterinary practice. J Am Vet Med Assoc 2000;217: 1195–200.
6. Tvedten H, Lilliehook I, Hillstrom A, et al. Plateletcrit is superior to platelet count for assessing platelet status in Cavalier King Charles Spaniels. Vet Clin Pathol 2008;37: 266–71.
7. Koplitz SL, Scott MA, Cohn LA. Effects of platelet clumping on platelet concentrations measured by use of impedance or buffy coat analysis in dogs. J Am Vet Med Assoc 2001;219:1552–6.
8. Norman EJ, Barron RC, Nash AS, et al. Prevalence of low automated platelet counts in cats: Comparison with prevalence of thrombocytopenia based on blood smear estimation. Vet Clin Pathol 2001;30:137–40.
9. Zelmanovic D, Hetherington EJ. Automated analysis of feline platelets in whole blood, including platelet count, mean platelet volume, and activation state. Vet Clin Pathol 1998;27:2–9.
10. Tvedten H, Grabski S, Frame L. Estimating platelets and leukocytes on canine blood smears. Vet Clin Pathol 1988;17:4–6.
11. Davis B, Toivio-Kinnucan M, Schuller S, et al. Mutation in beta-1 *tubulin* correlates with macrothrombocytopenia in Cavalier King Charles Spaniels. J Vet Intern Med 2008;22:540–5.
12. Papasouliotis K, Cue S, Crawford E, et al. Comparison of white blood cell differential percentages determined by the in-house LaserCyte hematology analyzer and a manual method. Vet Clin Pathol 2006;35:295–302.
13. Perkins P, Reagan W, Marweg L, et al. Evaluation of the Vet ABC-Diff hematology analyzer for performing hemograms on dog and cat blood. Vet Clin Pathol 1999;28: 120–1.
14. Schwendenwein I, Jolly M. Automated differentials by an impedance on-site hematology system. Vet Clin Pathol 2000;30:158.
15. Dewhurst EC, Crawford E, Cue S, et al. Analysis of canine and feline haemograms using the VetScan HMT analyzer. J Small An Pract 2003;44:443–8.
16. Welles EG, Hall AS, Carpenter DM. Canine complete blood counts: a comparison of four in-office instruments with the ADVIA 120 and manual differential counts. Vet Clin Pathol 2009;38:20–9.
17. Abaxis website: http://www.Abaxis.com.
18. Heska Corporation website: http://www.Heska.com.
19. scil website: http://www.scil.com.

Quality Management Recommendations for Automated and Manual In-House Hematology of Domestic Animals

Bente Flatland, DVM[a],*, Linda M. Vap, MT, DVM[b]

KEYWORDS

- Hematology • Point-of-care • Quality assurance
- Quality control • Veterinary

The term *point-of-care testing* (POCT) broadly refers to any laboratory testing performed outside the conventional reference laboratory and implies testing in close proximity to patients (aka "bedside," "near-patient," "decentralized," or "extralaboratory" testing).[1-3] In-house hematology testing has distinct advantages, including analysis of freshly drawn blood samples, short turnaround time for results, and the fact that in-house laboratory testing may provide a revenue stream. Additionally, blood smear review may be enjoyable for veterinarians and veterinary technicians interested in hematology and hematopathology. Considerations for and potential limitations of in-house hematology testing include the patient population served (eg, predominantly healthy vs emergency practice), direct and indirect costs of purchasing, using and maintaining in-house laboratory equipment, the need for personnel training and a commitment to ongoing quality management, and potential liability associated with issuing erroneous laboratory results.

Point-of-care analyzers (POCAs) are numerous and varied in complexity; analytical methods used in hematology POCA include centrifugation, impedance counter, and

The authors have nothing to disclose.

Recommendations made herein are adapted from a draft guideline for point-of-care testing in veterinary medicine, currently being written by the American Society for Veterinary Clinical Pathology (ASVCP) Quality Assurance and Laboratory Standards (QALS) Committee, and are used with permission of the ASVCP.

[a] Department of Biomedical and Diagnostic Sciences, College of Veterinary Medicine, University of Tennessee, 2407 River Drive, Knoxville, TN 37996, USA

[b] Department of Microbiology, Immunology, and Pathology, College of Veterinary Medicine and Biomedical Sciences, Colorado State University, 300 West Drake Road, Fort Collins, CO 80523-1644, USA

* Corresponding author.

E-mail address: bflatlan@utk.edu

Vet Clin Small Anim 42 (2012) 11–22

doi:10.1016/j.cvsm.2011.09.004

0195-5616/12/$ – see front matter © 2012 Elsevier Inc. All rights reserved.

vetsmall.theclinics.com

laser light-scatter systems.[4] (The reader is referred to article by Elizabeth G. Welles elsewhere in this issue for a complete discussion of available hematology instruments for the veterinary practice.) Factors that may influence selection of hematology POCA for a given veterinary hospital include the following:

- Direct and indirect costs
  - Instrument purchase vs lease
  - Reagent cost-per-billable test
    - Open container shelf-life
  - Quality control materials
    - Availability
    - Cost
    - Open container shelf-life
  - Proficiency testing
  - Maintenance/service contracts
  - Technical time
- Distinguishing test menu items
  - Differential: 3-part vs 5-part
  - Fibrinogen estimate, microfilaria detection (centrifugal only)
  - Erythrocyte indices (MCV by impedance or light scatter)
  - Mean platelet volume (MPV by impedance or light scatter)
  - Reticulocyte count (light scatter, estimate by centrifugal)
- Species capabilities
- Sample
  - Volume requirements (micro)
  - Type capabilities (some hematology POCA can also assay cavity fluids)
- Instrument
  - Size ("footprint")
  - Ease of operation and use of software
  - Turnaround time/throughput capability
  - Data management
    - Report format
    - Data storage and recall
    - Flags: operational, abnormal values, etc
    - Histograms or cytograms that aid data interpretation
  - Maintenance requirements
  - Analytical performance and quality control
- Health and safety considerations (including reagents, samples, and waste)
  - Infection control
- Customer support
  - Training and continuing education for instrument operators
  - Technical service provided by the manufacturer.

Generally speaking, hemic cells from birds, reptiles, and fish cannot be accurately enumerated using automated analyzers; this is due to the presence of nucleated red blood cells (RBCs) and thrombocytes in these species interfering with instrument's cell counting functions.[5] Hemocytometers and specialized pipette systems are used for exotic animal hematology; however, they are not covered this chapter. The reader is directed to the September 2008 edition of *Veterinary Clinics of North America: Exotic Animal Practice* in which hematology of these species is covered in detail.[6]

The following recommendations are not intended to be all-inclusive; rather, they provide a minimum standard for hematology quality assurance (QA) and maintenance of hematology POCA in the veterinary setting.

PERSONNEL TRAINING, HEALTH, AND SAFETY

Manufacturer's directions for instrument use and reagent handling and storage should be strictly followed. Qualified, adequately trained personnel should perform sample collection and handling as well as the making and evaluation of blood smears.

Working conditions for personnel performing CBCs should be comfortable and appropriate. Personnel should receive appropriate training from the hematology POCA instrument manufacturer, with periodic continuing education (provided by the manufacturer and/or veterinary organizations) as needed to maintain skills and knowledge. Personnel should receive appropriate safety and biohazard training for the handling and disposal of biologic materials (including information about transmission of potential infectious agents) and reagents. All training should be documented, and relevant local, state, and federal health and safety guidelines should be followed where applicable.[7]

MINIMIZING PREANALYTICAL ERROR

All patient samples should be clearly identified (eg, using patient name and/or identification number) and date/time of collection indicated on the tube. Blood sample CBCs in domestic animal species should be collected via direct venipuncture or, if collected from an intravenous line, after removal of sufficient contaminating fluid. Samples should be collected into potassium ethylenediaminetetraacetic acid (EDTA) (K_2EDTA or K_3EDTA) tubes, and tubes should not be underfilled (particularly if these contain liquid EDTA) or overfilled, which may result in clotting. Following collection, the sample should be thoroughly mixed with the anticoagulant by inverting the tube slowly at least 10 times.[8] Samples should be processed as soon as possible following collection. If a delay in analysis is anticipated, tubes of blood may be refrigerated at 4°C for up to 24 hours[8]; these should be brought to room temperature and gently, well mixed before analysis (by gentle manual inversion at least 50 times or several minutes on an automated blood mixer). Blood smears should be air-dried, and left unrefrigerated. Blood smears are best made immediately after blood collection and dried quickly to avoid crenation of cells. Smears that are shipped to outside laboratories for review should be protected from condensation, freezing, and formalin fumes.[7] Blood smears should be stained using a Romanowsky-family stain[8] that is fresh and uncontaminated by microorganisms.

Prior to analysis, blood samples should be visually inspected for gross clots. Clotted samples should not be analyzed, as cell counts will be inaccurate. If gross clots are not visible, the sample should be checked for small clots by gently stirring the sample with one or more clean, wooden applicator sticks; clots will adhere to the stick(s). Such small clots may plug tubing or apertures inside the POCA, affecting accuracy, particularly of platelet counts, and requiring instrument maintenance; if no small clots are found, the sample may be analyzed. Blood samples should be thoroughly mixed using gentle inversion immediately prior to analysis and making blood films. Any delay after sample collection may result in settling, particularly in ill animals, and automated results or cell distribution in the film will vary depending on the location of aliquot of blood removed from the sample tube.[9] Blood smears should be made carefully, and only smears of good to excellent quality should be examined. Blood smear technique is explained elsewhere.[9]

QUALITY ASSURANCE AND QUALITY CONTROL

QA considers all phases of the laboratory testing process and includes both nonstatistical QA procedures and quality control (QC, or statistical QC). Nonstatistical QA procedures include many common-sense procedures already performed in veterinary practices on a routine basis and help to minimize preanalytical, analytical, and postanalytical error. QC refers to analysis of quality control materials (QCM) and the statistical techniques applied to analysis of control data; QC helps to identify analytical error specifically.[10]

Nonstatistical QA for Automated and Manual Hematology

Nonstatistical QA procedures recommended for hematology and the management of hematology POCA include the following[7,11]:

- Provide and follow written standard operating procedure(s) [SOP(s)] for use and maintenance of hematology POCA and for performing related tasks, including sample acquisition, sample handling and storage, and the making of blood smears.
- Adequate personnel training (and documentation thereof)
- Inspection of hematocrit (Hct), packed cell volume (PCV), hemoglobin (Hgb), and mean cell (corpuscular) hemoglobin concentration (MCHC) results
- Microscopic evaluation of a well-made blood smear by an adequately trained individual
- Use of medical review criteria
- Use of repeat criteria
- Correlation of laboratory data with other clinical findings
- Documentation of POCA maintenance and repairs
- Documentation of maintenance and/or verification of:
  ○ Water quality and electrical power stability
  ○ Refrigerator, freezer, and water bath temperatures
  ○ Pipette volume
  ○ Centrifuge speed (or g force)
  ○ Microscopes.

Written SOPs ensure that all personnel performing CBCs and making blood smears adhere to the same procedures. SOPs should be reviewed and updated periodically (yearly is recommended), and a document control policy should be in place to ensure that outdated SOP versions are removed from circulation. Suggested SOP contents can be found in the American Society for Veterinary Clinical Pathology (ASVCP) Quality Assurance Guidelines; these guidelines are on the Society's website (http://www.asvcp.org/pubs/qas/index.cfm).[7] SOPs can also be used for personnel training; training and continuing education of personnel performing CBCs should be documented.

Hct is the percentage of blood volume composed of RBCs in the sample and is calculated by the POCA using the RBC concentration and mean cell volume (MCV).[12] PCV (or "spun hematocrit") is the percentage of blood volumes composed of RBCs in the sample as determined using a microhematocrit tube, centrifuge, and capillary tube reader.[12] Because a small amount of plasma and some platelets and leukocytes become trapped within the RBC column inside a microhematocrit tube, PCV may be slightly higher than Hct as reported by the POCA.[12] If concurrent PCV and Hct values disagree by greater than 3%, results should be investigated. Visual inspection of the capillary tube used to generate PCV is also helpful; color of the plasma layer may indicate lipemia, hemolysis, or icterus.

MCHC is calculated using Hgb concentration and Hct.[12] Assuming MCHC is in the range of 32 to 26 g/dL, the numerical value of the measured blood Hgb concentration should be approximately one-third of the Hct numerical value[12]; if this is not the case, results should be investigated. Hgb is measured via spectrophotometry and is therefore subject to interference by lipemia, markedly increased Heinz bodies, and (in some analytical systems) precipitation of globulin proteins.[12] Additionally, sample hemolysis increases MCHC because the proportion of free Hgb relative to intact RBCs in the sample is increased.[12] Increased MCHC is almost always an artifact and should prompt investigation of hemolysis, lipemia, or Heinz bodies.[12] If evidence for these artifacts is lacking, appropriate instrument operation should be confirmed with QCM and/or technical services should be contacted for assistance.

Microscopic evaluation of a well-made blood smear is an essential component of performing any CBC and should be performed in all cases by adequately trained personnel using good quality smears.[8] Blood smear examination need not be exhaustive or lengthy; rapid but complete examination of a blood smear and comparison of microscopic findings to numerical POCA data can be performed in a matter of minutes. Blood smear evaluation may identify the following problems, which may not or cannot be detected or reported by automated hematology analyzers: presence of nucleated RBCs (nRBCs), RBC poikilocytosis, Heinz bodies, neutrophil left shift, neutrophil toxic change, neoplastic cells, hemoparasites and other infectious organisms, platelet clumps, and large or giant platelets. The hematology POCA's automated differential WBC should be verified by microscopic examination of a blood smear. If more than 10 nRBCs/100 WBCs are identified, the automated total WBC count should be corrected,[8] and the absolute WBC differential results should be recalculated using the corrected total WBC count. If bands or abnormal leukocytes (eg, neoplastic cells) are identified, a manual WBC differential count should be performed and reported in place of any automated WBC differential count.

Medical review criteria are criteria used by personnel performing CBCs and blood smear evaluation that trigger review of a blood smear and concurrent CBC data by a veterinarian or board-certified veterinary clinical pathologist. Criteria may also be established to guide when automated differential WBC counts should be rejected in favor of manual WBC counts. Example manual differential and medical review criteria are presented in **Tables 1** and **2**, respectively.

Repeat criteria refers to criteria used by personnel performing CBCs that trigger repeat evaluation of the blood sample in question; these may overlap with medical review criteria. Example repeat criteria include presence of instrument error flags, results considered physiologically improbable (incompatible with life), or results that are inconsistent with other clinical findings.

CBC data should not be interpreted in a vacuum, and establishing that CBC findings correlate with other relevant clinical findings (physical examination, other laboratory data, imaging studies) in a given patient is important.[11] Results appearing clinically improbable (incompatible with other relevant clinical data) or physiologically improbable (incompatible with life) should be investigated.

Keeping an instrument log for the hematology POCA is recommended. Maintenance and quality control procedures should carried out as instructed by the manufacturer and results documented in the instrument log. Repairs and software upgrades should also be documented in such a log. In addition to maintaining the hematology POCA itself, additional relevant equipment that should be adequately maintained and monitored includes centrifuges, pipettes, refrigerators, and microscopes.

Table 1
Criteria for performing a manual WBC differential count

Presence of . . .	Suggested Cut-Off Value	Comments
Nucleated RBCs	If more than rare nRBC	Perform and report a manual differential count. Correct automated total WBC count for the number of nRBC if >10 nRBC/100 WBC. Recalculate absolute differential results using the corrected WBC count.
Neutrophil left shift	>1 band and/or earlier neutrophils forms (eg, metamyelocyte) observed	Perform and report a manual differential count, enumerating neutrophil forms (segmented, band, metamyelocyte, etc) separately. Note whether toxic change is present. Correct absolute differential results (eg, the neutrophils will now be split into bands and neutrophils).
Unclassified (unidentified) cells	Any	Perform and report a manual differential count, enumerating the unclassified cells in an "other" category. Describe morphology of the unclassified cells. Recalculate absolute differential results.
Subjective impression that automated WBC differential count may not be accurate	N/A	If for any reason the automated WBC differential count is suspect, perform a manual WBC differential count to verify it. Eg, is there is lack of clear distinction between cell types on histograms or cytograms.

Should You "Run Controls"? What Should You Do with Control Data?

The best way to determine whether a laboratory analyzer is performing adequately is to assay material having known analyte concentrations ("run controls"). Data resulting from analysis of such materials can then be examined and a determination made regarding whether POCA analytical performance is adequate (ie, suitable for analysis of patient samples). The purpose of performing quality control (QC) using materials having known analyte concentrations is to detect analytical error that *exceeds expected instrument performance, given stable operation in a routine setting*. At its most basic, the purpose of "running controls" is to detect faulty POCA operation that might lead to erroneous patient results.[10]

Materials having known analyte concentrations include calibrators and QCM. Calibrators, used to adjust how laboratory instruments measure, are available for some hematology POCA but will not be covered in these guidelines. Use of QCM is encouraged and is the best way to confirm proper function of the *entire hematology*

Table 2
Suggested criteria for medical review of blood smears and concurrent CBC data

Medical reviews should be performed by the attending veterinarian. Send blood smears and EDTA-anticoagulated whole blood to a board-certified clinical pathologist as needed to confirm abnormal findings.

Blood Smear	Criteria Triggering a Review
Background	Unusual background matrix Unusual background color Organisms or suspected organisms
Red Blood Cells	Moderate to marked poikilocytosis of any kind; moderate to severe anemias Reticulocytosis >300,000 cells/μL Any Heinz bodies in a non-feline species; >10% Heinz bodies in cats Any non-routine[a] inclusions (including organisms or suspected organisms) Basophilic stippling, siderocytes, or Howell-Jolly bodies in dog 10 nRBC/100 WBC in non-equine species; any nRBC in horses Abnormal MCV
White Blood Cells	Left shift of >5,000 bands/μL or any left shift with neutrophils forms less mature than bands; Leukopenia <3,000 WBC/μL Any left shift where immature neutrophil forms outnumber segmented neutrophils Leukocytosis >50,000 WBC/μL in non-ruminants; leukocytosis >30,000 WBC/μL in ruminants and horses Lymphocytosis >10,000 cells/μL; Monocytosis >4,000 cells/μL; Eosinophilia >4,000 cells/μL; Basophilia >1,000 cells/μL Any unclassified cells Any organisms or suspected organisms; Presence of vacuoles in non-monocytes and abnormal granulation in any leukocyte, other than toxic granulation in neutrophils)
Platelets	Platelet count >900,000 cells/μL (except pigs and ruminants); moderate to severe thrombocytopenia <100,000 cells/μL Abnormal MPV (if reported by instrument) Suspected inclusions or abnormal granulation

[a] Low numbers of Howell-Jolly bodies may be considered a "routine" RBC inclusion in cats and horses, but not dogs.

POCA system (instrument, reagents, and operator).[10] Commercial QCM are available for select veterinary hematology POCA. Hematology QCM are not as stable as those for chemistry analyzers; attention to shelf-life and proper handling and storage is critical. Most QCM require refrigerated storage; these should be brought to room temperature prior and mixed thoroughly (but gently) prior to use. Once a QCM tube or vial has been opened, accumulated material should be cleaned from the outside surfaces of the container opening prior to resealing to prevent drying and particles contaminating the vial when opened at a later time. Similarly, surfaces adjacent to the aspiration area should be kept clean to avoid particle buildup and potential sample or QCM contamination.

Daily QC (ie, analyzing QCM each day that the POCA is to be used for patient samples) is an ideal recommendation adopted from human medicine. This

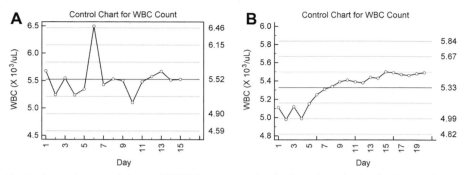

Fig. 1. Example control charts. (*A*) WBC concentration is plotted on the *y*-axis. Time in days is plotted on the *x*-axis. The mean (5.52 × 10³/μL) is represented by a solid line drawn parallel to the *x*-axis. Mean ±1 standard deviation, mean ±2 standard deviations, and mean ±3 standard deviations are represented by dashed lines drawn parallel to the *x*-axis. Traditionally, QC data points considered "unacceptable" on Levy-Jennings control charts are those falling outside mean ±2 standard deviations. On this chart, only one data point (day 6) is "out-of-control" using this rule. (Application of other statistical control rules may result in alternate control limits.) Unacceptable QC results should prompt trouble-shooting of the instrument, reagents, and operator. The manufacturer's technical representative should be contacted if obvious problems with reagents and operators have been ruled out and if the problem cannot be resolved with routine maintenance and operational procedures. (*B*) Control charts are also useful for evaluating data trends over time (eg, is there "drift" in a positive or negative direction?). Here, the mean is 5.33 × 10³/μL. A clear positive data trend is visible on this control chart; this drift should prompt troubleshooting, and the manufacturer's technical representative should be contacted if obvious problems with reagents and operators have been ruled out and if the problem cannot be resolved with routine maintenance and operational procedures.

recommendation may not be suitable for all veterinary clinics, depending upon the POCA analyzer type, clinic operating budget, and caseload. Generally, the lower the caseload, the more frequently QCM should be analyzed (with higher caseloads, aberrant trends in patient data may assist in detection of analytical error). Each veterinary practice using POCA must determine frequency of their QC based on these factors; at least daily QC is encouraged if possible. QC should be performed frequently enough that QCM are used cost-effectively and that POCA analytical error can be reliably detected.

A *control run* refers to one analysis (measurement) of a QCM. *Control data* refer to laboratory results generated by analysis of QCM. Control results should be recorded and archived. Results falling outside the QCM manufacturer's reported range (available in the QCM package insert) or those accompanied by instrument error flags should prompt investigation of the POCA itself, reagents, and/or instrument operators.

In addition recording and archiving numerical results in the POCA instrument log, control data may be graphed for visual inspection of trends over time. *Control charts*, which graph time on the *x*-axis and analyte concentration on the *y*-axis, are graphical displays of control data that show where QC data points fall in relation to the mean value. Control charts are very useful for spotting marked deviations from the mean as well as "drifts" over time that might prompt investigation of POCA function. The Westgard QC website[13] has an interactive tool demonstrating control charts. An example of a control chart is also provided in **Fig. 1**. The ability to construct and print out control charts is available with some POCA software packages.

What defines a "marked deviation" from the mean (ie, what are the "control limits" that define an unacceptable QC data point)? Traditionally (with Levy-Jennings control charts), data points falling outside ±2 standard deviations from the mean are considered "unacceptable" and should prompt investigation. Generic application of this rule has good probability for detecting analytical error; however, it may cause false rejection of a small percentage of acceptable control runs (resulting in increased expense if QCM are reanalyzed to verify an unacceptable result).[14] Today (at least in clinical pathology laboratories, where statistical QC using validated rules is more common), this traditional rule (aka the 1_{2s} rule) is more often thought of as a "warning" rule that should prompt investigation of control data using further statistical rules; generic application of 1_{2s} as the only control rule is no longer recommended when statistical QC using validated rules is possible.[15]

Comparing control results to QCM manufacturer's recommended ranges for that QCM is another way to determine whether control results are acceptable or unacceptable. POCA operators should ensure that the QCM used are designed for use with the instrument in question (ie, are appropriate for that analytical method and instrument model). Again, any control results falling outside manufacturer's limits or accompanied by instrument error flags should prompt investigation of POCA function. A data log should be maintained as a record of control results. POCA operators should be aware that this method of deciding whether control data are "acceptable" is less robust than statistical QC (see later).

What Is Statistical QC, and Is It Relevant to In-House Hematology?

Statistical QC refers to use of statistical rules (aka *control rules* or *Westgard rules*) to determine whether control results are acceptable ("in control") or unacceptable ("out of control"). The Levy-Jennings control chart rule, discussed above, is an example of a simple control rule; many different rules are possible. Statistical QC using a carefully chosen rule (or rule combination) is the most robust means of ascertaining whether control data are acceptable or unacceptable, because the process of choosing the statistical rules used to make this determination (a process called *QC validation*) takes into account (1) a particular instrument's inherent total analytical error and (2) a previously established benchmark of acceptable analytical performance (known as a *quality requirement*). Instrument analytical performance is a limiting factor and must be robust enough to allow this type of QC. Knowing a particular POCA's inherent total errors requires either obtaining minimum performance specifications from the instrument manufacturer or carrying out an instrument performance study to determine that POCA's imprecision (represented by coefficient of variation, or CV) and bias. Measured CV and bias are then used to calculate observed total error (TE_{obs}). Currently, in veterinary medicine, there is no consensus about quality requirement (often represented by allowable total error, or TEa) for commonly measured analytes in the major domestic species.

While used in many veterinary clinical pathology laboratories, statistical QC is not routinely used in veterinary private practice at this time. A major hurdle to its implementation is lack of training in laboratory quality management for veterinarians and veterinary technicians. Concern about the lack of laboratory quality management training in veterinary curricula has been expressed in prior published literature[10]; in the authors' experience, this deficit is still present today. Discussion among veterinary clinical pathologists serving as consultants to private veterinary practitioners identified that a lack of knowledge about what to do with control data is a commonly cited reason for why private practitioners do not use QCM routinely.[10] This knowledge gap may slowly narrow in future, as more continuing education and guidelines on this topic become available.

A second potential hurdle to implementation of statistical QC in veterinary private practice is the analytical performance capability of commonly used POCA. A recent study of biochemistry POCAs housed in various private practices found that analytical performance varies markedly, even among POCA of the same type.[16] For some instruments, for some analytes, analytical performance capability may not be robust enough such that desired quality requirements can be met and statistical QC applied.[16] It is also possible that the problem is not intrinsic to the instrument or the analyte being evaluated, but rather reflects a problem with assay reagents (eg, outdated, contaminated, improperly stored) or even instrument maintenance. Nevertheless, analytical performance capabilities of POCA available to veterinarians is an issue that requires further study and must ultimately be addressed by POCA manufacturers, with input from the veterinary community. Additionally, consensus within the veterinary community is needed regarding acceptable global quality goals for commonly measured analytes in the major domestic species.[16]

Statistical QC and a simple control rule *can* be used with biochemistry and hematology POCAs[16]; these programs are routinely used in commercial and university veterinary laboratories. Only by implementing such a program for hematology POCA in the private clinic setting can the practitioner assure his or her clients of the quality and reliability of the laboratory data generated. Successful implementation of statistical QC requires a firm commitment to quality and training in basic QC principles. Additional scientific studies are needed to document the implementation and benefits of statistical QC in veterinary private practice and to compare error detection ability and benefits of statistical QC procedures with "internal" (electronic) QC procedures found in some instruments.

PARTICIPATION IN EXTERNAL QUALITY ASSURANCE PROGRAMS

External quality assurance (EQA) programs (aka proficiency testing programs) are programs in which participants analyze aliquots of the same sample; frequency of testing varies between programs and modules within programs (eg, quarterly, biannually). Results are reported to the program organizers, who compile data from all participants and report these to the participating facilities with relevant statistics (means, standard deviations, etc).[17] In veterinary medicine, participation in an EQA program is voluntary (ie, not mandated by government regulation). The value of an EQA program is proportional to the number of participants.[17]

EQA programs can be an important way to monitor analytical performance and are particularly important for tests providing discrete categorical results, including CBCs.[17] EQA data may detect slowly developing analytical error that can be missed with in-house QC procedures.[17] An important consideration is that, for meaningful interpretation, a facility's laboratory results must be compared to those from an *appropriate peer group* (ie, must be compared to other practices or laboratories using the same analytical methodology).[7] Marked deviation from an appropriate peer group mean (or other benchmark of acceptable performance provided by the EQA program) should prompt investigation of the test in question (instrument, reagents, operator).[7] A limitation of proficiency testing for private practitioners using POCA is that current veterinary EQA programs are predominantly utilized by reference laboratories using large, sophisticated analyzers; thus an appropriate peer group using the same or similar analytical methods may be difficult for veterinary POCA users to find.

MINIMIZING POSTANALYTICAL ERROR

CBC data should be reported in a standard format decided upon by the individual veterinary hospital. Results should be communicated to the attending veterinarian and animal owner in a timely fashion.[7]

If any CBC results are known to be inaccurate, these should not be reported.[7] Automated platelet counts should not be reported if significant platelet clumping is observed on blood smear review. Many large clumps will falsely lower automated platelet counts. Unexpectedly low platelet counts (based on patient condition and other clinical information) should prompt evaluation of a blood smear to look for obvious platelet clumping. The authors have observed that presence, number, and size of platelet clumps are not always reproducible between smears made from the same blood sample. If large clumps are observed on smear review and/or a low automated platelet count (regardless of the degree of observed clumping) requires confirmation, a fresh blood sample should be drawn (using atraumatic venipuncture and conscientious sample handling) and analyzed.

If paper medical records are used, instrument print-outs should be archived in the patient's medical record. Instrument print-outs should be annotated with results of the blood smear review; annotations should be initialed and dated. Whether an automated or manual differential WBC count is used for patient management should be clear. If computerized medical records are used, CBC data, annotations, and comments should be added into the hospital information system for each patient. If numerical data are added manually (rather than by electronic download resulting from interface of the POCA with the hospital information system), a system should be in place to verify that no transcription errors have occurred.[7]

EDTA-anticoagulated whole blood samples may be stored for up to 24 hours at 4°C. Air-dried, stained blood smears may be stored indefinitely. Needles, syringes, blood samples, slides, and all reagents should be disposed of safely and appropriately in accordance with relevant government guidelines. Laboratory areas should be kept clean and tidy. Supplies and equipment should be inventoried regularly and replenished as needed.[7]

SUMMARY

In-house hematology testing has distinct advantages and requires an ongoing commitment to quality assurance. Hematology POCA should always be operated by qualified personnel who have received adequate instrument operational, safety, and biohazard training. Likewise, blood samples should be acquired and handled, and blood smears made, by adequately trained personnel. Nonstatistical QA procedures are vital to minimize all types of laboratory error (preanalytical, analytical, and postanalytical) and include many common sense procedures already performed in well-maintained veterinary practices. Blood smear review is a critical component of QA in hematology testing. Each veterinary practice using POCA must determine frequency of QC (ie, frequency of "running controls") based on factors such as POCA analyzer type, clinic operating budget, and caseload; at least daily QC is encouraged if possible. QC should be performed frequently enough that QCM are used cost-effectively and that POCA analytical error can be reliably detected. Unacceptable QC data (however defined) should prompt investigation of the POCA, reagents, and operator. Veterinarians and veterinary technicians are encouraged to pursue continuing education about laboratory quality management and to utilize relevant guidelines, such as those available from the ASVCP.

ACKNOWLEDGMENTS

The authors thank the faculty and staff of the Clinical Pathology Laboratory at the University of Tennessee for providing blood smear and medical review criteria.

REFERENCES

1. Kost GJ, editor. Goals, guidelines, and principles for point-of-care testing. In: Principles and practice of point-of-care testing. Philadelphia (PA): Lippincott Williams & Wilkins; 2002. p. 3.
2. Price CP, St. John A, Kricka LL, editors. Point of care testing: needs, opportunity, and innovation. 3rd edition. Washington, DC: AACC Press; 2010. p. 1, 27.
3. Medicines and Healthcare Products Regulatory Agency. February, 2010 MHRA Device Bulletin 2010(2): Management and use of IVD point of care test devices. Available at: http://www.mhra.gov.uk/Publications/Safetyguidance/DeviceBulletins/CON071082. Accessed June 9, 2011.
4. Weiser MG, Vap LM, Thrall MA. Perspectives and advances in in-clinic laboratory diagnostic capabilities: hematology and clinical chemistry. Vet Clin North Am 2007; 37:221–36.
5. Bounous D. Avian and reptile hematology. In: Ballard BM, Cheek R, editors. Exotic animal medicine for the veterinary technician. Ames (IA): Blackwell; 2003. p. 307.
6. Hadley TL, editor. Hematology and related disorders. Vet Clin Exot Anim 2008;11(3).
7. American Society for Veterinary Clinical Pathology. December, 2009. Quality assurance guidelines. Available at: http://www.asvcp.org/pubs/qas/index.cfm. Accessed June 9, 2011.
8. Stockham SL, Scott MA. Leukocytes. In: Fundamentals of veterinary clinical pathology. 3rd edition. Ames (IA): Blackwell; 2008. p. 53–106.
9. Lassen DL, Weiser G. Laboratory testing for veterinary medicine. In: Thrall's veterinary hematology and clinical chemistry. Ames (IA): Blackwell; 2004. p. 9–10.
10. Freeman KP, Evans EW, Lester S. Quality control for in-hospital veterinary laboratory testing. J Am Vet Med Assoc 1999;215:928–9.
11. Sacchini F, Freeman KP. Quality documentation challenges for veterinary clinical pathology laboratories. J Vet Diagn Invest 2008;20:266–73.
12. Stockham SL, Scott MA. Erythrocytes. In: Fundamentals of veterinary clinical pathology. 3rd edition. Ames (AI): Blackwell; 2008. p. 107–221.
13. Westgard QC online quality control plotter. Available at: http://tools.westgard.com/qcplotter.html. Accessed June 30, 2011.
14. Westgard JO. QC–The Westgard rules. In: Westgard JO, editor. Basic QC practices. 3rd edition. Madison (WI): Westgard QC; 2010. p. 81.
15. Westgard JO. QC–The chances of rejection. In: Westgard JO, editor. Basic QC practices. 3rd edition. Madison (WI): Westgard QC; 2010. p. 215–30.
16. Rishniw M, Pion PD, Maher T. The quality of veterinary in-clinic and reference laboratory biochemistry testing. Vet Clin Pathol, in press.
17. Bellamy JEC, Olexson DW. Monitoring for quality. In: Quality assurance handbook for veterinary laboratories. Ames (IA): Iowa State University Press; 2000. p. 33–6.

Bone Marrow Cytologic and Histologic Biopsies: Indications, Technique, and Evaluation

Rose E. Raskin, DVM, PhD*, Joanne B. Messick, VMD, PhD

KEYWORDS

- Bone marrow • Marrow cytology • Marrow histology
- Biopsy • Indications

Bone marrow evaluation is indicated when the routine examination of a blood smear has failed to provide an answer to the question: What is causing an observed hematologic abnormality? If the blood already clearly indicates an immune mediated hemolytic anemia or regenerative anemia for which an etiology is suspected/known, a bone marrow evaluation is likely superfluous. Similarly, an inflammatory response or leukocytosis for which a cause is suspected or known may not warrant a bone marrow evaluation.

SPECIFIC INDICATIONS FOR BONE MARROW EVALUATION

The most common indication for bone marrow evaluation is cytopenia of one, two, or all three hematopoietic cell lines for which an underlying etiology cannot be found.

- Nonregenerative anemia without evidence of polychromasia (reticulocytes). Persistent, poorly regenerative or nonregenerative anemia requires bone marrow examination particularly via a core biopsy to assess the severity and prognosis of various erythroid hypoplastic or aplastic conditions.
- Persistent neutropenia without a left shift or evidence of regeneration. Regeneration should involve a shift toward immaturity of the granulocytic line (ie, bands, metamyelocytes, and myelocytes) within 3 to 5 days following neutropenia.
- Thrombocytopenia is best evaluated by an assessment of the number and morphology of megakaryocytes via bone marrow core and aspirate biopsy. Levels as low as 10,000/μL often do not present a contraindication for bone marrow evaluation as bleeding is confined within the bone space. It is recommended that a

---

The authors have nothing to disclose.
Department of Comparative Pathobiology, Purdue University, School of Veterinary Medicine, 725 Harrison Street, West Lafayette, IN 47907, USA
* Corresponding author.
E-mail address: rraskin@purdue.edu

Vet Clin Small Anim 42 (2012) 23–42
doi:10.1016/j.cvsm.2011.10.001
0195-5616/12/$ – see front matter © 2012 Elsevier Inc. All rights reserved.

coagulation profile be performed first to rule out disseminated intravascular coagulopathy when thrombocytopenia is present.

- The presence of abnormal cell morphology in the blood will often warrant review of the marrow for evidence of leukemia. Dysplastic changes such as megaloblastic rubricytes, neutrophil hypersegmentation, or giant platelets may be subtle indicators of myelodysplastic syndrome or certain myeloid leukemias.
- The suspicion of marrow malignancy warrants bone marrow evaluation. Leukemia may be occult (ie, blast cells may be numerous in the bone marrow, but few or no blast cells are seen in the peripheral blood [subleukemic or aleukemic leukemia]).
- Unexplained elevations in blood cell numbers should suggest bone marrow evaluation. Note that relative erythrocytosis may result from splenic contraction, hypovolemia, physiological induced cardiac disease, and high-altitude hypoxia and in certain dog breeds (eg, greyhounds), all of which do not require bone marrow examination. Certain neoplasms can produce excessive erythropoietin (leading to erythrocytosis) or granulocyte and/or granulocyte-macrophage colony-stimulating factors (leading to leukocytosis) as a result of renal hypoxia or a paraneoplastic secretion. A reactive leukocytosis due to a nidus of inflammation is more common and should be excluded before pursuing the possibility of a paraneoplastic or neoplastic process to explain the elevation. Marked thrombocytosis can result from increased thrombopoietin or thrombopoietic cytokine stimulation, which may occur in chronic iron deficiency anemia and in various inflammatory/infectious conditions.[1] The possibility that persistent thrombocytosis may indicate an underlying myeloproliferative disorder such as a myelodysplastic syndrome or essential thrombocythemia must also be ruled out, particularly if an underlying etiology cannot be found. The latter may be independent of thrombopoietin stimulation; bone marrow examination in these conditions often reveals marked megakaryocytic hyperplasia with morphologic abnormality. Lymphocytosis may indicate antigenic stimulation but marked elevations in lymphoid cells should suggest possible malignancy. Chronic lymphocytic leukemia (CLL) of B-cell immunophenotype in the dog has significant infiltration of the bone marrow in contrast to CLL of T-cell origin, which circulates in peripheral blood but originates from the spleen.[2] T-CLL is more common than B-CLL in the dog compared to the human.
- Hypercalcemia may occur without obvious etiology such related to the presence of an anal mass or hyperparathyroidism. In these situations, occult lymphoid neoplasia with only bone marrow involvement should be considered.
- Focal lymphoma or plasma cell myeloma produces bone lysis and may only be recognized with early disease through core biopsy procedure.
- Hyperproteinemia with either a monoclonal or polyclonal gammopathy supports bone marrow evaluation for neoplasia or an infectious agent. Both B-CLL and plasma cell neoplasia may present with a monoclonal gammopathy. Systemic fungal and protozoal infectious agents such as *Histoplasma* and *Leishmania* may infiltrate the bone marrow and present with hyperglobulinemia. Others may not be visible but still result in gammopathy such as *Ehrlichia canis*.

Fever of unexplained origin often arises from immune-mediated causes but may also reflect a non–immune-mediated etiology where bone marrow evaluation becomes a useful diagnostic tool. Primary bone marrow abnormalities accounted for 22 of 101 canine cases of pyrexia of unknown origin, with myelodysplasia and lymphoid leukemia being most responsible.[3]

- Leukoerythroblastosis identified by concurrent immature granulocytes and nucleated red cells in circulation may indicate bone marrow damage caused by neoplastic infiltration of the bone marrow. While the presence of nucleated red cells in circulation may reflect bone marrow damage, the presence of a concurrent and significant left shift was key in supporting examination of the bone marrow leading to the discovery of a disseminated adenocarcinoma in a dog.[4]
- Therapeutic monitoring of chemotherapy administration and determination of clinical staging for malignancies such as lymphoma or mast cell tumor require bone marrow evaluation. Aspiration and core biopsies are recommended to determine changes in hematopoietic cell prevalence as well as the pattern of neoplastic cell infiltration. A focal type of metastasis is the most difficult to determine by blood smears or marrow aspirates alone. Core biopsy is useful to determine whether mast cells are in their normal perivascular location or abnormally in sheets of cells. Core biopsy examination of the bone marrow in canine lymphoma affords greater sensitivity than aspirate smears due to the manner of metastasis seen histologically.[5]
- Evaluation of iron stores is helpful in determining iron sequestration within macrophages. Marrow evaluation for iron in cats may be unproductive, because their bone marrow normally lacks discernible storage levels. Similarly, neonatal animals often rapidly use iron for erythropoiesis, and storage amounts are low. While both anemia of inflammatory disease and iron deficiency anemia in dogs present with low serum iron, there is a different appearance relative to iron stores within the bone marrow. Iron deficiency anemia has low to absent stores while anemia of inflammatory disease has normal to excessive amounts of hemosiderin in the bone marrow.[6]

CYTOLOGIC BIOPSY VERSUS HISTOLOGIC BIOPSY

Cytologic biopsy provides excellent morphological detail of bone marrow cells. It is relatively cheap and easy to perform and has a rapid turnaround time, providing diagnostic information within minutes of collection. The histologic biopsy provides similar information relative to cell types but more importantly allows architectural evaluation of fat and fibrous connective tissue relative to cellular content. Focal changes of the stroma and determination of overall cellularity are best appreciated by histologic biopsy samples. Such changes, which may be missed by aspiration biopsy alone, include inflammation, neoplasia, marrow necrosis, osteolysis, or myelofibrosis. For maximum information, the two techniques are concurrently performed and interpreted along with the complete blood count (CBC) data obtained within 1 day of the biopsy.

SITES OF BIOPSY
Antemortem

For small animals, site selection will be determined by the clinician's preference, age, body size, or condition of the animal.

Humerus

For obese or very muscular dogs, the craniolateral part of the greater tubercle of the humerus is the site preferred because of lack of muscle, fat, or substantial subcutaneous tissue in this region (**Fig. 1**). For humeral samples, both aspiration and core biopsy needles are directed posteromedial. The pronounced fascial covering of the bone permits the needle to slip easily; therefore patience is advised when inserting the

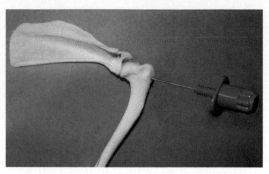

Fig. 1. Placement of the marrow biopsy needle is shown into the craniolateral part of the greater tubercle of the humerus. This site is preferred for obese and muscular adult dogs and cats.

needle into the bone. Lateral recumbency is preferred for collection. Young growing animals, typically less than 6 months of age should **not** be sampled in this location due to the proximity of the epiphyseal growth plate.

Ilium
For thin or nonobese dogs, the dorsal iliac crest is a popular location because it is readily accessible (**Fig. 2**). In small dogs and cats with a thin dorsal ilial crest, transilial samples for core samples are preferred over parallel placement of the needle within the ilium (**Fig. 3**). Patients may be positioned in sternal or lateral recumbency for ilial

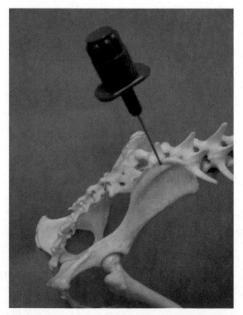

Fig. 2. The dorsal iliac crest is a popular location in thin or nonobese dogs, because it is readily accessible.

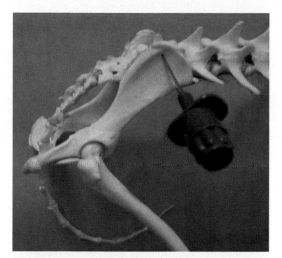

Fig. 3. One or more samples may be taken via a transilial procedure. This site may be helpful in young dogs and cats that have a dorsal ilial crest, too narrow to attempt parallel placement of the biopsy needle.

samples. The needle is introduced at the widest part of the dorsal ilium and directed ventromedial to conform to the concavity of the pelvic bone. If placed too laterally, the biopsy instrument may enter only cortical bone or slip off the sides into surrounding muscle or adipose tissue.

Femur
For small dogs and cats, penetration made just medial to the greater trochanter and parallel to the shaft of the proximal femur may be used to obtain marrow samples, but this area may be less accessible (**Fig. 4**). When obtaining femoral samples, avoid the sciatic nerve located medial and posterior to the greater trochanter. The animal is placed in lateral recumbency during the procedure. Large quantities of bone marrow may be obtained from this site. Bone trabeculae are minimal in this site, providing larger quantities, but the core biopsy may be more easily lost during collection related to the limited dense tissue available to retain the specimen.

Postmortem
Samples should be obtained within 30 minutes after death to ensure intact cell morphology as tissue breakdown is rapid at room or body temperature. Refrigeration, not freezing, is recommended to slow deterioration if a time delay is anticipated. Aspiration material is best obtained within minutes after death. If time delay prohibits aspiration collection, wedge sections from necropsy specimens using a scalpel blade should be taken from the metaphyseal region of long bones (femur or humerus) (**Fig. 5**). Avoid taking diaphyseal or mid-bone samples, especially in older animals, as there is likely to be much fat infiltration and the samples are less likely to be representative of active hematopoiesis within the bone marrow. Alternatively, tissue sections involving the costochondral joint of the ribs or the wing of the ilium may be used, depending on the size of the animal. Cytologic material from cut surfaces may be possible if collection is performed shortly after death but cellular detail is not likely to be optimum.

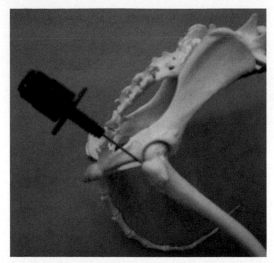

Fig. 4. The proximal femur may be most useful for small animals. Penetration is made just medial to the greater trochanter and parallel to the shaft of the samples, avoiding the sciatic nerve located more lateral and posterior.

PATIENT PREPARATION AND EQUIPMENT

Animals need not be placed under general anesthesia. Sedation with local anesthesia (eg, lidocaine) is often sufficient for aspiration and core biopsies. Pain relief medication may be given when indicated. The area is clipped and surgically scrubbed; then ½ to 2 mL of 2% lidocaine is infiltrated intradermally and deep to the periosteum. The area may be draped and sterile gloves are used. A stab incision is made in the skin with a No. 11 scalpel blade. It is recommended that aspiration biopsy be performed first, followed by core biopsy of the same bone. The core biopsy should be taken a

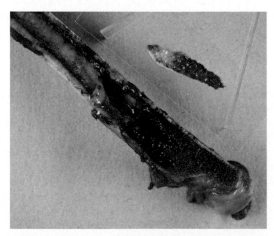

Fig. 5. Triangular wedge sections may be taken from necropsy specimens using a scalpel blade within the metaphyseal region of long bones (femur or humerus).

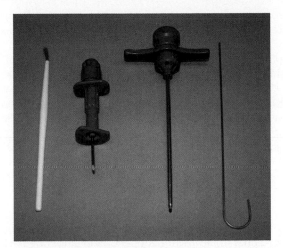

Fig. 6. Bone marrow biopsy equipment is shown. From left to right: paint brush, Illinois sternal aspiration biopsy needle, and a Jamshidi core biopsy needle along with its associated shepherd hook for specimen removal.

short distance away from the aspirate biopsy to avoid collecting the previously damaged tissue.

Bone marrow aspirate biopsy equipment and supplies are minimal (**Fig. 6**) consisting of a special biopsy needle,[a] 12-mL syringe, 5% EDTA solution, scalpel blade, and glass slides. Optionally, Petri dishes with hematocrit capillary tubes or glass pipettes are used to collect unit particles.

Core biopsy materials include a specialized biopsy needle,[b] scalpel blade, glass slides, and a tissue fixative (10% buffered formalin).

Postmortem cytologic and histologic collection materials consist of a fracturing technique such as a bone rongeur or a saw to assist in exposing the metaphyseal region. A cytologic sample can be acquired by gently scraping or brushing the medullary cavity with a hobby paint brush (**Fig. 6**). The acquired specimen can then be transferred to a glass slide by creating 2 or 3 linear streaks. Using the same exposed medullary cavity, a histologic sample is created with a No. 10 scalpel blade by cutting a triangular wedge within the spongy but firm tissue (see **Fig. 5**), which can be then placed into fixative fluid.

BIOPSY PROCEDURES
Aspirate Biopsy

The aspiration needle with stylet in place is passed through the skin incision to the bone. The needle is then rotated to penetrate the cortex several millimeters so that it becomes firmly embedded. Once embedded, the stylet is removed; the syringe containing EDTA is then attached to the needle, and quick, full, successive pulls are applied to the plunger to draw marrow into the syringe. Relax the pressure on the syringe plunger and remove the syringe and needle together. If direct smears are to

[a] Illinois sternal disposable needle, 15 to 18 gauge, 1 to 2 inches long; Cat. Nos. DIN1515X and DIN1518X, Cardinal Health, www.cardinal.com.
[b] Jamshidi biopsy/aspiration disposable needle, 11 to 13 gauge, 2 to 4 inches long; Cat. Nos. DJ2013X, DJ3513X, DJ4011X, Cardinal Health, www.cardinal.com.

be made, avoid excessive blood contamination. Touch a drop of marrow to the slide and quickly make your bone marrow preparations by either a "push" or "squash" technique.

A preferred method involves adding approximately 0.5 to 1 mL of 5% EDTA to the syringe before starting the procedure. Following collection of blood contaminated marrow, squirt it into a Petri dish or onto a slide and allow blood to drain off particles by tipping the dish or slide. Alternatively, marrow can be transferred to a glass slide so particles can adhere. Particles, which appear as tiny glistening flecks or granules, may be picked up with microhematocrit tubes or a glass pipette.

Following collection of a droplet, it is gently expelled onto a glass slide. Smears of the particles are best produced by the squash method. Extra smears should be made for in-house viewing or for special cytochemical or immunocytochemical stains.

Core Biopsy

The technique for acquiring a core biopsy is similar to the aspirate biopsy except that the stylet is removed prior to the instrument becoming embedded in bone. The needle is advanced about 1 cm by smooth twisting motion of the wrist until it is solidly embedded into the bone. To cut and retain the bone sample, the needle is sharply rotated in 360-degree revolutions in both clockwise and counterclockwise directions. The needle is withdrawn with a twisting motion. The section is removed from the Jamshidi biopsy needle by pushing the sample out the wider end with a probe that enters the narrower cutting end. The core biopsy may be rolled over a glass slide to allow exfoliation of marrow material before it is placed into the tissue fixative. The sample must remain in the fixative for a minimum of 2 to 3 hours. Following mild decalcification for 4 to 8 hours in formic acid/sodium citrate solution, sections of the bone marrow core are prepared and sent to a histopathologist for evaluation. Recommended thickness involves 3-μm hematoxylin and eosin (H&E) sections as well as sections for reticulin and immunohistochemistry stains. Formalin materials should be kept separate (not even close by) from aspirate smears to avoid fixation artifacts to the cytologic preparations. If mailing, send aspirate and core biopsy materials in separate boxes.

Biopsy Complications

Rare complications are encountered during bone marrow aspiration or core biopsy. Tissue injury is minimal unless the sciatic nerve is damaged when obtaining a femoral sample. Excessive bleeding is rarely encountered, even in markedly thrombocytopenic patients. Rare reports have described tumor seeding of hematopoietic neoplasms in humans as a result of bone marrow biopsy attempts. No such cases have been reported in animals.

TECHNICAL ASPECTS OF BONE MARROW PROCESSING
Storage of Bone Marrow Aspiration Samples

Bone marrow samples should be processed as quickly as possible after collection. The best results are obtained when films are prepared within 2 hours of their collection. For short-term storage (<8 hours), it is recommended that marrow samples be kept dry and cooled at 4°C; however, storage at room temperature (25°C) is acceptable. Prior to the making of bone marrow films, the sample should be gently and completely mixed by inversion a minimum of 15 to 20 times. Degenerative changes such as cytoplasmic vacuolization, nuclear lobation or fragmentation, and apoptotic changes are often caused by prolong or inappropriate sample storage.

Processing and Staining of Bone Marrow Films

To avoid artifactual changes, bone marrow films also must be rapidly and completely air dried before they are fixed and stained. Slow drying of the marrow preparations causes cell to contract or shrink, whereas excessive water in methanol fixing solution (>3%) can lead to cellular swelling and distorted morphology. In the latter scenario, the cellular features will not be "crisp," nuclear contents may appears to leak into the cytoplasm, a feature in erythroblasts that may be misinterpreted as dyserythropoiesis, and artificial cytoplasmic vacuolation may occur.

Prior to shipping (or delivery) the marrow sample and unstained films to the laboratory, the adequacy of the marrow preparations should be evaluated on a stained preparation. Bone marrow films can be stained with a Romanowsky stain, such as May-Grünwald-Giemsa, Wright-Giemsa, or aqueous-based Wright. Because of their thickness, aspirate smears require a longer staining period with Romanowsky-type stains than blood films. Rapid evaluation of the marrow smear can be made within minutes of collection to ensure adequate material has been obtained. Once stained, a cover slip may be applied. All slides, stained and unstained, should be labeled with date and patient identifying information.

COMPLETE MARROW EVALUATION

For a complete marrow evaluation (CME), testing should include a CBC, bone marrow aspirate, and bone marrow biopsy. A CBC gives excellent quantitative and morphologic information; it should be collected at the same time or within 24 hours of the bone marrow aspirate. Careful review of the blood film by the pathologist reading the aspirate is strongly recommended as it may provide additional information to support marrow findings or help to direct marrow evaluations. Depending on the CBC findings, it may be also useful to obtain a current reticulocyte count, particularly for determining whether erythroid hyperplasia is associated with effective or ineffective erythropoiesis.

The bone marrow aspirate allows excellent morphologic evaluation of cells, differential count and myeloid:erythroid (M:E) ratio. However, if the cellularity of a bone marrow aspirate is low, the finding may be due to "real" pathology or just hemodilution of the sample. A histologic section of a biopsy sample gives the best quantitative information on the cellularity of the marrow as well as revealing myelofibrosis, architectural patterns, and focal lesions. Neglecting one or two parts of the CME often leaves unanswered questions and performing a test several days after the other may also leave some questions. It is recommended that all three tests be done and at the same time.

Assessing Bone Marrow Films

A guideline for the assessment of bone marrow aspirate cytology is shown in **Box 1**. Marrow films should first be examined under low power (×10 objective). The number of particles and overall degree of cellularity, megakaryocyte numbers, as well as presence of low numbers of abnormal cells such as carcinoma cells or focal accumulations of round cells, are assessed at this power. For normocellular marrow particles, the hematopoietic cells should be piled up on the stroma of the spicules, but vacuoles of fat are still present; the overall cellularity should be greater than 25% but less than 75%. Hypocellular marrow has readily visible stromal cells and abundant fat (>75% of the particles area is fat) with few hematopoietic cells. On the other hand, hypercellular marrow contains no or rare fat vacuoles and an abundance of cells (>75% of the particles are composed of cells). An absence of particles in films of the

---

Box 1
Steps in assessing bone marrow aspiration cytology

1. Particles and/or overall degree of cellularity
2. Content of particles
   a. Iron stores
   b. Megakaryocytes
   c. Stromal cells
   d. Hematopoietic cells
   e. Other cells
3. Myeloid:erythroid ratio (M:E ratio)
4. Megakaryocytic lineage
   a. Numbers
   b. Sequence and completeness of maturation
   c. Dysplasia
5. Erythroid lineage
   a. Sequence and completeness of maturation
   b. Dysplasia
6. Myeloid lineage
   a. Sequence and completeness of maturation
   b. Dysplasia
7. % Blasts
   a. Of all nucleated cells
   b. Of the nonerythroid lineage
8. Other cells
   a. Lymphocytes
   b. Plasma cells
   c. Histiocytic cells
   d. Mast cells
   e. Neoplastic cells (nonhematopoietic)
9. Morphologic interpretation: must have a recent CBC
10. Comments

---

bone marrow aspirate may preclude valid estimation of cellularity and megakaryocyte number in most instances. Megakaryocytes are often identified within or very near the particles and estimates of their numbers are quite subjective. If more than a few megakaryocytes are found, then the number is designated as "adequate"; if almost none are present, then decreased; if many are present, then increased.

A systematic assessment of the content of particles and a differential count from which the M:E ratio can be calculated are made using the ×40 or ×50 objectives. Since the marrow film is minimally diluted by peripheral blood in the "trails" of cells

Table 1
Differential cell counts from bone marrow for the dog and cat

CELL TYPE	DOG	CAT
Myeloblasts (%)	0.4–1.1	0–0.4
Promyelocytes (%)	1.1–2.3	0–3.0
Myelocyte neutrophils (%)	3.1–6.1	0.6–8.0
Metamyelocyte neutrophils (%)	5.3–8.8	4.4–13.2
Band neutrophils (%)	12.7–17.2	12.8–16.6
Segmented neutrophils (%)	13.8–24.2	6.8–22.0
Eosinophils (%)	1.8–5.6	0.8–3.2
Basophils (%)	0–0.8	0–0.4
Rubriblasts (%)	0.2–1.1	0–0.8
Prorubricytes (%)	0.9–2.2	0–1.6
Basophilic rubricytes (%)	3.7–10.0	1.6–6.2
Polychromatic rubricytes (%)	15.5–25.1	8.6–23.2
Metarubricytes (%)	9.2–16.4	1.0–10.4
Granulocytic to Erythroid Ratio or M:E	0.9–1.8	1.2–2.2
Lymphocytes (%)	1.7–4.9	11.6–21.6
Plasma cells (%)	0.6–2.4	0.2–1.8
Monocytes (%)	0.4–2.0	0.2–1.6
Macrophages (%)	0–0.4	0–0.2
Mast cells	Rare	Rare

Data from Harvey JW. Atlas of veterinary hematology. Philadelphia: WB Saunders; 2001.

adjacent to the particles, the differential counts should be performed in these areas. At the very least, several hundred cells should be counted; granulocytes, nucleated erythroid cells, lymphocytes, plasma cells, and other cells are enumerated. The majority of cells in a marrow smear are differentiating granulocytes, monocytes, and erythroid cells. In normal marrow, neutrophils are the most numerous with monocytes, eosinophils, and basophils collectively accounting for only 5% to 10% of the total myelomonocytic cells. The marrow report should indicate the relative number of granulocytic and erythroid cells in the form of an M:E ratio. In health, the M:E ratio is approximately 1 but can range from 2 to 0.5, depending on the species (**Table 1**). The balance and completeness of maturation in the three hematopoietic cell lines should be assessed. In each series, cells in the late stages of differentiation, the postmitotic pool, should be far more numerous (approximately 85% of the total cells in that series) than the immature stages. A 500-cell differential with all cell types enumerated on several different bone marrow films should be performed if marrow features indicate the possibility of an acute leukemia or myelodysplastic syndrome.

Abnormally high numbers of nonhematopoietic cells, such as plasma cells, lymphocytes, macrophages, and mast cells, in marrow should be noted and reported. It is important to recognize that the accumulation of cells of one particular lineage may be focal; scanning the blood film at low power as well as examining multiple blood films at higher magnifications is necessary to be certain these areas are not missed. Lymphocytes and plasma cells and macrophages are commonly present in low number, scattered throughout the marrow and collectively are fewer than approximately 10% of all the nucleated cells (see **Table 1**). In the cat, small/mature lymphocytes may represent up to 20% of all the cells. These cells are also slightly more numerous in immature animals than in adult animals.

Fine cytological details of hematopoietic or other cells should be assessed using an oil immersion ×100 objective. Differentiating hematopoietic cells in all series should be evaluated for morphologic evidence of disturbed maturation, such as dysplastic and toxic changes, and left shift. Toxic changes are apparent only in neutrophils and are associated with stimulated granulocytopoiesis, particularly in inflammation. Dysplastic change or (morphologic evidence of abnormal maturation) in erythroid cells and megakaryocytes most commonly are associated with neoplastic disorders of hematopoiesis-myelodysplastic syndromes and acute myeloid leukemias. A pronounced left shift in a series can represent a "maturation block," which can result from destruction of cells in later stages of maturation or from intrinsic defect in regulation of differentiation (hematopoietic neoplasia), or can represent a transient stage in a wave of regeneration after acute injury to marrow, such as myelotoxic drug, acute radiation, or feline panleukopenia infection. Feline leukemia virus (FeLV) infection in cats causes a wide range of dysplastic changes in hematopoietic cells and/or alterations in their numbers—these findings are often disparate, ranging from nonregenerative anemia to erythremic myelosis, neutropenia to leukemia, and thrombocytopenia to megakaryocytic leukemia. Thus, it is strongly recommended that any cat with a hematologic disorder should be tested for FeLV as well as feline immunodeficiency virus (FIV) infection.

Stainable Iron

The quantitative and qualitative assessment of cells in Romanowsky-stained films should be followed by the evaluation of marrow iron stores. While imprecise, the amount of hemosiderin (stainable iron) in marrow helps to support a diagnose iron deficiency anemia (absence) or anemia of inflammation (increased). Adult dogs, horses, and cows should have hemosiderin; however, cats normally have no stainable iron in marrow.

Assessing Bone Marrow Histology

The components involved in bone marrow histology are cortical and trabecular bone and stroma, vasculature, sinus wall layers, nerves, hematopoietic cells, and non-hematopoietic interstitial cells. Refer to **Boxes 2** and **3** for a checklist and list of histochemical stains used to assess bone marrow histologic specimens.

Connective Tissue Elements

Young animals generally present with hypercellular bone marrow, defined as having greater than 75% cellular elements with the remainder of the space occupied by adipose tissue, if present. As the animal ages or when hematopoiesis decreases with disease, fat cells, fibrous tissue, necrosis, or metastatic tumor cells often replace normal cellular elements. The adventitial-reticular (A-R) cell or stromal cell that lines most marrow sinuses influences the change in adipose or fibrous tissue content. The A-R cell will project its cell processes into hematopoietic cords for support and produce reticulin (argentiphilic) fibers during early bone marrow injury. Fibroblasts that produce collagen may also arise from the A-R cells during severe marrow injury or in response to cytokines (platelet-derived growth factor, transforming growth factor-β) released from monocytes and neoplastic megakaryocytes. Reticular cells stain alkaline phosphatase positive and produce interleukin-7. Actin and stem cell factor are expressed by these cells. Ultrastructurally, microtubules, microfilaments,

---

Box 2
Checklist for bone marrow histologic evaluation

1. Sample integrity; contour/quantity of bone and presence of other elements e.g., muscle.

2. Overall cellularity of hematopoietic elements relative to fat content; estimate proportion.

3. Number of megakaryocytes in high power field ($\times$40 or $\times$50 oil), their distribution, and general maturity.

4. Cellular patterns in core biopsy (focal or diffuse)

   a. Focal infiltrates with high density areas within adipose

   b. Metastatic populations typically found in paratrabecular location

5. Cell types

   a. Normal heterogeneity of cell types

   b. Monomorphism of a cell type

6. Maturation sequence of granulocytes and erythroid precursors

   a. Majority cells are normally late-stage forms (segmented granulocytes, metarubricytes)

   b. Maturation arrest at any stage? All stages seen?

7 Estimation of myeloid:erythroid ratio comparing granulocytes and erythroid precursors.

8 Iron content may be noted if increased when viewed under H&E staining as coarse orange-brown granules within macrophages; best evaluated with Prussian blue stain. Erythrophagocytosis when noted should be reported.

9 Provide a morphologic interpretation and compare the biopsy findings to the peripheral blood results to see if an appropriate bone marrow response is present. Best if the CBC is performed within 24 hours of bone marrow biopsy.

---

and intermediate filaments are commonly found to provide structural support. Connected to the cortex is a meshwork of trabecular bone that forms the support for the hematopoietic compartment. It is lined by endosteum along with osteoblasts and osteoclasts that are prominent in young animals or actively remodeled bone. It is thought that the paratrabecular area exerts an inductive effect on granulopoiesis since myeloblasts are most prominent in this area.

Vasculature

The vascular supply to the bone marrow arises from two sources. A minor source occurs from the nutrient artery, which enters the midshaft through the cortex dividing

---

Box 3
Suggested additional histochemical stains for bone marrow evaluation

Giemsa—eosinophils, mast cells; highlights erythroid precursors especially late stages

Periodic acid–Schiff (PAS)—granulocytes, histiocytic, megakaryocytic, and plasma cells

Prussian blue—hemosiderin deposits

Argentiphilic stain—reticulin fibers

Trichrome—collagen fibers

into ascending and descending medullary arteries from which form the radial arteries. The radial arteries enter through the cortex along the endosteum leading into cortical capillaries, which communicate with capillaries coming from the major source, namely periosteal and muscular arterioles. From these capillaries, blood flows into terminal sinuses within the marrow space. The sinuses are lined by a thin interrupted basement membrane visible with PAS staining. Facing the lumen is a continuous layer of endothelium joined by junctional complexes that reacts with anti-CD34, the stem cell marker. Small apertures in the endothelium allow for cell passage into the lumen from the interstitium. Hypoxia or erythropoietin influences produce wider apertures leading to the early release of precursor erythroid cells. Returning blood drains into a central sinus that exits through the nutrient foramen. Associated with the blood vessels are vasomotor nerves that may react to the discomfort caused by bone marrow aspiration.

Hematopoietic Elements

The major cellular component consists of hematopoietic elements and generally accounts for 25% to 75% of the marrow space. Hematopoiesis occurs in an organized fashion within the marrow.

Granulopoiesis occurs primarily adjacent to trabeculae and is easily visualized with the use of PAS stain. The myeloblasts have large round to oval vesicular nuclei with often a single large nucleolus. As they mature, metamyelocytes and later stages crawl away from this site and may be found anywhere in the interstitium. PAS will stain all stages of granulocytes; however, it is more intense in the myelocyte and later forms. For the monocytic cells, monocytes and macrophages stain more intensely with PAS compared with the promonocyte stage.

Erythropoiesis is evident as erythroblastic islands that contain a central macrophage. These islands are found adjacent to the sinus endothelium. In this location, erythroblasts can mature by pitting the nucleus of the metarubricyte and releasing the remaining polychromatic erythrocyte through openings in the endothelium into the sinus lumen. An exception to this location is found in the avian and reptilian species, whereby erythroblasts line the inside of sinus and all developing stages progress toward the center of the sinus for release into circulation.

Thrombopoiesis, similar to erythropoiesis, occurs adjacent to the sinus so that megakaryocytes can extend their cytoplasmic processes directly into the sinus lumen and fragment into platelets.

Lymphopoiesis is based on their B or T immunophenotype. Small follicles or nodules of B- lymphocytes have been found in people, dogs, and cats. These are small well-differentiated lymphocytes that may respond with formation of a germinal center and demonstration of centrally located immunoblasts. In the cat, these are more prominent in the femur and in conditions such as FIV infection. T-lymphocytes and plasma cells may be concentrated around radial arteries.

Other cells such as mast cells are located perivascular and adjacent to lymphoid nodules. These are in low numbers and scattered individually, not in sheets.

Mononuclear Phagocytes and Iron

Macrophages are present in low numbers often associated with erythroblastic islands as "nurse cells" and may be quite evident with ingested iron or hemosiderin. Additionally, during pathologic conditions such as immune-mediated hemolysis, some infections, histiocytic malignancies, and benign histiocytic proliferations, macrophages may display prominent erythrophagocytosis.

Young animals will have more rapid red cell turnover and therefore less deposits of iron in their marrow compared with adult animals. Species differences also exist, as for example scattered Prussian blue–positive granules within macrophages are found normally in the dog but are generally absent in the cat, except under pathologic conditions. Ferritin represents a better gauge of body iron content but this minimally stains with Prussian blue unless present in aggregates. Acidic chelating agents, which are present in the decalcifier reduce stainable iron. In these circumstances, review of a cytologic preparation will help determine iron content.

Interpretation of Marrow Findings

The interpretation of bone marrow aspiration and histology should provide quantitative information as well as a morphologic assessment of individual cells and cell lines. Most of the bone marrow abnormalities relate to the overall cellularity and/or presence of cell types. **Table 2** lists disorders to consider based on the cell numbers or morphologic appearance of cells in the blood and cellularity, morphologic abnormalities, or stromal changes in the bone marrow. An explanation of the terms often used when interpreting the aspirate is provided next.

Erythroid, myeloid, and *megakaryocytic hyperplasia* are terms that indicate increased numbers of precursor stages of red cells, granulocytes/monocytes, and platelets, respectively. This is the expected marrow response to loss or destruction of these mature cells from the peripheral circulation. If the response is effective, increased numbers of the end product should be evident in blood (ie, reticulocytosis, rising white blood cells, hematocrit, and/or platelet count).

The bone marrow under conditions of strong regeneration is characteristically hyperplastic such as following recovery from feline panleukopenia. The regeneration may be anticipated from examination of the peripheral blood with the presence of macrocytic polychromatic erythrocytes, left-shifted granulocytes, or megaplatelets. The bone marrow may be hyperplastic relative to megakaryocyte numbers in consumptive or destructive platelet disorders such as subacute to chronic disseminated intravascular coagulopathy or immune-mediated thrombocytopenia. Immune-mediated destruction of platelets has been associated with drug therapy and various neoplasms (mast cell, hemangiosarcoma, mixed mammary tumor, or nasal adenocarcinoma).[7] Therefore, bone marrow hyperplasia may be expected in the presence of these conditions. Granulocytic hyperplasia as a paraneoplastic syndrome has been documented in several tumors.[8]

Neoplasia refers to new or uncontrolled cell growth that within the bone marrow can arise primarily from hemolymphatic tissue or secondarily from metastasis of a nonhematopoietic tumor. Common malignancies that metastasize include lymphoma, mast cell tumor, and various carcinomas.[4] Primary malignancies include acute or chronic lymphoid or myeloid leukemias. Acute myeloid leukemia (AML) is applied to the situation in which the hematopoietic precursors are arrested in an early stage of development. The mechanism of this arrest is believed to involve the activation of abnormal genes through genetic abnormalities. The presence of greater than 20% blast cells in the bone marrow is strongly supportive of an interpretation of AML; however, clinical and laboratory information is essential to distinguish this from an exuberant hyperplastic response.

Dysplasia refers to abnormal growth of cells. Cytologically, these abnormalities include asynchronous maturation of the nucleus and cytoplasm resulting in megaloblastic erythroid precursors, dwarf megakaryocytes, or abnormally segmented neutrophils. Dysplasia may affect one cell line (eg, erythroid, as occurs in lead toxicity or poodle macrocytosis) or two or more cell lines may be affected as may occur with nutritional deficiencies or drug-induced toxicosis.[9] These secondary myelodysplastic cases should be distinguished from the primary myelodysplastic syndrome.[10]

Table 2
Selected causes of bone marrow disorders based on blood and bone marrow examination

	Peripheral Blood Examination		
Cytopenia	Hematocytosis	Dysplastic Cells	Blast Cells
	Bone Marrow Evaluation		
Aplasia/Hypoplasia	Hyperplasia	Myelodysplasia	Neoplasia
Infections:	Infections:	Myelodysplastic syndrome	Primary lymphoid leukemia
Viral	Bacterial		Primary myeloid leukemia
Rickettsial	Mycoplasmal	Drug-induced dysplasia	Metastatic neoplasia
Protozoal	Rickettsial	Lead toxicosis	
Fungal	Protozoal	Infections:	
Drugs or chemicals	Fungal	FeLV	
Hyperestrogenism	FIV (early)	FIV	
Organ failure	Parvovirus (recovery)	Nutritional deficiencies	
Chronic disease/inflammation	Immune-mediated damage	Pelger-Huet anomaly	
Endocrine disorders	Iron deficiency	Macrocytosis (poodles)	
Irradiation	Oxidative injury	Myeloid neoplasia	
Hereditary cytopenia	Zinc toxicosis		
Nutritional deficiencies	Hereditary enzyme deficiency		
Myelophthisis	Parasitic infections		
Myelofibrosis	Allergic reactions		
Marrow necrosis	Inflammation/hypersensitivity		
Immune-mediated damage	Paraneoplastic syndrome		
	Mature lymphoid leukemia		
	Myeloproliferative neoplasia		
	Plasma cell neoplasia		

Abbreviations: FIV, feline immunodeficiency virus; FeLV, feline leukemia virus.

Myelodysplastic syndrome (MDS) is a term used to designate a group of disorders characterized by peripheral blood cytopenias; however, the marrow is either hyper-cellular or normocellular for the corresponding cell lineage and there is morphologic evidence of dysplasia in one or more cell lines. Blast cell forms compose less than 20% of nucleated cells.[11] It is believed that normal blood cell maturation, differenti-ation, function, and survival are impaired, leading to the development of peripheral blood pancytopenia; patients may be at increased risk to transform to AML.[12] Primary MDSs are irreversible acquired developmental disorders of bone marrow stem cells unrelated to concurrent disease, nutritional deficiency, or drug-induced toxicosis.[10] MDSs may be divided into two subtypes (MDS-refractory cytopenia and MDS-excess blasts) depending on the percentage of blast cells in the bone marrow.[13] Cases of MDS-excess blasts, those with 5% or greater percentage of myeloblasts, demon-strate shorter survival and poor response to treatment.[10] MDS is sometimes referred to as *preleukemia* as patients with this syndrome often suffer from chronic debilitation that may continue unchanged or evolve into acute leukemia. The cause is often unknown, but the condition has been associated with FeLV infections.[14]

Ineffective erythropoiesis, granulocytopoiesis, and *megakaryocytopoiesis* are terms applied to the situation in which there is hyperplasia of a cell line in marrow but persistence of the corresponding cytopenia in blood with no evidence of a cause of peripheral loss. Intramedullary death of precursor cells, usually by apoptosis, is inferred from this finding; the most common cause is immune-mediated destruction of precursor cells.[15]

Erythroid, myeloid, and/or *megakaryocytic hypoplasia* are terms applied to the situation in which there are fewer precursor cells than appropriate for the number of mature cells in peripheral blood. For example, the absence of erythroid hyperplasia in an anemic patient would be called erythroid hypoplasia denoting some degree of suppression of erythropoiesis. While the number of erythroid cells in marrow from patients with anemia of inflammatory disease or renal failure may be within normal limits for a nonanemic animal, it is hypoplastic in light of a low hematocrit. Dogs with Sertoli cell tumors may have severe bone marrow hypoplasia due to suppressive effects of estrogen produced by the tumor.[16] Hypoplasia may also result with the effects of infectious agents including viruses (eg, FeLV, FIV, feline coronavirus, feline parvovirus, canine parvovirus, canine distemper virus), rickettsia, protozoa, and fungi. Drugs are often responsible for bone marrow damage and include anticonvulsants, antineoplastic agents, estrogen, and antibiotics such as chloramphenicol and trim-ethoprim-sulfadiazine.[17] Patients with endocrine disturbances, chronic renal failure, or intestinal malabsorption may have hypoplasia of the erythroid line alone.[18] Hypoplasia of granulocytic lines can result from various infections and toxic insults.[19] Animals admitted for tumor resection and receiving antineoplastic agents should be evaluated for the presence of drug-related myelosuppression. Less common causes involve hereditary disorders, marrow necrosis, immune-mediated disease, myeloph-thisis, and irradiation. Cytologically, when the hematocrit or CBC is not provided but the marrow particles appear hypocellular with more fat than cells and there is an increased M:E, one is not certain whether erythroid production is less than expected. In this case it can be said that there is a relative erythroid hypoplasia compared to the granulocytic response.

Aplastic anemia is a term applied to the situation in which the marrow is devoid of hematopoietic cells and has been replaced by fat. Destruction or suppression of multipotential hematopoietic stem cells is implicated by this finding. Causative mechanisms may include myelotoxic substances, immune-mediated mechanisms, and some infectious diseases (eg, canine ehrlichiosis).[20,21] Selective absence of one cell line with normal production of cells in the other two lines is called *pure red cell aplasia, pure white cell aplasia,* or *amegakaryocytosis.*[22] Immune-mediated attack (eg, young cats with pure red cell aplasia) on committed progenitor cells of the affected series is the apparent cause in most cases.[23]

Plasmacytosis, lymphocytosis, histiocytosis, and *mastocytosis* are descriptive terms for increased numbers of plasma cells, lymphocytes, macrophages, and mast cells in marrow samples. Whether the increase is reactive or neoplastic must be determined in each case from other clinical and laboratory findings. When marrow injury is mild, with minimal cell destruction, a reactive response usually occurs. *Reactivity* is a nonspecific immune response involving an increase in such cells as plasma cells, mast cells, macrophages, and eosinophils. B-cell hyperplasia has been associated with FIV infection in cats.[24]

Necrosis and *myelofibrosis* are morphologic changes associated with bone marrow destruction with subsequent healing response. Infection, drugs, chemicals, neoplasia, radiation, or immune destruction may damage the bone marrow. When the insult is severe enough to damage the microcirculation, causing ischemia or directly destroying the hematopoietic cells, permanent and irreversible necrosis may occur.[25] The prognosis is generally poor because long-term supportive care is necessary. If necrosis or marrow injury is moderate, attempts to repair the affected area may result in increased numbers of reticulin and collagen fibers, a condition termed *myelofibrosis*. This is considered a secondary response and may be reversible.[26] In both necrosis and myelofibrosis, bone marrow aspirates often contain particles with low cellularity, much blood contamination, and occasional fibrocytes present. For this reason, a core biopsy sample obtained concurrently with the aspirate biopsy is necessary for confirmation of these conditions. In some cases, the suspicion of connective tissue infiltration may need to be confirmed with special histochemical stains. The peripheral blood may reveal few changes or show severe cytopenias.

Hemosiderosis is considered when iron stores accumulate within macrophages thus appearing as dense aggregates with large coarse granules that react strongly with Prussian blue stain. The accumulation implies increased erythrocyte destruction or ineffective erythropoiesis. This situation is present in cases with anemia of chronic disease related to decreased iron utilization or with pure red cell aplasia related to immune-mediated destruction of erythroid precursors. Increased hemosiderin levels have also been associated with feline myelofibrosis and myelodysplastic conditions.[27]

Reporting Bone Marrow Findings

Key features of the CBC and blood film, as well as bone marrow cytologic and histologic findings should be included in the final report. The white cell count, hemoglobin concentration, and red cell indices (MCV and MCHC), and platelet count should be routinely reported and for some patients, the reticulocyte count or chemistry abnormalities (eg, increased globulins) should be provided. The body of the report should include an assessment of cellularity, a systematic description of each cell lineage and their sequence of maturation, the M:E ratio, and evaluation of marrow iron stores. The presence of abnormal marrow components, including abnormal cells or cell numbers and matrix material, should be also described. The presence of focal lesions, identified only in the histologic sections must also be included in the final bone marrow report. If the patient has a previous bone marrow aspiration, comparison should be provided with previous findings to assess disease progress or response to treatment. While it is possible that a definitive diagnosis can be made based on the marrow aspirate, if it cannot, a list of additional tests (eg, immunophenotyping, protein electrophoresis, and infectious disease testing) should be provided.

It is also important for the pathologist to relate what his/her level of certainty is in the diagnosis. For example, varying levels of confidence are provided by the following statements: the findings are consistent with an AML; the marrow features are suggestive for, but are not alone conclusive of a diagnosis of AML; the marrow aspiration cytology supports a diagnosis of AML, however it is essential to assess these findings in light of clinical and other laboratory data; or marrow aspiration cytology does not support a diagnosis of AML. Finally, if a bone marrow aspirate yields only peripheral blood or cellularity is too low for an adequate evaluate, this should be reported so that it become part of the patient's record.

REFERENCES

1. Rizzo F, Tappin SW, Tasker S. Thrombocytosis in cats: a retrospective study of 51 cases (2000–2005). J Fel Med Surg 2007;9:319–25.
2. Vernau W, Moore PF. An immunophenotypic study of canine leukemias and preliminary asessment of clonality by polymerase chain reaction. Vet Immunol Immunopathol 1999;69:145–64.
3. Dunn KJ, Dunn JK. Diagnostic investigations in 101 dogs with pyrexia of unknown origin. J Sm An Pract 1998;39:574–80.
4. Henson KL, Alleman AR, Fox LE, et al. Diagnosis of disseminated adenocarcinoma by bone marrow aspiration in a dog with leukoerythroblastosis and fever of unknown origin. Vet Clin Pathol 1998;27:80–4.
5. Raskin RE, Krehbiel JD. Prevalence of leukemic blood and bone marrow in dogs with multicentric lymphoma. J Am Vet Med Assoc 1989;194:1427–9.
6. Weiss DJ. A retrospective study of the incidence and the classification of bone marrow disorders in the dog at a veterinary teaching hospital (1996-2004). J Vet Intern Med 2006;20:955–61.
7. Helfand SC, Couto CG, Madewell BR. Immune-mediated thrombocytopenia associated with solid tumors in dogs. J Am Anim Hosp Assoc 1985;21:787–94.
8. Sharkey LC, Rosol TJ, Gröne A, et al. Production of granulocyte colony-stimulating factor and granulocyte-macrophage colony-stimulating factor by carcinomas in a dog and a cat with paraneoplastic leukocytosis. J Vet Intern Med 1996;10:405–8.
9. Alleman AR, Harvey JW. The morphologic effects of vincristine sulfate on canine bone marrow cells. Vet Clin Pathol 1993;22:36–41.
10. Weiss DJ, Smith SA. Primary myelodysplastic syndromes of dogs: a report of 12 cases. J Vet Intern Med 2000;14:491–4.
11. Vardiman JW, Brunning RD, Arber DA, et al. Introduction and overview of the classification of the myeloid neoplasms. In: Swerdlow SH, Campo E, Harris NL, et al, editors. WHO classification of tumours of haematopoietic and lymphoid tissues. Lyon (France): IARC; 2008. p. 18–30.
12. Weiss DJ. Recognition and classification of dysmyelopoiesis in the dog: a review. J Vet Intern Med 2005;19:147–54.
13. Raskin RE. Myelopoiesis and myeloproliferative disorders. Vet Clin North Am Sm An Pract 1996;26:1023–42.
14. Breuer W, Hermanns W, Thiele J. Myelodysplastic syndrome (MDS), acute myeloid leukaemia (AML) and chronic myeloproliferative disorder (CMPD) in cats. J Comp Pathol 1999;121:203–16.
15. Stokol T, Blue JT, French TW. Idiopathic pure red cell aplasia and nonregenerative immune-mediated anemia in dogs: 43 cases (1988-1999). J Am Vet Med Assoc 2000;216:1429–36.

16. Sherding RG, Wilson GP, Kociba GJ. Bone marrow hypoplasia in eight dogs with Sertoli cell tumor. J Am Vet Med Assoc 1981;178:497–501.

17. Fox LE, Ford S, Alleman AR, et al. Aplastic anemia associated with prolonged high-dose trimethoprim-sulfadiazine administration in two dogs. Vet Clin Pathol 1993;22:89–92.

18. Fyfe JC, Jezyk PF, Giger U, et al. Inherited selective malabsorption of vitamin B12 in giant schnauzers. J Am Anim Hosp Assoc 1989;25:533–9.

19. Brown MR, Rogers KS. Neutropenia in dogs and cats: a retrospective study of 261 cases. J Am Anim Hosp Assoc 2001;37:131–9.

20. Weiss DJ, Evanson OA. A retrospective study of feline pancytopenia. Comp Haematol Int 2000;10:50–5.

21. Weiss DJ, Evanson OA, Sykes J. A retrospective study of canine pancytopenia. Vet Clin Pathol 1999;28:83–8.

22. Brazzell JL, Weiss DJ. A retrospective study of aplastic pancytopenia in the dog: 9 cases (1996-2003). Vet Clin Pathol 2006;35:413–7.

23. Stokol T, Blue JT. Pure red cell aplasia in cats: 9 cases (1989-1997). J Am Vet Med Assoc 1999;214:75–9.

24. Shelton GH, Abkowitz JL, Linenberger ML, et al. Chronic leukopenia associated with feline immunodeficiency virus infection in a cat. J Am Vet Med Assoc 1989;194:253–5.

25. Hoenig M. Six dogs with features compatible with myelonecrosis and myelofibrosis. J Am Anim Hosp Assoc 1989;25:335–9.

26. Villiers EJ, Dunn JK. Clinicopathological features of seven cases of canine myelofibrosis and the possible relationship between the histological findings and prognosis. Vet Rec 1999;145:222–8.

27. Blue JT. Myelofibrosis in cats with myelodysplastic syndrome and acute myelogenous leukemia. Vet Pathol 1988;25:154–60.

Coombs' Testing and Its Diagnostic Significance in Dogs and Cats

K. Jane Wardrop, DVM, MS

KEYWORDS

- Blood • IMHA • Coombs' test • Antiglobulin test
- Hematology

The Coombs' test, also known as the antiglobulin test, is used to detect antibody and complement on the surface of red blood cells (RBCs). The test was developed by the veterinarian Robin R.A. Coombs in 1945, and was originally used to detect antibodies against antigens in the human Rh blood group system.[1,2] It is used most often in veterinary medicine to aid in the diagnosis of immune-mediated hemolytic anemia (IMHA). An extensive review of the Coombs' test in veterinary medicine has been previously published.[3] The current article provides a brief overview and in addition focuses on more recent studies, particularly those examining test performance, diagnostic significance, and alternate technologies.

TEST METHODOLOGY

The antiglobulin reagents used in the Coombs' test are species-specific and are generally produced in rabbits or goats. Polyvalent reagents contain a combination of anti-IgG, anti-IgM and anti-C3 and can detect immunoglobulin and complement on the surface of RBCs. Monovalent reagents are directed against individual immunoglobulins (Ig) or complement (generally C3 or C3b). The reagents are typically adsorbed with normal RBCs from the target species to remove any heterologous antibodies that may be present. The activity or agglutinating potential of polyvalent and monovalent reagents can vary, dependent on their mode of preparation.

Two forms of the antiglobulin test can be used in veterinary medicine. The direct antiglobulin test (DAT) detects Ig and/or complement that is bound to patient RBCs, and is frequently used in the diagnosis of IMHA (**Fig. 1**). The indirect antiglobulin test (IAT) detects the presence of unbound antibody in the serum and is infrequently used in veterinary medicine, being reserved for commercial blood typing and occasionally

The author has nothing to disclose.
Department of Veterinary Clinical Sciences, College of Veterinary Medicine, Washington State University, Pullman, WA 99164, USA
E-mail address: kjw@vetmed.wsu.edu

Vet Clin Small Anim 42 (2012) 43–51
doi:10.1016/j.cvsm.2011.09.005
0195-5616/12/$ – see front matter © 2012 Elsevier Inc. All rights reserved.

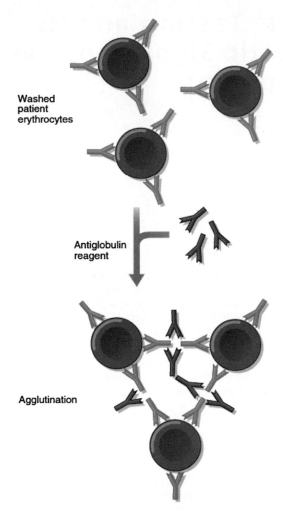

Fig. 1. Principle of the Coombs' test. Antiglobulin reagent reacts with immunoglobulin or complement bound to RBCs, forming a lattice that appears as agglutination. (*From* Day MJ. Immune-mediated anemias in the dog. In: Weiss DJ, Wardrop KJ, editors. Schalm's veterinary hematology. 6th edition. Ames (IA): Wiley-Blackwell; 2010. p. 216–25; with permission.)

used for crossmatching. Standard procedures for the DAT and IAT using tubes are described in **Tables 1** and **2**. The test can also be performed in microtiter plates, which use smaller volumes of reagent and RBCs per well and allow for a greater number of tests and dilutions of antiglobulin reagent to be performed. Typically, one or more wells of the microtiter plates contain the negative reagent control and the remaining wells contain a washed suspension of RBCs and antiglobulin reagent at increasing dilutions. Following incubation, wells are considered negative if they contain a button of RBCs that stream when the plate is tilted. Positive wells have a matte formation that does not stream. The term "full Coombs test" has been used to describe a Coombs' test performed in microtiter plates, fully titrated with both polyvalent and monovalent reagents and tested at both 4°C and 37°C.[4,5]

Table 1
Direct antiglobulin test (DAT) tube technique
1. Place 1–2 drops of a 2%–5% RBC suspension in a 10 or 12 × 75 mm test tube.
2. Wash 3–4 times with normal saline or with phosphate-buffered saline (PBS). Thoroughly decant the last wash residual, in order to avoid dilution or neutralization of the antiglobulin reagent.
3. Immediately add antiglobulin reagent in amounts and as diluted per manufacturer's guidelines. Prepare a negative control tube by adding saline instead of reagent to a tube.
4. Incubate tubes according to manufacturer's directions.
5. Centrifuge, gently dislodge red cell button and record agglutination reactions observed as the cells come off the button. If no agglutination is apparent, a small amount of the tube contents can be placed on a slide and examined microscopically.
6. If available, add IgG-sensitized red cells to nonreactive (unagglutinated) tests to serve as a positive control. Centrifuge and examine for agglutination.
7. If a positive DAT is obtained, monospecific reagents (if available for the species) can be used to determine whether immunoglobulin or complement (or both) are present. Freshly washed cells must be used for this step.

Modified from Wardrop KJ. The Coombs' test in veterinary medicine: past, present, future. Vet Clin Pathol 2005;34:325–34; with permission.

TEST PERFORMANCE

Sensitivity of the traditional tube direct Coombs' test for the detection of IMHA has been problematic, with sensitivity as low as 48% previously reported in dogs.[6] False negative test results may be secondary to factors such as incomplete washing of RBCs, insufficient RBC-bound antibody, elution of Ig or C3, or to a prozone effect.[3,7] Negative tests can also occur in those cases of nonregenerative immune-mediated anemias where antibodies only recognize epitopes expressed on RBC precursors, rather than on circulating RBCs.[8,9]

Recent studies have focused on enhancing the sensitivity of the direct Coombs' test through use of monovalent reagents, performing the test at both 37°C and 4°C, and using microtiter plates with more dilutions to avoid a prozone effect (also see

Table 2
Indirect antiglobulin test (IAT) tube technique
1. Place 2 drops of patient serum or plasma into appropriately labeled tubes.
2. Add 1 drop washed 2%–5% saline-suspended donor RBC to each tube and mix.
3. Centrifuge and observe for hemolysis and/or agglutination.
4. Incubate at 37°C for 30–60 minutes.
5. Centrifuge and observe for hemolysis and agglutination.
6. Wash cells 3–4 times with saline and completely decant the final wash.
7. Immediately add antiglobulin reagent in amounts and as diluted per manufacturer's guidelines. Mix well.
8. Centrifuge and observe for macroscopic and microscopic agglutination.
9. Confirm the validity of negative tests by adding IgG-coated red cells.

Modified from Wardrop KJ. The Coombs' test in veterinary medicine: past, present, future. Vet Clin Pathol 2005;34:325–34; with permission.

section on Diagnostic Significance).[5,7,10] The prozone effect is caused by a relative excess of antiglobulin in relation to antigen (Ig or C3 on RBCs) at lower antisera dilutions. The relative excess of antiglobulin results in decreased cross-linking of RBCs, causing a failure to agglutinate at low antisera dilutions. At higher antisera dilutions, the proportion of antiglobulin to antigen becomes appropriate for agglutination to take place, and a positive result is evident.

One study in dogs determined the effect of dilutions and use of monovalent reagents on test sensitivity.[7] The study evaluated 65 blood samples submitted for canine Coombs' testing over a 2½ year period. Of these 65 samples, 28 (43%) of 65 were from dogs classified as IMHA positive based on specific inclusion criteria, and 37 (57%) of 65 were from dogs classified as IMHA negative. Both polyvalent and monovalent reagents were used, and tests were performed at several dilutions in microtiter plates at 37°C. Differences were noted between results obtained by a commercially obtained polyvalent Coombs' reagent (61% sensitivity, 100% specificity) and results obtained by reagent that was obtained from another commercial source, but further prepared or modified on site (82% sensitivity, 95% specificity). The use of monovalent antisera in this study did not result in enhanced sensitivity compared to use of the single polyvalent antisera prepared or modified on site. When monovalent reagents were used, the majority of patients positive with both polyvalent reagents were also positive using anti-IgG antiserum. The use of increased dilutions of antisera beyond what was recommended by manufacturers (ie, 1:2 to 1:8) resulted in 6 Coombs' positive results that would have been missed at lower dilutions. The highest dilution at which the Coombs' test initially became positive was 1:64 for the modified reagent and 1:128 for the commercial reagent. Thus the use of multiple antisera dilutions increased test sensitivity. The study also pointed out the differences that can occur between Coombs' reagents.

The use of both 37°C and 4°C incubation in the Coombs' test is controversial. Early studies pointed out that nonpathogenic cold reactive antibodies can exist in healthy animals, yielding a low titer, positive reaction in the 4°C Coombs' test (≤1:8 for dogs and 1:2 for cats).[11,12] Recent studies, however, have suggested that enhanced sensitivity can result from cold incubation. Incubation temperature had an effect on sensitivity in a study of 65 Coombs' test–positive dogs with primary and secondary IMHA.[5] Eleven (17%) of the 65 dogs were negative when tested with polyvalent Coombs' reagent at 37°C alone. Six of these 11 became positive when the polyvalent Coombs' reagent at 4°C was used. Use of the monovalent reagents anti-IgM and anti-C3 at 4°C added the remaining 5 dogs (4 and 1 dogs, respectively; 1 dog was also positive using anti-IgM at 37°C). The majority (73%) of those dogs negative at 37°C with the polyvalent Coombs' reagent had underlying or concurrent disease of a nonimmune nature. The association of reactivity at 4°C with additional supportive evidence of hemolysis suggested that the reactivity was significant, and that antibodies binding to RBC at temperatures of 0° to 4°C may be a cause of hemolytic disease. The study conclusion was that optimum performance of the canine Coombs' test was at both 4°C and 37°C, with both polyvalent and monovalent antisera. A similar conclusion was reached in a recent study of IMHA in cats, where persistent autoagglutination was noted in some cats at 4°C.[10]

DIAGNOSTIC SIGNIFICANCE OF THE COOMBS' TEST IN DOGS

The use of the Coombs' test as an aid in the diagnosis of IMHA in dogs was first described by Miller and coworkers in 1954, and subsequently by Lewis and colleagues in 1963.[13,14] Despite problems with sensitivity (see Test Performance), the test does have diagnostic value for IMHA. As an example, one large, retrospective study looked at 151 dogs with IMHA not associated with underlying infectious or neoplastic disease. Coombs' testing was done using polyvalent antisera in microtiter plates at 37°C. The direct Coombs' test was positive in 58 (77%) of 75 dogs tested (dogs with overt autoagglutination were not tested).[15]

Another study looked at the clinical significance of the pattern of Coombs' test reactivity in dogs with IMHA, and whether the pattern varied between dogs with primary IMHA compared to dogs with secondary IMHA.[5] Sixty-five anemic dogs with positive Coombs' test results were included. Inclusion criteria for IMHA included a PCV of 30% or less, evidence of hemolysis, and adequate clinical investigation to diagnose or exclude underlying or concurrent disease. Coombs' testing was performed in microtiter plates at 37°C and at 4°C with both polyvalent rabbit anti-canine Coombs' reagent (specificity for canine IgG, IgM, and C3) and monovalent rabbit anti-canine IgG (Fc), rabbit anti-canine IgM (Fc) and goat anti-canine C3. Forty-six of the 65 dogs were diagnosed with primary IMHA, with 5 dogs of these dogs also showing signs of concurrent immune-mediated disease (thrombocytopenia, IBD, glomerulonephritis). The remaining 19 dogs had underlying or concurrent disease of a nonimmune nature (secondary IMHA). The dogs with primary IMHA were more likely to be positive when tested with the polyvalent antiserum or anti-dog IgG than were the dogs with secondary IMHA and less likely to be positive with anti-dog IgM alone. More dogs with secondary IMHA than with primary IMHA were positive at 4°C with anti-dog IgM. The study could not confirm that low titers or C3 alone were more consistent with secondary IMHA. Interestingly, a positive IgM titer has been associated with a negative effect on survival in dogs with IMHA, based on one study using only monovalent reagents.[16]

Care should be taken to not use the Coombs' test alone to diagnose IMHA. Any positive test should be interpreted in the presence of clinical and hematologic evidence for IMHA. One early study examined the diagnostic significance of the DAT performed in 371 anemic dogs (anemic from any cause).[12] In this study, the DAT was positive in 134 dogs using monovalent reagents. Interestingly, only 37 of these positive anemic dogs had clinical evidence of hemolysis induced by primary IMHA, with most being positive for IgG or IgG and C3b. Positive anemic dogs without evidence of hemolytic disease tended to be positive for C3b alone, and included dogs with infections, inflammatory disorders, and myeloproliferative and lymphoproliferative diseases.

DIAGNOSTIC SIGNIFICANCE OF THE COOMBS' TEST IN CATS

In cats, DAT positive hemolytic anemia was first described in 1973 by Scott and colleagues, who looked at 7 cases of feline IMHA, 6 of which had positive Coombs' test results.[17] Subsequent studies have looked at the significance of the Coombs' test in both anemic and nonanemic cats. In one early study, a DAT was performed on 20 anemic and 20 nonanemic, healthy cats. Sixteen of the 20 anemic cats were DAT positive. Eleven of the 16 were FeLV positive, and the remaining 5 positive cats had inflammatory disease or hemoplasmosis. Interestingly, 9 of the nonanemic cats showed a weakly positive result. Conservative interpretation of a positive test in the absence of hemolysis was recommended.[11]

Other, more recent studies looking at Coombs' testing in both anemic and nonanemic cats have also been performed. In a study of anemia of inflammatory disease in cats with abscesses, pyothorax, or fat necrosis, Coombs' test results (using monovalent reagents against IgG, IgM, and C3b) were negative for 8 cats, and positive (IgG) for 1 cat with pyothorax.[18]

Kohn performed the direct Coombs' test in 78 anemic and 14 nonanemic cats to determine its diagnostic significance.[19] Monovalent reagents (IgG, IgM, and C3b) and both 4°C and 37°C incubation temperatures were used. The IgG and IgM antisera was diluted from 1:20 to 1:640. The dilution of C3b ranged from 1:10 to 1:320. Tests were performed in round bottomed, 96 well microtiter plates, and the RBC suspension was incubated with antisera for 90 minutes at 4°C or 37°C. The test was negative in all 14 nonanemic cats (5 healthy and 9 sick nonanemic) and in 55 cats with different types of anemia (eg, blood loss anemia, anemia from chronic renal failure, anemia associated with neoplastic or inflammatory disease, hemolytic anemia due to hypophosphatemia or Heinz bodies). Of the 23 remaining anemic cats, 5 had persistent agglutination (Coombs' test could not be performed) and 18 cats had a positive Coombs' test. Most of these cats were either positive for IgG, or for both IgG and IgM. Based on additional clinical and laboratory criteria, these 23 cats were judged to have either primary (19 cats) or secondary (4 cats) IMHA. The Coombs' positive cats were positive at both 4°C and at 37°C, suggesting that the Coombs' test only needed to be performed at one temperature. Results showed that the Coombs' test was very useful in the diagnosis of immune-mediated anemia in cats, and that an immune-mediated component of hemolytic anemia in Coombs' negative cats was unlikely.

Tasker also performed Coombs' testing in 60 anemic and 60 nonanemic cats.[10] The 60 nonanemic cats used in the study had a variety of diseases, with only 1 cat deemed clinically well. Eleven of the 60 anemic cats used in the study were determined to have IMHA, as evidenced by the presence of anemia, evidence of hemolysis, lack of evidence of other causes, and response to immunosuppressive therapy. Serial dilutions of reagent (1:5 to 1:10,240) and polyvalent and monovalent (anti-feline IgG, IgM, and IgA) antisera were used. Testing was performed in U-bottom 96 well plates. Plates were incubated for 1 hour at either 4°C or 37°C.

In Coombs' testing with polyvalent antiserum at 37°C, 15 (12.5%) of the 120 cats gave positive results, including 13 anemic cats and 2 nonanemic cats with pancreatitis. Nine of the 11 IMHA cats showed a positive result. Autoagglutination in the PBS control wells at 37°C was not seen in any cat. When Coombs' testing was performed at 4°C, 13 (21.7%) of the 60 anemic cats had persistent autoagglutination in PBS control wells, which precluded determination of Coombs' test titers. All 11 IMHA cats had positive results at 4° C, with 9 of 11 showing persistent autoagglutination (no Coombs reagent) at 4°C and 2 of the 11 showing positive Coombs' reactions at 4°C with polyvalent antiserum (titers of 20 or 160), IgM antiserum (titers of 20 or 40) and IgG antiserum (titer of 640, one cat only). Of the 2 IMHA cats that were only positive at 4°C, one showed persistent autoagglutination and the other was positive with IgM antiserum. Cats that showed persistent agglutination at 4°C were more likely to be Coombs' positive (any antisera at any titer) at 37°C than to be negative. The study showed that cats with IMHA were more likely to have persistent cold autoagglutination and show positive Coombs' test results at 37°C, suggesting that cats suspected of having IMHA should be evaluated for persistent autoagglutination at 4°C as well as performing Coombs' testing at 37°C. In addition, testing always needed to be interpreted in parallel with documentation of hemolysis in anemic cats.

Positive Coombs' tests and IMHA have been reported in association with infectious agents in cats. FeLV infection has been shown to be a common underlying disease in retrospective studies of cats with IMHA.[11,17,20] IMHA can also occur in cats experimentally or naturally infected with Mycoplasma haemofelis.[20-22]

In a recent study where cats were experimentally infected with Mycoplasma haemofelis, Candidatus M haemominutum, or Candidatus M turicensis, only those cats infected with M haemofelis (10 cats) developed both anemia (often severe) and RBC-bound antibodies.[22] Coombs' testing was performed at 4°C and 37°C with both polyvalent feline Coombs' reagent (against feline IgG, IgM, IgA, and C3) and with monovalent reagents against IgG and IgM. All 10 cats developed cold-reactive antibodies (cold agglutinins), with either persistent autoagglutination or Coombs' positivity at 4°C observed. Eight of the cats also showed evidence of warm reactive antibodies, which appeared after the cold-reactive antibodies, when the anemia was fully established. In 3 cats, only warm reactive antibodies were identified at the latest time points (≥50 days postinfection). RBC-bound antibodies reactive at 4°C (IgM and IgG) appeared 8 to 22 days postinfection and persisted for 2 to 4 weeks. RBC-bound antibodies reactive at 37°C (primarily IgG) developed between 22 to 29 days postinfection and persisted for 1 to 5 weeks. A prozone effect for monovalent IgG was observed in one cat, where agglutination was not observed until a higher dilution of antibody (≥1:640) was performed.

The pathophysiologic role of the cold-reactive antibodies in this study was unclear, but they did appear shortly after the hemoglobin values began to fall. This suggested insensitivity of the Coombs' test early in the course of the disease or the presence of other factors, such as direct organism damage to the RBC before formation of cold-reactive antibodies. The cold-reactive antibodies were thought to be consistent with the presence of IgG or IgM antibodies that eluted from the surface of the RBCs at physiologic temperatures in vitro. Complement deposition onto RBCs could occur at lower temperatures of the peripheral circulation, even if the initiating antibodies then dissociated from the RBCs at higher body temperatures. The cold agglutinins detected in the *M haemofelis*–infected cats were not active at room temperature (18°C to 20°C), which suggested a narrow range of thermal activity. The study demonstrated that *M haemofelis* resulted in a severe anemia and a positive Coombs' test, with development of both cold and warm reactive RBC-bound antibodies.

ALTERNATE TECHNOLOGIES FOR ANTIGLOBULIN TESTS

Alternate tests for detection of RBC-bound immunoglobulin or complement have been developed. Most of the alternate technology associated with antiglobulin testing has been designed to either increase the sensitivity of the test or to lessen the subjectivity associated with assessment of degrees of agglutination. Enzyme-linked antiglobulin tests appear to enhance sensitivity but are difficult to perform and also decrease the specificity for IMHA.[23,24] Flow cytometry has been shown to be a sensitive diagnostic technique for IMHA in dogs, with some decrease in specificity.[25,26]

One prospective study used flow cytometry to determine the overall prevalence of immunoglobulin bound to RBC in healthy and sick dogs and to evaluate the sensitivity and specificity of flow cytometry for the diagnosis of IMHA. Blood samples from 292 dogs, including 147 anemic and 145 nonanemic (31 normal) animals, were analyzed. Among the nonanemic dogs, 8.3% had RBC antibodies detected by flow cytometry, and positive test results were more common in dogs with infectious disease and neoplasia. Among the 147 anemic dogs, 26 (17.7%) had anti-RBC antibodies (IgG or IgG and IgM). Seventeen (77%) of 22 dogs with IMHA (based on inclusion criteria of anemia, evidence of regeneration, and evidence of RBC destruction) had anti-RBC antibodies.[27] Another study compared flow cytometric detection of IgG bound to RBC of anemic dogs to microtiter plate detection, using 2 different anti-IgG reagents at 4°C and 37°C. The flow cytometric method was more sensitive, but differences between the 2 reagents used were also noted.[28] Flow cytometry for detection of anti-RBC antibodies is a potentially useful technique; however, the test currently lacks standardization between laboratories and necessitates the use of a flow cytometer.

Antiglobulin gel tests incorporate antiglobulin into a gel matrix and have been used for both direct and indirect antiglobulin testing in humans.[29–32] An RBC suspension is dispensed into the reaction chamber of the microtube containing the gel, and the tubes are incubated and centrifuged. Any RBC agglutinates become trapped and remain stable in the gel, while free RBCs pass through and form a button at the bottom of the tube. The end point reactions are more stable than conventional tube agglutination reactions. Gel antiglobulin tests have been previously used in the dog, for both direct and indirect testing.[33] These gels are no longer commercially available.

SUMMARY

The Coombs' test can detect both immunoglobulin and complement on the surface of RBCs, and as such can be of value as an aid in the diagnosis of IMHA. Techniques that may improve sensitivity include use of monovalent reagents, increased dilutions of antiglobulin to avoid a prozone effect, and testing at 4°C. These techniques are not without controversy, and positive tests should always be interpreted in the presence of other clinical and hematologic evidence for IMHA. Alternate techniques, such as flow cytometry, can improve detection of RBC-bound immunoglobulin, but require a flow cytometer and further standardization between laboratories.

REFERENCES

1. Coombs RRA. Historical note: past, present and future of the antiglobulin test. Vox Sang 1998;74:67–73.
2. Coombs RRA. Immunohematology: reminiscences and reflections. Transf Med 1994; 4:185–93.
3. Wardrop KJ. The Coombs' test in veterinary medicine: past, present, future. Vet Clin Pathol 2005;34:325–34.
4. Day MJ. Immune-mediated anemias in the dog. In: Weiss DJ, Wardrop KJ, editors. Schalm's veterinary hematology. 6th edition. Ames (IA): Wiley-Blackwell; 2010. p. 216–25.
5. Warman SM, Murray JK, Ridyard A, et al. Pattern of Coombs' test reactivity has diagnostic significance in dogs with immune-mediated haemolytic anaemia. J Small An Pract 2008;49:525–30.
6. Jones DRE, Gruffydd-Jones TJ, Stokes CR, et al. Investigation into factors influencing performance of the canine antiglobulin test. Res Vet Sci 1990;48:53–8.
7. Overmann JA, Sharkey LC, Weiss DJ, et al. Performance of 2 microtiter canine Coombs' tests. Vet Clin Pathol 2007;36:179–83.
8. Stokal T, Blue JT. Pure red cell aplasia in cats: 9 cases (1989-1997). J Am Vet Med Assoc 1999;9:530–9.
9. Abrams-Ogg ACG, Wood RD, Cheung A. Idiopathic non-regenerative anemia in cats: a retrospective study [abstract]. J Vet Intern Med 2007;21:624.
10. Tasker S, Murray JK, Knowles TG, et al. Coombs', haemoplasma and retrovirus testing in feline anaemia. J Small Anim Pract 2010;51:192–9.
11. Dunn JK, Searcy GP, Hirsch VM. The diagnostic significance of a positive direct antiglobulin test in anemic cats. Can J Comp Med 1984;48:349–53.
12. Slappendel RJ. The diagnostic significance of the direct antiglobulin test (DAT) in anemic dogs. Vet Immunol Immunopathol 1979;1:49–59.
13. Miller G, Swisher SN, Young LE. A case of autoimmune hemolytic anemia in a dog. Clin Res Proc 1954;260–1.
14. Lewis RM, Henry WB Jr, Thornton GW, et al. A syndrome of autoimmune hemolytic anemia and thrombocytopenia in dogs. Proc Am Vet Med Assoc 1963:140–63.
15. Weinkle TK, Center SA, Randolph JF, et al. Evaluation of prognostic factors, survival rates, and treatment protocols for immune-mediated hemolytic anemia in dogs: 151 cases (1993–2002). J Am Vet Med Assoc 2005;226:1869–80.

16. Piek CJ, Junius G, Dekker A, et al. Idiopathic immune-mediated hemolytic anemia: Treatment outcome and prognostic factors in 149 dogs. J Vet Intern Med 2008;22: 366–73.

17. Scott DW, Schultz RD, Post JE, et al. Autoimmune hemolytic anemia in the cat. J Am Anim Hosp Assoc 1973;9:530–9.

18. Ottenjann M, Weingart C, Arndt G, et al. Characterization of the anemia of inflammatory disease in cats with abscesses, pyothorax, or fat necrosis. J Vet Intern Med 2006;20:1143–50.

19. Kohn B, Weingart C, Eckmann V, et al. Primary immune-mediated hemolytic anemia in 19 cats: diagnosis, therapy, and outcome (1998-2004). J Vet Intern Med 2006;20: 159 66.

20. Werner LL, Gorman NT. Immune mediated disorders in cats. Vet ClinNorth Am Small Anim Pract 1984;14:1039–64.

21. Zulty JC, Kociba GJ. Cold agglutinins in cats with haemobartonellosis. J Am Vet Med Assoc 1990;196:907–10.

22. Tasker S, Peters IR, Papasouliotis K, et al. Description of outcomes of experimental infection with feline haemoplasmas: copy numbers, haematology, Coombs' testing and blood glucose concentrations. Vet Microbiol 2009;139:323–32.

23. Barker RN, Gruffydd-Jones TJ, Elson CJ. Red cell-bound immunoglobulins and complement measured by an enzyme-linked antiglobulin test in dogs with autoimmune haemolysis or other anaemias. Res Vet Sci 1993;54:170–8.

24. Jones DRE, Gruffydd-Jones TJ, Stokes CR, et al. Use of a direct enzyme-linked antiglobulin test for laboratory diagnosis of immune-mediated hemolytic anemia in dogs. Am J Vet Res 1992;53:457–65.

25. Wilkerson MJ, Davis E, Shuman W, et al. Isotype-specific antibodies in horses and dogs with immune-mediated hemolytic anemia. J Vet Intern Med 2000;14:190–6.

26. Quigley KA, Chelack BJ, Haines DM, et al. Application of a direct flow cytometric erythrocyte immunofluorescence assay in dogs with immune-mediated hemolytic anemia and comparison to the direct antiglobulin test. J Vet Diagn Invest 2001;13: 297–300.

27. Morley P, Mathes M, Guth A, et al. Anti-erythrocyte antibodies and disease associations in anemic and nonanemic dogs. J Vet Intern Med 2008;22:886–92.

28. Kucinskiene G, Schuberth HJ, Leibold W, et al. Flow cytometric evaluation of bound IgG on erythrocytes of anaemic dogs. Vet J 2005;169:303–7.

29. Nathalang O, Chuansumrit A, Prayoonwiwat W, et al. Comparison between the conventional tube technique and the gel technique in direct antiglobulin tests. Vox Sang 1997;72:169–71.

30. Novaretti MCZ, Jens E, Pagliarini T, et al. Comparison of conventional tube test technique and gel microcolumn assay for direct antiglobulin test: a large study. J Clin Lab Anal 2004;18:255–8.

31. Bromilow IM, Eggington JA, Owen GA, et al. Red cell antibody screening and identification: a comparison of two column technology methods. Br J Biomed Sci 1993;50:329–33.

32. Pinkerton PH, Ward J, Chan R, et al. An evaluation of a gel technique for antibody screening compared with a conventional tube method. Transf Med 1993;3:275–9.

33. Kessler RJ, Reese J, Chang D, et al. Dog erythrocyte antigens 1.1, 1.2, 3, 4, 7, and *Dal* blood typing and crossmatching by gel column technique. Vet Clin Pathol 2010;39: 306–16.

Principles and Applications of Flow Cytometry and Cell Sorting in Companion Animal Medicine

Melinda J. Wilkerson, DVM, MS, PhD

KEYWORDS

- Flow cytometry • Fluorochrome • Immunophenotyping
- Cluster of differentiation antigens • Lymphocyte subset
- Fluorescent activated cell sorting • Immune-mediated disorders

Flow cytometry is a powerful tool in the clinical and research setting for defining the characteristics of cells or particles utilizing the light scattering properties of analyzed cells or particles and fluorescence emissions of targeted antibodies or cellular probes. Flow cytometry has evolved over the past 60 years from single-parameter instruments (Coulter Counter) which detected the size of cells and was incorporated into hematology analyzers,[1] to sophistocated instruments that measure up to 14 parameters simultaneously (eg, Becton Dickinson's FACSAria). The insertion of flow cytometry technology into hematology instruments replaced the labor intensive methods of manual counting of erythrocytes and leukocytes with a hemacytometer. The first fluorescent activated cell sorter (FACS) was described by Max Fulwyler in 1965.[2] Although the first clinical flow cytometers were introduced in human medical centers in the 1980s and were used by researchers to define lymphocyte subsets in animal models of human disease,[3] it was nearly 15 to 20 years later before flow cytometers become a part of diagnostic testing in veterinary medicine.[4–6]

BASIC PRINCIPLES AND ESSENTIAL COMPONENTS OF FLOW CYTOMETER INSTUMENTATION

Flow cytometry is defined as an instrument that measures characteristics of cells or particles in a fluid stream as they pass through a light source (laser). The power of flow cytometers is the capacity to measure multiple parameters of not only cells but also chromosomes, proteins or nucleic acids that are attached to a particle (eg, microsphere) as long as the particles or cells are suspended in a fluid.[7] Fluorescent

The author has nothing to disclose.
Department of Diagnostic Medicine/Pathobiology, College of Veterinary Medicine, Kansas State University, 340 Coles Hall, 1800 Denison Avenue, Manhattan, KS 66506, USA
E-mail address: wilkersn@vet.k-state.edu

Vet Clin Small Anim 42 (2012) 53–71
doi:10.1016/j.cvsm.2011.09.012   **vetsmall.theclinics.com**

activated cell sorters are flow cytometers that have the capacity to separate or sort fluorescent-labeled cells from a mixed cell population. Most bench top flow cytometers including hematology analyzers cannot sort cells and are dedicated to analytical methods that measure light scatter and emitted fluorscent light.

The major components of flow cytometers and cell sorters consist of fluidics, optics (excitation and collection), an electronic network, and a computer. The fluidics direct a liquid stream containing particles through the focused light source. The excitation (laser) focuses the light source on the cells/particles, where collection optics (filters and mirrors) directs the light scatter or fluorescent light of the particle to an electronic network. The electronic network detects the light signals coming from the particle as it passes through the light beam and then converts the signals to a digital readout that is proportional to light intensity. The computer records the digital signals from the electronic detectors, allowing the operator to analyse the data and place it in one of several outputs (eg, histograms, dot plots, contour plots, density plots).[8] An example of a common bench top analyzer with capability of four-color analysis is the FACSCalibur (Becton Dickinson, San Jose, CA, USA) (**Fig. 1**A). The Beckman Coulter MoFlo XDP (see **Fig. 1**B) is an example of a high-speed cell sorter equipped with three lasers and collection optics and electronic configuration for six-color analysis and sorting capability. A brief explanation of each of the essential components of flow cytometers and activated cell sorters will be provided. The use of these instruments is limited to the academic institutions, pharmaceutical companies, or reference laboratories because of their substantial cost ($50,000 to $150,000 for bench top flow cytometers and $350,000 to $500,000 for high speed cell sorters). This sophisticated technology also requires a highly trained technician to operate, analyze the samples, and maintain the equipment, and for clinical samples a trained veterinary pathologist to interpret the data.

FLUIDICS

The fluidic system is composed of a reservoir of phosphate-buffered saline (sheath fluid) and pressurized lines that inject the sheath fluid into a flow chamber where the laser beams interrogate the cells of the sample (**Fig. 2**, gray box). A pressurized air line also injects the suspended cells in the sample tube into the flow cell (see **Fig. 2**, inset A). Because there is a pressure differential between the sheath fluid and sample stream, the sample stream becomes a central core in the sheath fluid stream, referred to as coxial flow, and serves to aline the sample cells in single file through the laser beam, thus ensuring uniform illumination of a cell, one cell at a time (see **Fig. 2**, inset A). The rate at which the cells in the core sample stream are injected into the laser beam can be adjusted by the operator. High flow rates are common for most applications (eg, immunophenotyping of mammalian cells), whereas slow flow rates are essential for quantitation of DNA content in fluorescent-stained nuclei. The slow flow rate reduces the size of the sample stream increasing the uniformity and accuracy of the illumination of the nuclei by the laser beam.[8]

EXCITATION AND COLLECTION OPTICS

The optical bench of the flow cytometer consists of a laser (excitation optics) and a series of lenses and filters (collection optics) to collect side angle scatter and the various fluorescent signals of excited fluorochromes. Lasers produce light by energizing electrons to high energy orbitals with high voltage electricity, when the electrons fall back into their lower energy orbitals, photons of light is created. The applied voltage maintains the electrons in excited orbitals within a tube contacting

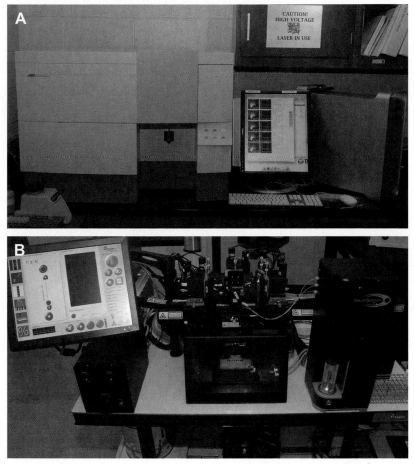

Fig. 1. (*A*) A typical bench top analytical flow cytometer (FACSCalibur, Becton Dickinson, San Jose, CA, USA) interfaced with a Macintosh Pro computer. (*B*) The MoFlo XDP (Beckman Coulter, Brea, CA, USA) is a fluorescent activated cell sorter. The sampler apparatus to the right (Smart-Sampler) samples the cells, the sorting chamber is in the center of the slide, the detectors and electronics are located behind the sort chamber, and a monitor (left section of the slide) provides a magnified image of the sample stream for the operator to manipulate.

mirrors that causes the photons to oscillate back and forth, amplifying the signal. The laser light is focused into an elliptical beam 60 μm in diameter by a focusing lens. The sample stream will span 50 to 150 μm in diameter depending on the adjustment of the flow rate by the operator. Flow cytometers may have a variety of laser configurations that dictate the types of fluorochromes that can be excited. Many synthetic (eg, fluorescein isothiocynate [FITC]) and natural fluorochrome dyes including algae and phytoplanktons are excited by the argon laser (a common laser with an excitation wavelength of 488 nm) resulting in emission of light at a higher wavelength (eg, the argon laser excits FITC to emit in the green spectrum, 535 nm, phycoerythrin is excited to emit in the orange spectrum, 585 nm, and propidium iodide is excited to emit light in the red spectrum, 630 nm). Many flow cytometers and sorters have additional lasers including ultraviolet that excite UV (300 to 400 nm) sensitive

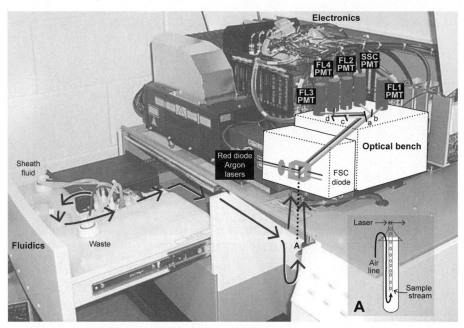

Fig. 2. Essential components of the bench top flow cytometer (FACSCalibur) include the fluidics (sheath fluid and waste resevoir), optical bench including excitation optics (lasers) and collection optics (*a, b, c,* and *d*), and the electronic network including photo diode for FSC and detectors (SSC, FL1, FL2, FL3, and FL4 PMTs) for side angle scatter and 4-fluorescent wavelengths. Red arrows represent the pressurized flow of the sheath fluid to the flow chamber (*gray box* where lasers interegate cells). (*A*) Inset of the sample tube. Differential pressures between the sheath fluid and sample stream form a coxial flow whereby the cells enter the laser beam in single file.

fluorochromes or the red diode which excites fluorochromes of the far red (630 nm) range. The FACSCalibur has a two-laser (argon and red diode) and four-color detector system in which dyes in the green, orange, and red emission spectra are excited by the argon laser and detected by three photomultipier tubes (PMT) referred to as FL1, FL2, and FL3 (see **Fig. 2**), whereas a red diode laser excites far red dyes that are detected by the FL4 PMT (see **Fig. 2**). Dichroic mirrors, long pass, short pass, and band pass filters split and separate the various wavelengths of light to direct them to the appropriate detectors (see **Fig. 2**a–d).

DETECTING PROPERTIES OF CELLS WITH LIGHT SCATTER AND FLUORESCENCE

When the laser beam interrogrates the cell, two types of light scatter occurs: forward-angle scatter (FSC) and side-angle scatter (SSC) (**Fig. 3**A). Forward angle scatter is the light that has diffracted around the cell and is proportional to cell size. Side-angle scatter is 90-degree angle scatter and proportional to the internal complexity (granularity or nuclear lobularity) of the cell. Note that fluorescent light from labeling of surface antigens via fluorescent-labeled antibodies or DNA by a nucleic acid stain, propidium dye, is reflected at the same angle as side-angle scatter (see **Fig. 3**A). The unique light scatter properties of cells is used to distinguish subpopulations of cells based on their size and internal complexity (**Fig. 3**B) and is

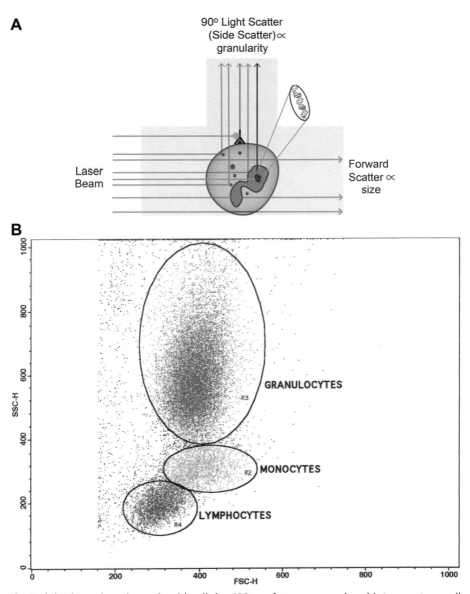

Fig. 3. (*A*) When a laser beam (eg, blue light, 488 nm, from an argon laser) interrogates a cell, light scatters around the cell referred to as forward angle scatter and is proporational to size. Nonfluorescent light that is scattered at a 90-degree angle is side-angle and proportional to internal complexity contributed by the degree of granularity and nucler lobularity. The green line of light represents fluoresence of an excited green fluorochrome conjugated to an antibody bound to a surface antigen. DNA dyes, like propidium iodide, have affinity for nucleic acids and will fluoresce in the red spectrum (600 to630 nm) (represented by the *red line*) following excitation by the argon laser. Both green and the red fluorescence is collected by detectors (FL1, FL2, or FL3) positioned at 90 degrees to the laser. (*B*) Scatter plot (SSC-H vs FSC-H) of peripheral blood leukocytes from a healthy dog. Lymphocytes (Region 4, *red gate*) have the lowest forward and side scatter indicating their small size and low complexity, whereas monocytes are intermediate (R2 or *green gate*), and granulocytes are most complex (R3 or *pink gate*).

intregral to the leukocyte differential counts performed by laser-based clinical hematology analyzers. Dedicated flow cytometers also differentiate cellular parameters further by using fluorescently labeled antibodies to surface antigens (eg, cluster differentiation molecules) and to internal structures/organelles (eg, nucleic acids or mitochondrial membrane potential) to determine the DNA content, viability, or activation state of subsets of cells.

The light scatter signals and fluorescent emissions from the excitation of fluorescent dyes are converted to electronic voltage pulses by an electronic network that includes a photodiode to convert forward light scatter and photomultiplier tubes to convert side scatter and fluorescent light. The voltage pulses are converted to a digital output and transferred to a computer for manipulation by the operator.[8] The operator can amplify or reduce the light scatter signals to fit the type of cells analyzed by the cytometer, eg, signals from fluorescent-tagged bacteria can be amplified, whereas fluorescent signals of labeled tumor cells can be reduced. Unlike sorters, the cells in bench top analytical flow cytometers are removed under vacuum into a waste resevoir after the analysis has occurred.

It is important for the user to know the laser, filter, and detector configuration in flow cytometer when choosing fluorochrome-labeled probes for cellular studies. For example, rhodamine is a commonly used dye in fluorescent microscopy; however, it is excited by the 514-nm line of the argon laser and not the 488-nm line. The latter is the more common tuning for argon lasers in flow cytometers.[8] Knowing the capability of the flow cytometer prior to purchasing the fluorochromes will reduce the cost, labor, and frustration of the user.

PRINCIPLES OF CELL SORTING

FACSs have the capacity to isolate subpopulations of fluorescent-tagged cells into a variety of collection vessels including tubes and 96-well plates or onto glass slides. FACS systems use a principle of electrostatic deflection of charged droplets, similar to that used in ink-jet printers.[9] In this system, the cells are ejected into air in a stream of sheath fluid. To be able to charge individual fluorescent cells, a droplet needs to be formed. These instruments contain a nozzle tip that oscillates the sample core at a very high frequency (eg, 30,000 cycles per second) resulting in a stream that breaks into droplets. A diagram of the essential sorting components of the MoFlo XDP is illustrated in **Fig. 4**. Cells are ejected from the vibrating nozzle in individual droplets, then they pass through one or more laser beams, allowing the information about the cells to be gathered. Once the operator selects the fluorescent cell of interest using a computer, the tagged cells in the drop will be charged by a charging electrode as they pass through the laser beam. Thereafter, positively charged droplets are deflected toward a platinum plate of negative charge, negatively charged droplets are deflected toward the positively charged platinum plate, and uncharged droplets are collected into a waste container. Although the new cell sorters are more compact, they still require dedicated trained personel; especially to align the laser beams, calculate the charge delay between the analysis point and the break off point of the droplet, and maintain the equipment.

The power of the cell sorter is the ability to collect a specific subpopulation of cells or rare cells from a heterogeneous source of cells (eg, stem cells from bone marrow). Particular cells tagged with fluorescent dyes can be sorted under aspectic conditions for expansion in culture, to detect DNA or RNA gene expression analysis by polymerase chain reaction, for functional assays, or for transplantation into animal patients. In additional to mammalian and plant cells, flow sorters can sort sperm, yeast, bacteria, subcellular organelles, or chromosomes.[9]

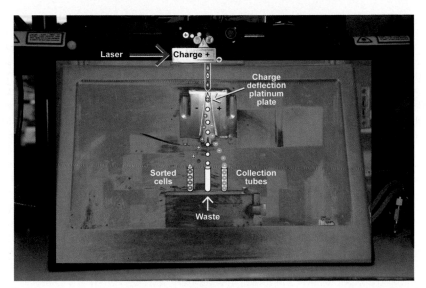

Fig. 4. Diagram of sort chamber components of the MoFlo XDP sorter including laser, charging electrode , droplet formation, charge deflection platinium plates, and collection tubes.

SAMPLE PREPARATION AND PROCESSING

Sample collection and preparation may vary depending on the type of flow cytometry application. For example, lymphocytes or granulocytes can be isolated from whole blood prior to labeling with fluorescent probes using density gradients appropriate for the cell and the species of interest.[10] Although these methods are labor intensive, they may be necessary to isolate certain populations of cells for further studies in culture. Diagnostic samples include whole blood, tissue aspirates or biopsies, and body cavity fluid samples. In these cases, the cells of interest can be selected using gating strategies that highlight the cells based on their unique light scatter or fluorescent properties. For immunophenotyping applications of leukocytes, whole blood can be collected in EDTA-K2, avoiding activation, cell death, or aggregation that can occur when cells are isolated over density gradients. A mixture of fluorescent-labeled antibodies are then added directly to the whole blood. Erythrocytes are removed by addition of a lysis buffer. Bone marrow collected in EDTA can be analyzed by flow cytometry methods in a similar manner.[11–14] Needle biopsies of solid tissues (lymph nodes) provide adequate cellularity and should be placed in a tube with saline and 2% to 5% serum. For platelet analysis, platelet-rich plasma is prepared by low speed centrifugation of EDTA anticoagulated whole blood. Since platelets are readily activated, various platelet function inhibitors can be added.[15] A major consideration of proper labeling and analysis of cells by flow cytometry is having adequate number of cells in the preparations. As a rule, preparations need to have approximately 1 to 2 million cells per milliliter.[10] The concentration of the cells in the preparations will dictate how many antibodies or flurosecent probes are applied to the cells and how many cells are analyzed. For certain samples that have limited cell concentrations (eg, cerebrospinal fluid), the number of antibody labels applied to the cell preparations can be abreviated; plus, the number of cells analyzed can be reduced from a typical analysis of 10,000 cells to either 5000 or 2000 as long as each labeled preparation is analyzed consistently.

There are a multitude of flow cytometric applications for analysis of blood cells, tissue cells, and cultured cells that involve labeling the cell surface or internal antigens, determining cellular health with viability assays, and measuring cellular processes by using probes for subcellular organelles or lipophilic dyes for proliferation assays. Protocols for these assays and instructional CDs can be found at several commercial and academic websites including http://www.invitrogen.com/site/us/en/home/Applications/Cell-and-Tissue-Analysis/Flow-Cytometry/Flow-Cytometry-Microbiology-Assays.html and http://www.cyto.purdue.edu/flowcyt/cdseries.htm. For clinical assays, common methods of sample processing involve incubation of the cells, typically 20 minutes, with a monoclonal or polyclonal antibody that is specific to the cellular antigen of interest. To label intracellular antigens, the cells are permeabilized with a permeabilizing agent (eg, saponin), which allows the antibody to enter the cell. Fluorescent-conjugated antibodies to the species-specific antigen of interest is then added to the cells, incubated, washed, and analyzed fairly quickly. However, the availability of fluroscent-lableled antibodies to antigens in veteirnary species is limited. The reader is referred to a partial list of references that have used species-specific and cross-reactive antibodies in veterinary species.[16] In many cases, directly conjugated primary antibodies are not available; therefore, fluorescent-labeled secondary antibodies are required, which adds an additional incubation and washing step to the sample processing. Samples need to be labeled at the proper concentrations and inspected for clumping. Cell or nuclear clumps can be removed from samples by poring the sample through filtered caps with a 30-μm pore that fit onto the top of special flow cytometry sample tubes and vortexed. Protocols to perform the sample analysis will be dependent on the type of fluorochromes the users chooses, the capability of the instrument, and the experience of the operator. The reader is referred to many excellent reviews and resources on cell preparation, fluorochromes, and analysis.[17–20]

APPLICATIONS IN SMALL ANIMAL MEDICINE
Automated Hematology Analyzer

Several automated hematology analyzers use excitation optics to enumerate erythrocytes, platelets, platelet size, and leukocytes based on light scatter. These include the CELL DYN (Abbott Laboratories, Abbott Park, IL, USA), ADVIA (GMA, Ramsey, MN, USA), and SYSMEX (Mundelein, IL, USA), LASERCYTE (IDEXX, Westbrook, ME, USA). Even though many of these automated analyzers have species-specific settings, the automated differential has not replaced the manual method due to inccurate monocyte, eosinophils, and basophil assignments in many domestic animals species.[21,22] Other applications include determination of red blood cell indices, leukocytes in body fluids, and predicting leukemic cell lineages in peripheral blood of dogs and cats.[23–26]

Testing for Immune-Mediated Hematologic Disease

Immune-mediated hematologic diseases including immune-mediated hemolytic anemia (IMHA), immune-mediated thrombocytopenia (IMT), and immune-mediated neutropenia occur with some frequency in dogs and cats. Laboratory diagnosis of immune-mediated cytopenias typically involve detection of antibody directed against cellular antigens. Although direct agglutination based tests (eg, Coombs' test for IMHA) are available to detect antibody and complement on the surface of erythrocytes the sensitivity is low in comparison to newer flow cytometry assays. In two studies, the sensitivity of the flow assay to detect IMHA in dogs was 92% to 100% compared to the Coombs' test (53% to 58%). In contrast, the specifiicity of the two assays were similar (87.5% to 100%).[27,28] This increased sensitivity is most likely due to the ability of the flow cytometry assay to detect fewer cells coated with antibody since it is not dependent on agglutination. Moreover, flow cytometry assays can identify the immunoglobulin class(es) bound to the cell. The downside of its increased sensitivity is the potential to detect nonspecific reactions (nonpathogenic binding of antibodies to aged cells, absorption of antibodies to the cell surface); this is a common issue with antibody tests in general.[29] Platelets easily suffer from nonspecific binding by cytoplasmic and plasma derived antibodies following prolonged storage; to minimize this effect, samples for surface associated platelet IgG testing should be processed and analyzed within 24 hours of collection.[15,30-32] An example of a dot-plot analysis of platelets and erythrocytes (**Fig. 5**) generated from a dog with Evan's syndrome illustrates the detection of IgG on the surface of a population of platelets (see **Fig. 5C**) and IgG, IgM, and rare IgA on the surface of erythrocytes (see **Fig. 5E–G**). The advantage to this assay is that it is quantiative and detects the proportion of antibody-coated cells, so that the practitioner can monitor the degree of affected cells over time following treatment. Reticulated platelets (immature platelets) and reticulo-cytes can be detected by flow cytometery with the use of a nuclei acid stain, thiazole orange that stains the RNA (see **Fig. 5H and I**). Determining the presence of reticulated platelets in cases of IMT provides a reasonable assessment of thrombo-poiesis in dogs that have regenerative thrombocytopenia secondary to IMT or drug-induced thrombocytopenia.[32-34]

In the author's experience, direct flow cytometry assays to demonstrate antineu-trophil antibodies have not been rewarding. We have observed reactivity of healthy dog neutrophils with a $F(ab')_2$ fragment of fluoresent-conjugated anti-dog IgG, indicating that healthy neutrophils have IgG bound to their surfaces via Fc receptors. An indirect flow cytometry anti-neutrophil antibody test, however, has been described to be useful in dogs with immune-mediated neutropenia. In this assay, the patient's serum is incubated with paraformaldehyde-fixed neutrophils from a healthy donor dog. A fluorescein-conjugated rabbit anti-dog IgG is then added to the mixture.[35] In 12 dogs with neutropenia, the test was positive for five of six dogs with a clinical diagnosis of immune-mediated neutropenia and negative in six of six dogs with neutropenia associated with other diseases.[36]

Diagnosis of Immunodeficiencies, Immune Disorders, and Thrombopathies

The enumeration of T-cell subsets (CD4 and CD8) by flow cytometry to monitor the progression of acquired immunodeficiency syndrome (AIDS) in humans with human immunodeficiency virus (HIV) infection became the most commonly performed application of flow cytometry in human diagnostic laboratories[37] and drove the commercialization and implementation of bench top analytical flow cytometers into hospitals. In companion animals, lymphocyte subset analysis has been useful in diagnosing dogs with immune deficiencies such as severe combined immunodefi-ciency,[38,39] monitoring the progression of AIDS in cats infected with feline immuno-deficiency virus, whereby decreases in CD4 T cells and CD4:CD8 occur over time,[40] and CD4:CD8 subset changes in dogs with deep pyoderma, systemic lupus erythem-atosus, and leishmaniasis.[41] Lymphocyte subset analysis was reported to be useful in monitoring dogs with symptoms of systemic lupus erythematosus, in which increased CD4:CD8 ratio was associated with the active disease and reversion of this ratio occurred after successful immunotherapy.[42] Flow cytometry has been used to identify defects in adhesion molecules (CD18) in dogs with leukocyte adhesion

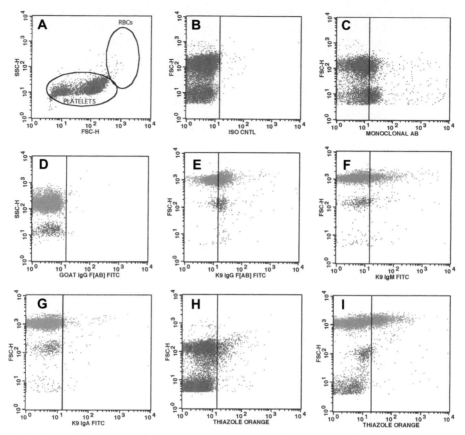

Fig. 5. Dog with Evan's syndrome. Dot-plot output of platelets (in *red*). (*A*) Scatter plot. (*B*) Isotype control antibody to determine nonspecific binding. (*C*) Detection of IgG on the surface of the two populations of platelets. Dot-plot output of erythrocytes (in *green*). (*D*) Negative control antibody. (*E*) Detection of erythrocytes coated with IgG by anti-canine IgG-FITC. (*F*) Detection of erythrocytes coated with IgM by anti-canine IgM-FITC. (*G*) Detection of rare erythrocytes with IgA by anti-canine IgA-FTIC. Thiazole orange staining of reticulated platelets (*H*) and reticulocytes (*I*). Vertical line separates nonfluorescent cells from cells labeled with fluorescent conjugated antibody or thiazole orange dye.

deficiency,[43] defects in platelet glycoprotein complex IIb-III that lead to Glanzmann thrombasthenia,[44] and alternations in the exposure of platelet phosphatylserine that leads to defective procoagulant activity in dogs with Scott syndrome.[45]

Determining the Lineage of Hemolymphoid Neoplasia

There are several reviews of the applications of flow cytometry and immunophenotyping to characterize hemolymphoid neoplasms in veterinary species.[46–48] Immunophenotyping is a laboratory procedure in which a panel of antibodies specific to certain lineage specific or lineage associated antigens is used to identify the lineage of leukemic blood cells or classify a lymphoma as either T or B cell. In the case of leukemic cells, immunophenotyping can define the cell lineage and the stage of cell maturation, which provides prognostic information to the veterinary oncologist. Prior to immunophenotyping methods, cytologic and histopathologic evaluations of the cells on blood films, aspirates, or biopsies were the principal methods to classify the neoplasm. It become readily apparent from extensive studies that cytologic evalua-tion alone was not sufficient in distinquishing lymphoid cells from myelod blasts.[49] The discovery of monoclonal antibody (MAb) technology[50] led the way to MAbs that react with molecules expressed by hematopoietic lineages and lymphoid subsets. International workshops were held to exchange species-specific MAbs and to compare their reactivity with cells and cell proteins from veterinary species.[16] Molecules that were recognized by a cluster of MAbs were assigned a "cluster of differentiation" (CD), number creating a standard nomenclature for classifying the protein specificity of the MAbs across species. The availability of MAbs to lineage-specific or lineage-associated CD molecules has allowed immunophenotyping meth-ods using flow cyotmetry to become an important diagnostic tool in veteirnary oncology. Although established antibody panels used for immunophenotypic char-acterization of human hemolymphoid neoplasias can involve over 20 antibodies for each lineage (B-lymphocytes, T-lymphocytes, natural killer cells, myeloid lineage, and plasma cells),[51] the limited availability of well-characterized reagents reduces the number and of lineage-specific CD markers that can be assessed in veterinary species. **Table 1** lists the most important CD antigens and others, their distribution on various stages and maturation states of leukocytes, and the type of hemolymphoid neoplasia in which thery are found. Until more reagents are available, the panel for cats is less comprehensive. The antibody panel can be abbreviated if the cellular concentration of the sample is low. Details of each CD antigen and other surface molecules listed in **Table 1** will not be discussed in detail but can be found in other reviews.[16,52] Samples that lend well to immunophenotyping include peripheral blood,

Table 1
Cluster differentiation molecule panel suggested for immunophenotyping of samples from hemic neoplasias

CD Molecule	Cellular Distribution	Hemolymphoid Neoplasia
CD45	All leukocytes	Not expressed in eyrthroid leukemias
CD34	Stem cell	Acute leukemia
CD14	Monocytes	Monocytic leukemias
CD11b	Granulocytes, monocytes	Myelomonocytic, myeolid leukemias
Myeloperoxidase	Myeloid lineage	Myeloid and myelomonocytic leukemias
CD11c	Dendritic cells	Dendritic cell leukemias
CD1a	Dendritic cells Cortical thymocytes	Dendritic cell leukemias, immature T cells
CD3	T cells	T-cell lymphoma
CD4	T help cell	T-cell lymphoma
CD8	Cytotoxic T cell	T-cell lymphoma
CD79a	Pro–B cell through plasma cell	B-cell lymphoma Plasma cell if negative for other B-cell antigens
MHC II	Mature B cell	B-cell lymphoma
CD21	Mature B cell	B-cell lymphoma
Surface IgM	Immature B cell	B-cell lymphoma
Surface IgG	Mature B cell	B-cell lymphoma

A

B

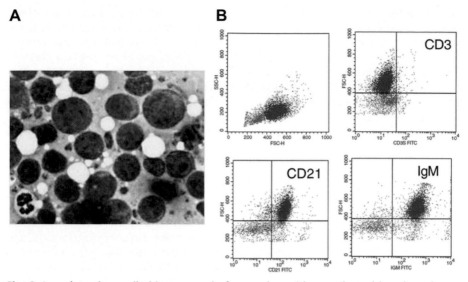

Fig. 6. Lymph node needle biopsy sample from a dog with an enlarged lymph node was prepared for cytologic assessment (Wright Giemsa stain, *A*) and immunophenotyping (*B*). The cells were monomorphic with immature chromatin patterns and prominent nucleoli (*A*). Scatter plot (*left* plot) of the sample indicates the presence of a small population (*green gate*) and a large population (*pink gate*). Large lymphocytes in the preparation were negative for CD3 and positive for CD21 and surface IgM consistent with a B-cell lymphoma. Horizontal line separates the small populations from the large populations. Vertical lines separate the nonfluorescent cells from those labeled with antibody.

body cavity fluids, bone marrow, cerebrospinal fluid if the cellular concentration is sufficient, and solid tissue aspirates (principally lymphoid tissues).[17]

Samples from lymphocytic neoplasias are probed with antibodies that are specific for T-lymphocyte antigens including CD3, CD4, and CD8; B-lymphocyte antigens CD79a, CD21, surface IgM and IgG; and major histocompatobility complex II (MHC II). CD3 and CD79a are lineage specific for T- and B-lymphocytes, whereas the other CD antigens are lineage associated with some infidelity of expression on other leukocytes or neoplasias.[53,54] Detection of CD79a expression by flow cytometry should be interpreted with caution because of nonspecific staining of the nucleus and is more commonly used in formalin-fixed tissues.[46] **Figs. 6** and **7** illustrate how an abbreviated panel of essential combinations of T- and B-lymphocyte antibodies can identify a B-cell lymphoma (CD21[+] and IgM[+]) or a T-cell lymphoma (CD3[+] and CD4[+]). Both lymphomas have a monomorphic appearance with immature chromatin patterns (**Figs. 6**A and **7**A) and nucleoli that are more apparent in the B-cell lymphoma (see **Fig. 6**A). The cells that shift to the right of the vertical line in each plot represent those expressing the antigen of interest. The scatter plot (SSC-H vs FSC-H) illustrates how the operator can place color gates on the populations of cells that vary in size (see **Figs. 6**B and **7**B). Note in the B-cell lymphoma case, the small lymphocytes (green) do not express CD21 or surface IgM and dimly express CD3, most likely representing the resident population of healthy T cells in the lymph node needle biopsy sample (see **Fig. 6**B). In contrast, in **Fig. 7**B large lymphocytes express T-cell antigens CD3 and CD4 typical of a T-cell lymphoma. Identifying large CD21[+] B-lymphocytes in dogs with lymphocytosis is important because it is associated with

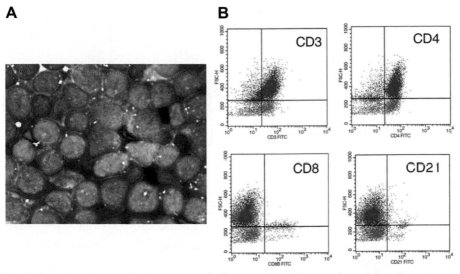

Fig. 7. Lymph node needle biopsy sample from a dog with an enlarged lymph node was prepared for cytologic assessment (Wright-Giemsa, *A*) and immunophenotyping (*B*). The cells were monomorphic with immature chromatin patterns (*A*). Scatter plot (*left* plot) of the sample indicates the presence of a small population (*green gate*) and a large population (*pink gate*). The majority of cells in the preparation expressed CD3 and CD4 but were negative for CD8 and CD21 consistent with a T-cell lymphoma. Few cells of intermediate to small size expressed CD8 or CD21. Horizontal line separates the small populations from the large populations. Vertical lines separate the nonfluorescent cells from those labeled with antibody.

shorter survival times.[55] Immunophenotyping analysis of lymphoid neoplasia samples is not done without cytopathologic assessment by a board-certified veterinary pathologist. In some cases, polymerase chain reaction for antigen rearrangment (PARR test) is necessary to confirm the presence of a clonal population.[56-58] Furthermore, histopathologic assessment of the affected lymphoid tissue is important for staging and classification of canine malignant lymphomas.[59] Myeloid or nonlymphocytic leukemia samples require, in addition to the panel of antibodies listed for lymphocytes, CD45, CD34, CD14, and CD11b or myeloperoxidase to distinguish acute leukemias (CD34$^+$) from chronic leukemias and myeloid (CD11b$^+$, myeloperoxidase$^+$) or monocytic (CD14$^+$) from lymphocytic cells. **Fig. 8** illustrates the cytologic morphology and part of the flow cytometry immunophenotyping profile of leukemic blood cells in a dog with marked leukocytosis. The cells had round, reniform to partially lobulated nuclei (see **Fig. 8**A) and expressed a combination of monocytic (CD14), myeloid (CD11b), and stem cell (CD34) antigens (see **Fig. 8**B) most compatible with a myelomonocytic acute leukemia.

Determination of DNA Content and Ploidy of Tumors

A range of fluorescent dyes are available that have loose binding affinity for nuclei acids. Propidium idodide is the most common dye used to determine the DNA content and S-phase fraction of tumor cells because it is excited by the argon laser. Since this dye is not permenant and has affinity for both DNA and RNA, the cells are incubated in a solution containing a detergent to lyse the cell membrane and RNase

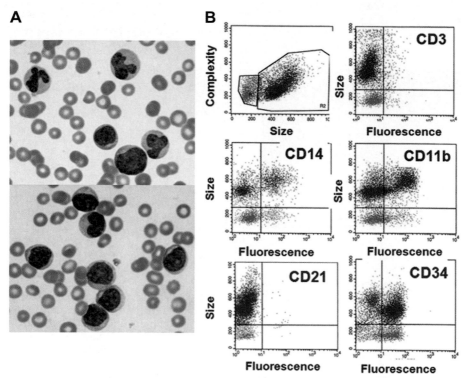

Fig. 8. Blood from a dog with leukemia (leukocyte concentration of 220,000/μL) was prepared for cytologic assessment (Wright-Giesma stain, *A*) and immunophenotyping (*B*). The leukocytes had pale blue cytoplasms with variably shaped round, reniform, to moderately lobulated nuclei. Scatter plot (*top left* plot) of the sample indicates the presence of a small population (*green gate*) and a large population (*pink gate*) of low complexity. The majority of the large cells expressed CD14, CD11b, and CD34 and were negative for CD3 and CD21 consistent with an acute myelomonocytic phenotype. Horizontal line separates the small populations from the large populations. Vertical lines separate the nonfluorescent cells from those labeled with antibody.

to digest RNA.[60] Most somatic cells in organisms have diploid DNA (2N) or two copies of each chromosome. Cells under going meiosis have half the chromosome content (haploid), whereas apoptotic cells are hypodiploid with less than 2N DNA. Tumor cells that are not diploid may have an abnormal number of chromosomes that lead to an anueploid cell. Flow cytometric analysis of nuclear DNA content will demonstrate histogram peaks for nuclei of the sample that is in phases of the cell cycle including G0/G1, S-phase, and G2/M. If the nuclei are diploid and not replicating, the nuclei should all fall into a single narrow histogram peak representing the quiescent G0/G1 phase of the cell cycle. If the cells are replicating, the G2/M peak (representing the G2/mitosis phase) will appear twice the distance from the G0/G1 peak, indicating a population of 4N or tetraploid nuclei. The S-phase will be the area under the curve between G0/G and G2/M fractions. If the cell is aneuploid, then extra peaks will appear in the plot. Several studies have noted no correlation with detection of aneuploidy or S-phase fractions in canine lymphomas and transitional cell carcinomas,[61,62] whereas others have reported poor prognosis for tumors that have aneuploidy and high S-phase fractions.[63–66] Because the DNA staining reflects the total DNA per sample, it may not detect chomromosomal translocations, insertions, or deletions if these abnormal nuclei are infrequent and diluted by diploid nuclei.[46,60]

FUTURE APPLICATIONS

Future applications of flow cytometry in veterinary medicine are many and limited only by the availability of reagents and the imagination of diagnostician. One future application is the use of microspheres that can be placed in high throughput multiplexing formats (Luminex technology; Luminex Corp, Austin, TX, USA) to measure numerous analytes, nucleic acid sequences, or antibodies in a single tube of patient serum. This technology uses microspheres that are internally dyed with varying proportions of red and infrared fluorescence such that each microsphere will have distinct spectral properties that separate it from another microsphere. Proteins or nuclei acids can be conjugated to the microspheres through chemical reactions. These protein-coated microspheres are incubated with patient serum to bind up patient antibodies that are specific to the proteins. A flurorescent-labeled secondary antibody is used to detect the patient's antibody. Since each microsphere as a separate spectral property, each bead can be conjugated with a different protein to identify a panel of autoimmune antibodies.[67] For example, a panel of proteins or nuclei acid substances can be conjugated to a collection of microspheres to screen canine serum for autoantibodies to DNA- or nucleic acid–associated proteins that may be useful in diagnosing dogs with autoimmune diseases.[68] Alternately, the microspheres may have nuclei acids attached to them that will react with antisense strands of pathogenic viruses[69] or antibodies that can detect panels of cytokines.[70]

SUMMARY

Flow cyotmetry measures multiple characteristic of single cells using light scatter properties and fluorescence properties of fluorescent probes with specificity to cellular constituents. The use of flow cytometry in the veterinary clinical laborary has become more routine in veteirnary diagnostic laboratories and institutions (http://www.vet.k-state.edu/depts/dmp/service/immunology/index.htm), and reference laboratories. The most common applications in small animal medicine includes quantitation of erythrocytes and leukocytes in automated hemology instruments, detection of antibodies to erythrocytes and platelets in cases of immune-mediated diseases, immunophenotyping of leukocytes and lymphocytes in immunodeficiency syndromes, or leukemias and lymphomas. DNA content analysis to identify aneuploidy or replicating cells in tumor preparations has not gained routine acceptance because of the variability of prognostic results. Other applications including cell sorting and multiplexing using microspheres are potential assays of the future once they become validated and the instrumentation footprint becomes more and more compact, less expensive, and easier to use.

ACKNOWLEDGMENTS

The authors would like to thank Mal Hoover, board-certified medical illustrator, for her efforts in preparing the expert illustrations for this article.

REFERENCES

1. Coulter WH. High speed automatic blood cell counter and size analyzer. Proc Natl Electronics Conf 1956:1034–40.

2. Herzenberg LA, Parks D, Sahaf B, et al. The history and future of the fluorescence activated cell sorter and flow cytometry: a view from Stanford. Clin Chem 2002;48: 1819–27.
3. Wilkerson MJ, Davis WC, Cheevers WP. Peripheral blood and synovial fluid mononuclear cell phenotypes in lentivirus induced arthritis. J Rheumatol 1995;22:8–15.
4. Kristensen AT, Weiss DJ, Klausner JS, et al. Comparison of microscopic and flow cytometric detection of platelet antibody in dogs suspected of having immune-mediated thrombocytopenia. Am J Vet Res 1994;55:1111–4.
5. Lewis DC, McVey DS, Shuman WS, et al. Development and characterization of a flow cytometric assay for detection of platelet-bound immunoglobulin G in dogs. Am J Vet Res 1995;56:1555–8.
6. Wilkerson MJ, Davis E, Shuman W, et al. Isotype-specific antibodies in horses and dogs with immune-mediated hemolytic anemia. J Vet Intern Med 2000;14:190–6.
7. Macey MG. Principles of flow cytometry. In: Macey MG, editor. Flow cytometry: principles and applications. Totowa (NJ): Humana Press; 2010. p. 1–15.
8. Longobardi Given A. Flow cytometry, first principles. New York: Wiley-Liss; 2004.
9. Davies D. Cell sorting by flow cytometry. In: Macey MG, editor. Flow cytometry: principles and applications. Totowa (NJ): Humana Press; 2010. p. 257–76.
10. Davis WC, Davis JE, Hamilton MJ. Use of monoclonal antibodies and flow cytometry to cluster and analyze leukocyte differentiation molecules. Monoclonal antibody protocols. Totowa (NJ): Humana Press; 1995. p. 149–76.
11. Weiss DJ. Determination of differential cell counts in feline bone marrow by use of flow cytometry. Am J Vet Res 2001;62:474–8.
12. Weiss DJ, Blauvelt M, Sykes J, et al. Flow cytometric evaluation of canine bone marrow differential cell counts. Vet Clin Pathol 2000;29:97–104.
13. Weiss DJ. Evaluation of proliferative disorders in canine bone marrow by use of flow cytometric scatter plots and monoclonal antibodies. Vet Pathol 2001;38:512–8.
14. Weiss DJ. Flow cytometric and immunophenotypic evaluation of acute lymphocytic leukemia in dog bone marrow. J Vet Intern Med 2001;15:589–94.
15. Scott MA, Kaiser L, Davis JM, et al. Development of a sensitive immunoradiometric assay for detection of platelet surface-associated immunoglobulins in thrombocytopenic dogs. Am J Vet Res 2002;63:124–9.
16. Wilkerson MJ. Cluster differentiation (CD) antigens. In: Weiss DJW, Wilkerson MJ, editors. Schalm's veterinary hematology. 6th edition. Ames (IA): Wiley Blackwell; 2010. p. 20–6.
17. Weiss DJ, Wilkerson MJ. Flow cytometry. In: Weiss DJW, Wilkerson MJ, editors. Schalm's Veterinary hematology. 6th edition. Ames (IA): Wiley-Blackwell; 2010. p. 1074–81.
18. McCarty DA. Cell preparation. In: Macey MG, editor. Flow cytometry: principles and applications. Totowa (NJ): Humana Press; 2010. p. 17–58.
19. McCarty DA. Fluorochromes and fluorescence. In: Macey MG, editor. Flow cytometry: principles and applications. Totowa (NJ): Humana Press; 2010. p. 59–112.
20. Lowdell MW. Experimental design, data analysis, and fluroescence quantitation. In: Macey MG, editor. Flow cytometry: principles and applications. Totowa (NJ): Humana Press; 2010. p. 133–45.
21. Tvedten HW, Korcal D. Automated differential leukocyte count in horses, cattle, and cats using the Technicon H-1E hematology system. Vet Clin Pathol 1996;25:14–22.
22. Tvedten HW, Haines C. Canine automated differential leukocyte count: study using a hematology analyzer system. Vet Clin Pathol 1994;23:90–6.

23. Gorman ME, Villarroel A, Tornquist SJ, et al. Comparison between manual and automated total nucleated cell counts using the ADVIA 120 for pleural and peritoneal fluid samples from dogs, cats, horses, and alpacas. Vet Clin Pathol 2009;38:388–91.

24. Becker M, Bauer N, Moritz A. Automated flow cytometric cell count and differentiation of canine cerebrospinal fluid cells using the ADVIA 2120. Vet Clin Pathol 2008;37: 344–52.

25. Bauer N, Moritz A. Evaluation of three methods for measurement of hemoglobin and calculated hemoglobin parameters with the ADVIA 2120 and ADVIA 120 in dogs, cats, and horses. Vet Clin Pathol 2008;37:173–9.

26. Fernandes PJ, Modiano JF, Wojcieszyn J, et al. Use of the Cell-Dyn 3500 to predict leukemic cell lineage in peripheral blood of dogs and cats. Vet Clin Pathol 2002;31: 167–82.

27. Wilkerson MJ, Meyers KM, Wardrop KJ. Anti-A isoagglutinins in two blood type B cats are IgG and IgM. Vet Clin Pathol 1991;20:10–4.

28. Quigley KA, Chelack BJ, Haines DM, et al. Application of a direct flow cytometric erythrocyte immunofluorescence assay in dogs with immune-mediated hemolytic anemia and comparison to the direct antiglobulin test. J Vet Diagn Invest 2001;13: 297–300.

29. Scott MA. Immune-mediated thrombocytopenia. In: Feldman BF, Zinkl JG, Jain NC, editors. Schalm's veterinary hematology. Philadelphia: Lippincott Williams & Wilkins; 2000. p. 478–86.

30. Lewis DC, Meyers KM. Effect of anticoagulant and blood storage time on platelet-bound antibody concentrations in clinically normal dogs. Am J Vet Res 1994;55: 602–5.

31. Wilkerson MJ, Shuman W. Alterations in normal canine platelets during storage in EDTA anticoagulated blood. Vet Clin Pathol 2001;30:107–13.

32. Wilkerson MJ, Shuman W, Swist S, et al. Platelet size, platelet surface-associated IgG, and reticulated platelets in dogs with immune-mediated thrombocytopenia. Vet Clin Pathol 2001;30:141–9.

33. Weiss JD, Townsend E. Evaluation of reticulated platelets in dogs. Comp Haemat Int 1998;8:166–70.

34. Smith R III, Thomas JS. Quantitation of reticulated platelets in healthy dogs and in nonthrombocytopenic dogs with clinical disease. Vet Clin Pathol 2002;31:26–32.

35. Weiss DJ. An indirect flow cytometric test for detection of anti-neutrophil antibodies in dogs. Am J Vet Res 2007;68:464–7.

36. Weiss DJ. Evaluation of antineutrophil IgG antibodies in persistently neutropenic dogs. J Vet Intern Med 2007;21:440–4.

37. McCoy JP Jr, Keren DF. Current practices in clinical flow cytometry. A practice survey by the American Society of Clinical Pathologists. Am J Clin Pathol 1999;111:161–8.

38. Meek K, Kienker L, Dallas C, et al. SCID in Jack Russell terriers: a new animal model of DNA-PKcs deficiency. J Immunol 2001;167:2142–50.

39. Felsburg PJ, Hartnett BJ, Henthorn PS, et al. Canine X-linked severe combined immunodeficiency. Vet Immunol Immunopathol 1999;69:127–35.

40. Tompkins MB, Tompkins WA. Lentivirus-induced immune dysregulation. Vet Immunol Immunopathol 2008;123:45–55.

41. Chabanne L, Bonnefont C, Bernaud J, et al. Clinical applications of flow cytometry and cell immunophenotyping to companion animals (dog and cat). Methods Cell Sci 2000;22:199–207.

42. Chabanne L, Fournel C, Caux C, et al. Abnormalities of lymphocyte subsets in canine systemic lupus erythematosus. Autoimmunity 1995;22:1–8.

43. Bauer TR Jr, Gu YC, Creevy KE, et al. Leukocyte adhesion deficiency in children and Irish setter dogs. Pediatr Res 2004;55:363–7.
44. Boudreaux MK, Lipscomb DL. Clinical, biochemical, and molecular aspects of Glanzmann's thrombasthenia in humans and dogs. Vet Pathol 2001;38:249–60.
45. Brooks MB, Catalfamo JL, Brown HA, et al. A hereditary bleeding disorder of dogs caused by a lack of platelet procoagulant activity. Blood 2002;99:2434–41.
46. Reggeti F, Bienzle D. Flow cytometry in veterinary oncology. Vet Pathol 2011;48: 223–35.
47. Culmsee K, Nolte I. Flow cytometry and its application in small animal oncology. Methods Cell Sci 2002;24:49–54.
48. Tarrant JM. The role of flow cytometry in companion animal diagnostic medicine. Vet J 2005;170:278–88.
49. Vernau W, Moore PF. An immunophenotypic study of canine leukemias and preliminary assessment of clonality by polymerase chain reaction. Vet Immunol Immunopathol 1999;69:145–64.
50. Kohler G, Milstein C. Continuous cultures of fused cells secreting antibody of predefined specificity. Nature 1975;256:495–7.
51. Wood BL, Arroz M, Barnett D, et al. 2006 Bethesda International Consensus recommendations on the immunophenotypic analysis of hematolymphoid neoplasia by flow cytometry: optimal reagents and reporting for the flow cytometric diagnosis of hematopoietic neoplasia. Cytometry B Clin Cytom 2007;72(Suppl 1):S14–22.
52. Moore PF, Vernau W, Feldman BF, et al. Lymphocytes: Differentiation molecules in diagnosis and prognosis. In: Schalm's veterinary hematology. Philadelphia: Lippincott Williams & Wilkins; 2004. p. 247–55.
53. Wilkerson MJ, Dolce K, Koopman T, et al. Lineage differentiation of canine lymphoma/leukemias and aberrant expression of CD molecules. Vet Immunol Immunopathol 2005;106:179–96.
54. Moore PF, Rossitto PV, Danilenko DM, et al. Monoclonal antibodies specific for canine CD4 and CD8 define functional T-lymphocyte subsets and high-density expression of CD4 by canine neutrophils. Tissue Antigens 1992;40:75–85.
55. Williams MJ, Avery AC, Lana SE, et al. Canine lymphoproliferative disease characterized by lymphocytosis: immunophenotypic markers of prognosis. J Vet Intern Med 2008;22:596–601.
56. Avery A. Molecular diagnostics of hematologic malignancies. Top Comp Anim Med 2009;24:144–50.
57. Avery PR, Avery AC. Molecular methods to distinguish reactive and neoplastic lymphocyte expansions and their importance in transitional neoplastic states. Vet Clin Pathol 2004;33:196–207.
58. Burnett RC, Vernau W, Modiano JF, et al. Diagnosis of canine lymphoid neoplasia using clonal rearrangements of antigen receptor genes. Vet Pathol 2003;40:32–41.
59. Valli VE, San Myint M, Barthel A, et al. Classification of canine malignant lymphomas according to the World Health Organization criteria. Vet Pathol 2011;48:198–211.
60. Longobardi Givan A. DNA in life and death. Flow cytometry first principles. New York: John Wiley & Sons; 2001. p. 123–58.
61. Teske E, Rutteman GR, Kuipers-Dijkshoorn NJ, et al. DNA ploidy and cell kinetic characteristics in canine non-Hodgkin's lymphoma. Exp Hematol 1993;21:579–84.
62. Clemo FA, DeNicola DB, Carlton WW, et al. Flow cytometric DNA ploidy analysis in canine transitional cell carcinoma of urinary bladders. Vet Pathol 1994;31:207–15.
63. Ayl RD, Couto CG, Hammer AS, et al. Correlation of DNA ploidy to tumor histologic grade, clinical variables, and survival in dogs with mast cell tumors. Vet Pathol 1992;29:386–90.

64. Bolon B, Calderwood Mays MB, Hall BJ. Characteristics of canine melanomas and comparison of histology and DNA ploidy to their biologic behavior. Vet Pathol 1990;27:96–102.
65. Hellmen E, Bergstrom R, Holmberg L, et al. Prognostic factors in canine mammary tumors: a multivariate study of 202 consecutive cases. Vet Pathol 1993;30:20–7.
66. Fox MH, Armstrong LW, Withrow SJ, et al. Comparison of DNA aneuploidy of primary and metastatic spontaneous canine osteosarcomas. Cancer Res 1990;50:6176–8.
67. Shovman O, Gilburd B, Zandman-Goddard G, et al. Multiplexed AtheNA multi-lyte immunoassay for ANA screening in autoimmune diseases. Autoimmunity 2005;38:105–9.
68. Paul S, Wilkerson MJ, Shuman W, et al. Development and evaluation of a flow cytometry microsphere assay to detect anti-histone antibody in dogs. Vet Immunol Immunopathol 2005;107:315–25.
69. Defoort JP, Martin M, Casano B, et al. Simultaneous detection of multiplex-amplified human immunodeficiency virus type 1 RNA, hepatitis C virus RNA, and hepatitis B virus DNA using a flow cytometer microsphere-based hybridization assay. J Clin Microbiol 2000;38:1066–71.
70. Wagner B, Freer H. Development of a bead-based multiplex assay for simultaneous quantification of cytokines in horses. Vet Immunol Immunopathol 2009;127:242–8.

Hemolytic Anemia in Dogs and Cats Due to Erythrocyte Enzyme Deficiencies

Jennifer L. Owen, DVM, PhD, John W. Harvey, DVM, PhD*

KEYWORDS

• Hemolytic anemia • Erythrocyte • Pyruvate kinase deficiency
• Phosphofructokinase deficiency • Dogs • Cats

Mature mammalian erythrocytes or red blood cells (RBCs) circulate in the blood for several months despite limited synthetic capacities and repeated exposure to mechanical and metabolic insults. RBCs do not have nuclei, so they cannot synthesize nucleic acids or proteins. In addition, the loss of mitochondria during the maturation of reticulocytes prevents the generation of adenosine triphosphate (ATP) by the Krebs cycle and oxidation phosphorylation. However, erythrocytes still require energy in the form of ATP for maintenance of shape, deformability, active membrane transport, and the synthesis of glutathione.[1] Thus, mature erythrocytes depend solely on anaerobic glycolysis or the Embden-Meyerhof pathway for ATP generation (**Fig. 1**). Consequently, deficiencies of rate-controlling enzymes required for anaerobic glycolysis can have significant effects on erythrocyte function and survival, leading to hemolytic anemia.[1]

DIFFERENTIAL DIAGNOSIS

Congenital deficiencies of rate-controlling enzymes involved in anaerobic glycolysis such as phosphofructokinase (PFK) and pyruvate kinase (PK) result in hemolytic anemia with a regenerative bone marrow response characterized by a reticulocytosis and polychromasia. These enzyme deficiencies must be differentiated from more common causes of hemolytic anemia including primary or idiopathic immune-mediated hemolytic anemia (IMHA) or IMHA secondary to another underlying cause such as hemotrophic parasites (eg, *Mycoplasma haemocanis, Mycoplasma haemofelis, Babesia canis, Babesia gibsoni, Cytauxzoon felis,* or *Bartonella* spp), other infectious agents, neoplasia, or drug/chemical/toxin exposure. Congenital enzyme-deficient animals should be Coombs' test negative,

The authors have nothing to disclose.
Department of Physiological Sciences, University of Florida College of Veterinary Medicine, Gainesville, FL 32610, USA
* Corresponding author. 1600 SW Archer Road, PO Box 100144, Gainesville, FL 32610-0144.
E-mail address: jwharvey@ufl.edu

Vet Clin Small Anim 42 (2012) 73–84
doi:10.1016/j.cvsm.2011.09.006
0195-5616/12/$ – see front matter © 2012 Elsevier Inc. All rights reserved.

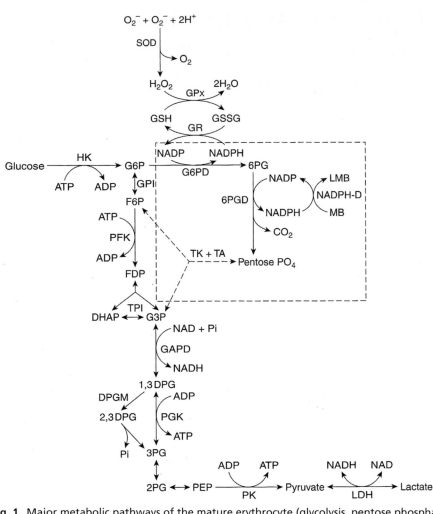

Fig. 1. Major metabolic pathways of the mature erythrocyte (glycolysis, pentose phosphate pathway, and 2,3-bisphosphoglycertate metabolism). The dotted lines surround pentose phosphate pathway reactions shown in abbreviated form. 1,3DPG, 1,3-diphosphoglycerate; 2,3DPG, 2,3-diphosphoglycerate; 2PG, 2-phosphoglycerate; 3PG, 3-phosphoglycerate; 6PGD, 6-phosphogluconate dehydrogenase; ADP, adenosine diphosphate; ATP, adenosine triphosphate; DHAP, dihydroxyacetone phosphate; DPGM, diphosphoglycerate mutase; F6P, fructose-6-phosphate; FDP, fructose-1,6-diphosphate; G3P, glyceraldehyde-3-phosphate; G6P, glucose-6-phosphate; G6PD, glucose-6-phosphate dehydrogenase; GAPD, glyceraldehyde-3-phosphate dehydrogenase; GPI, glucose phosphate isomerase; GPx, glutathione peroxidase; GR, glutathione reductase; GSH, reduced glutathione; GSSG, oxidized glutathione; HK, hexokinase; LDH, lactate dehydrogenase; MPGM, monophosphoglycerate mutase; NAD, nicotinamide adenine dinucleotide; NADH, reduced nicotinamide adenine dinucleotide; NADP, nicotinamide adenine dinucleotide phosphate; NADPH, reduced nicotinamide adenine dinucleotide phosphate; PEP, phosphoenolpyruvate; PFK, phosphofructokinase; PGK, phosphoglycerate kinase; Pi, inorganic phosphate; PK, pyruvate kinase; SOD, superoxide dismutase; TA, transaldolase; TK, transketolase; TPI, triosephosphate isomerase. (*From* Harvey JW. The erythrocyte: physiology, metabolism and biochemical disorders. In: Kaneko JJ, Harvey JW, Bruss ML, editors. Clinical biochemistry of domestic animals. 6th edition. San Diego (CA): Academic Press; 2008. p. 173–240; with permission.)

test negative for antinuclear antibodies (ANAs), lack Heinz bodies and intracellular or epicellular erythrocyte parasites on stained blood films, be polymerase chain reaction (PCR)- or sero-negative for tick-borne organisms, have no history of recent vaccination, drug administration or exposure to toxins, and lack evidence of microangiopathy caused by disseminated intravascular coagulation, heartworm disease, glomerulonephritis, vasculitis, lymphoma, hemangiosarcoma, or other tumors. Congenital disorders are often recognized in young animals but may not be recognized for several years in some patients. With the exception of PFK-deficient dogs in an exercise-induced hemolytic crisis, most animals that have congenital hemolytic anemia have a prolonged clinical course of low-grade, chronic hemolysis, rather than an acute presentation.

PYRUVATE KINASE DEFICIENCY IN DOGS AND CATS

Congenital hemolytic anemia resulting from erythrocyte PK deficiency occurs in many breeds of dogs and is the more common enzymopathy of the 2 that will be discussed in this review. PK deficiency was initially recognized in Basenji[2–4] and beagle dogs,[5–7] but it also occurs in West Highland white terriers,[8] Cairn terriers,[9] miniature poodles, chihuahuas, pugs, dachshunds, and toy American Eskimo dogs.[10,11] Because PK catalyzes an important rate-controlling, ATP-generating step in glycolysis, energy metabolism is markedly impaired in PK-deficient erythrocytes, resulting in a shortened erythrocyte life span and hemolytic anemia.[2,12] This deficiency is transmitted as an autosomal recessive trait. Heterozygous dogs exhibit no clinical signs, but homozygous dogs may present with decreased exercise tolerance, tachycardia, systolic heart murmurs, pale mucous membranes, and splenomegaly. Icterus is rarely observed.

Dogs with PK deficiency have a regenerative anemia, which because of the marked reticulocytosis, is macrocytic and hypochromic. In general, the mean cell volume (MCV) is between 86 fL and 105 fL, mean corpuscular hemoglobin content (MCHC) is between 25 g/dL and 32 g/dL, and the hematocrit (Hct) is between 17% and 28% (**Table 1**). The uncorrected reticulocyte percentage is between 12% and 66%, and the absolute reticulocyte count is between $0.5 \times 10^6/\mu L$ and $1.5 \times 10^6/\mu L$. However, the Hct and reticulocyte count will decrease as the disease sequelae of myelofibrosis and osteosclerosis become severe.[13] Leukocyte counts are generally normal or slightly increased with a mature neutrophilia. Platelet counts are usually within the reference interval or slightly increased, and moderate to marked polychromasia, anisocytosis, and frequent nucleated erythrocytes are recognized on stained blood films.[10,11] Echinocytes may be observed in low numbers in blood films,[7,14] but marked poikilocytosis with schistocytes and acanthocytes has only been recognized in

Table 1			
Comparison (mean ± SD) of Hct, uncorrected reticulocyte percentage, and erythrocyte 2,3-DPG concentration in normal, pyruvate kinase (PK)- and phosphofructokinase (PFK)-deficient dogs			
Dogs	Hct, %	Reticulocytes, %	2,3-DPG, mmol/L
Normal (n = 59)	48 ± 5	0.4 ± 0.4	6.0 ± 0.6
PK deficient (n = 8)	21 ± 3	40 ± 12	8.8 ± 0.8
PFK deficient (n = 20)	39 ± 3	19 ± 9	2.3 ± 0.6

From Harvey JW. Pathogenesis, laboratory diagnosis, and clinical implications of erythrocyte deficiencies in dogs, cats, and horses. Vet Clin Pathol 2006;35:144–56; with permission.

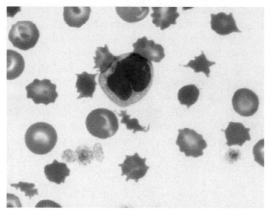

Fig. 2. Poikilocytosis in blood from a pyruvate kinase–deficient Cairn terrier after splenectomy (Wright's-Giemsa stain, original magnification ×100). (*From* Harvey JW. Pathogenesis, laboratory diagnosis, and clinical implications of erythrocyte deficiencies in dogs, cats, and horses. Vet Clin Pathol 2006;35:144–56; with permission.)

PK-deficient dogs after splenectomy (**Fig. 2**)[7,9]; presumably the spleen had previously removed these fragmented erythrocytes from the circulation.

Four different PK isoforms are produced by alternate splicing of products from 2 different genes. The *PKLR* gene encodes for the liver (L) and the RBC (R) isoenzymes of PK, while the *PKM* gene encodes for the muscle (M_1 and M_2) isoforms. The M_2 isozyme is normally present in many fetal and adult tissues, including erythroid precursor cells.[15–17] Reticulocytes in normal dogs contain some M_2-type PK, but the R-type PK predominates. Reticulocytes also typically have much higher PK activity than do mature erythrocytes.[18,19] Mature erythrocytes normally contain only R-type PK and no M_2-type PK.[20]

Erythrocytes of affected dogs lack the normal adult R isozyme of PK but have persistence of the M_2 isoform. Diagnosis of PK deficiency can be made in some dogs by measuring total RBC PK activity, but most affected dogs have normal or increased activity because of this persistent expression of the M_2 isoenzyme not normally present in mature RBCs. Erythrocytes in heterozygous dogs have approximately half of the normal PK activity, while erythrocytes in most homozygous dogs have normal or increased PK activity.[8,21] Consequently, the finding of PK activity within or slightly above the reference interval in a dog with marked reticulocytosis is highly suggestive of PK deficiency.

PK activity in hemolysates from affected dogs decreases rapidly when samples are kept at room temperature.[22] Because of this inherent M_2 isozyme lability, a heat stability test may also be used to aid in the diagnosis of PK deficiency in dogs.[23] Assuming that the M_2-isozyme is also unstable in vivo, its rapid loss of activity could explain the shortened life span of erythrocytes in affected dogs.[12] Additional assays including electrophoresis of isozymes, immunoblotting, enzyme immunoprecipitation, and measurement of erythrocyte glycolytic intermediates have also been used to diagnose PK deficiency in dogs in which the total enzyme activity was not decreased.[2,9,23]

Because the defect in glycolysis occurs distal to the diphosphoglycerate shunt (see **Fig. 1**), erythrocytes from PK-deficient dogs have increased concentrations of 2,3-diphosphoglycerate (2,3-DPG), a molecule that binds to deoxyhemoglobin and facilitates oxygen release from hemoglobin (**Table 1**).[1] Thus, the blood oxygen affinity of PK-deficient dogs is lower (P_{50} is higher) than that of normal dogs as a consequence of increased 2,3-DPG.[24] This decreased hemoglobin oxygen affinity should promote oxygen delivery to the tissues and help compensate for the persistent anemia, thereby improving the clinical signs of severe anemia in these patients.

Prolonged hemolytic anemia in these dogs results in excessive absorption of iron from the intestine, even in the face of increased plasma iron concentrations.[25] Hemosiderosis, hemochromatosis, and fibrosis develop in the liver of PK-deficient dogs secondary to the progressive iron overload.[4,26,27] Hepatic iron overload also occurs as a late complication in PK deficiency in humans.[28] A unique feature of PK deficiency in dogs is the progressive development of myelofibrosis and osteosclerosis that can be seen on radiographs of the long bones. It is proposed that the marrow fibrosis, like the cirrhosis, occurs in response to damage caused by iron overload.[27] However, extremely high pharmacologic doses of recombinant human erythropoietin elicited both marked erythropoiesis and myelofibrosis in experimental dogs, suggesting that factors associated with marked erythropoiesis might also contribute to the development of myelofibrosis.[29] Affected dogs generally die between 1 and 5 years of age because of bone marrow and/or liver failure.[10,27]

The defect in Basenji dogs is the result of a single nucleotide deletion in the R-type PK gene.[17] Unfortunately, different mutations in the R-type PK gene have been identified in other dog breeds.[10,30] Consequently, different DNA-based diagnostic assays must be validated for each affected dog breed. DNA-based tests for PK deficiency are available for multiple breeds of dogs at PennGen Laboratories, University of Pennsylvania.[31]

Erythrocyte PK deficiency has also been characterized in Abyssinian, Somali, and domestic shorthair cats.[32–35] Clinical signs were not recognized in a majority of cats detected by genetic screening, but some cats exhibit lethargy, pale mucous membranes, intermittent diarrhea, and inappetence. Icterus is a rare finding; however, a marked lymphocytosis and hyperglobulinemia can be seen.[35] Affected cats have intermittent mild to moderate, slightly macrocytic-hypochromic anemia, although severe anemia may be present terminally. Reticulocyte counts are slightly to markedly increased.[35] Splenectomy may reduce the severity of the anemia. In contrast to dogs in which the anemia is typically first recognized in young animals, some cats are not diagnosed until they are of advanced age.[10] Total erythrocyte PK activity is markedly reduced in deficient cats, with no evidence of the persistent M_2 isozyme reported in dogs,[32] and all PK-deficient cats identified thus far have had the same mutation.[10,33] Also in contrast to dogs, myelofibrosis and osteosclerosis have not been recognized in cats.[10]

PHOSPHOFRUCTOKINASE DEFICIENCY IN DOGS

As an important rate-controlling enzyme in glycolysis, quantitative and qualitative alterations in PFK can result in significantly altered states of energy metabolism in erythrocytes and in intensely exercising skeletal muscle, both of which depend heavily on glucose metabolism.[1] PFK composition is controlled by three separate genetic loci that code for muscle-type (M), liver-type (L), and platelet-type (P) subunits, and random tetramerization of the subunits produces various homo- or heterotetramer isozymes.[36] The PFK subunit composition in a given tissue is determined by the amounts of each subunit synthesized in that tissue. PFK in erythrocytes from normal adult dogs consists of ≥80% M-type subunits, with lower amounts of P- and L-type subunits. PFK from normal dog muscle is composed almost exclusively of M-type subunits.[37]

PFK deficiency is another autosomal recessive trait that is less common than the aforementioned PK deficiency and is seen in English Springer spaniels, American cocker spaniels, and mixed-breed dogs.[38–40] It has also recently been described in Whippet littermates and distantly related Wachtelhunds (German spaniels).[41,42] Native M-type subunits are not present in tissue from homozygous PFK-deficient dogs, but small amounts of a structurally unstable truncated M-type subunit are present.[37,43] A single nonsense mutation occurs in the M-type gene of most deficient dogs, causing rapid degradation of the unstable truncated M-PFK protein and total deficiency of the normal M-type subunit.[44] The recently reported PFK deficiency in Wachtelhunds is due to a different mutation that has yet to be identified.[41] As would be expected from the subunit composition of normal erythrocytes and muscle, total erythrocyte PFK activity is generally about 20% of normal and there is nearly a complete absence of PFK activity in muscle.[39,45]

The concentration of 2,3-DPG is low because it is formed below the PFK reaction (**Fig. 1**). 2,3-DPG is the major impermeant anion in canine erythrocytes and is normally present in much higher concentrations within erythrocytes than all other phosphorylated intermediates and all adenine nucleotides combined. Consequently, a substantial decrease in 2,3-DPG concentration results in a higher intracellular pH,[46] leading to increased alkaline fragility of affected erythrocytes. The low 2,3-DPG concentration also results in increased oxygen affinity of hemoglobin (P_{50} is lower) in affected canine erythrocytes. This increased oxygen affinity results in tissue hypoxia, stimulating erythropoiesis and leading to a reticulocytosis, even without a significant anemia (see **Table 1**).[39,40,47]

Homozygously affected dogs have persistent compensated hemolytic anemia and sporadic episodes of intravascular hemolysis with hemoglobinuria, although hemoglobinuria has not been recognized in all dogs (especially females) diagnosed with this defect. Erythrocyte life spans are markedly shortened and serum haptoglobin concentrations are generally low, even during steady-state conditions, indicating that increased erythrocyte destruction and some degree of intravascular hemolysis occur even when hemoglobinuria is not observed.[48,49]

Hyperbilirubinuria is persistent in affected adult male dogs but is variable in affected female dogs and pups. This may be related to the unique ability of the kidneys of male dogs to reabsorb filtered hemoglobin in the proximal tubules, catabolize it, and excrete the formed bilirubin into the tubular lumen.[50] Reabsorption and degradation of filtered hemoglobin is also demonstrated by hemosiderosis in proximal tubular epithelial cells.

Animals usually appear normal between episodes of intravascular hemolysis, although decreased muscle mass is sometimes recognized. Clinical findings that typically occur during hemolytic crises include lethargy, weakness, pale or icteric mucous membranes, mild hepatosplenomegaly, and fever as high as 41°C.[10,11,39] In general, HCTs are between 30% and 45%, except during hemolytic crises when the Hct may decrease to as low as 12%. The anemia is macrocytic, hypochromic with an MCV between 80 fL and 90 fL and an MCHC between 30 g/dL and 33 g/dL. A strong regenerative response is seen; uncorrected reticulocyte percentages are generally between 10% and 30%, and absolute reticulocyte counts are between $0.5 \times 10^6/\mu L$ and $1.5 \times 10^6/\mu L$.[39,49] Compared to healthy dogs, stable PFK-deficient dogs have slightly, but significantly, increased serum concentrations of potassium, magnesium, calcium, urea, total protein, and total globulins and increased serum activity of aspartate aminotransferase (AST). Mean serum concentrations of bilirubin, iron, and ferritin, and activities of alkaline phosphatase (ALP), lactate dehydrogenase (LDH), and creatine kinase (CK) in PFK-deficient dogs were at least twice those of healthy dogs. Serum concentrations of bilirubin and potassium, and CK activity may be higher during hemolytic crises.[39] In contrast, serum concentrations of creatinine and albumin are slightly, but significantly, lower in stable PFK-deficient dogs compared to healthy dogs.[49]

Hemolytic crises occur secondarily to hyperventilation-induced alkalemia in affected dogs, as PFK-deficient erythrocytes are extremely alkaline-fragile compared to normal erythrocytes in dogs.[39] Normal canine erythrocytes are more alkaline-fragile than those of humans and other mammals studied.[51,52] The even greater alkaline fragility of PFK-deficient canine erythrocytes results from decreased 2,3-DPG concentration (see **Table 1**).[53]

Normal and PFK-deficient newborn dogs have erythrocyte PFK activities that are about 3 times that of normal adult dogs.[54] Consequently, hematologic findings in affected dogs are similar to those of normal dogs at birth. This high neonatal PFK activity results from the presence of large amounts of the L-type subunit of PFK, which accounts for only about 2% of normal adult canine erythrocyte PFK subunit content.[37,54] The amount of L-type subunit and the total PFK activity in erythrocytes decrease during the first 6 to 8 weeks of life in normal and affected pups. The M-type subunit is low at birth in all dogs but increases as the L-type decreases in normal dogs. These changes in PFK composition are explained by the replacement of erythrocytes formed in the fetus with those formed after birth.[54]

PFK activity in skeletal muscle of affected dogs is only about 1% of that of normal dogs.[55,56] Myopathy is the most prominent clinical feature of human M-type PFK deficiency. Affected dogs appear to tire more easily than normal dogs, and in vivo studies of PFK-deficient dogs indicate diminished muscle function. However, deficient dogs generally exhibit less evidence of myopathy than is observed in affected humans.[57–59] Muscle wasting is sometimes recognized in dogs and muscle cramping rarely occurs.[58] The limited signs of myopathy in most dogs is explained by the fact that canine skeletal muscle is less dependent on anaerobic glycolysis than is human skeletal muscle because dogs lack the classic fast-twitch glycolytic (type IIB) muscle fibers.[60] However, 2 Whippet littermates were recently described to have marked exertional myopathy similar to that seen in humans. In addition, these dogs also demonstrated signs of cardiac disease such as persistent tachycardia, murmurs and rising serum concentrations of N-terminal pro-B-type natriuretic peptide (NT-proBNP).[42] Severe progressive myopathy has also been documented in an 11-year-old PFK-deficient dog that had amylopectin-like polysaccharide deposits in skeletal muscle[61]; however, similar abnormal polysaccharide deposits have been identified in type I muscle fibers of other adult PFK-deficient dogs without severe progressive myopathy.[62]

After the high levels of neonatal L-type PFK have decreased, homozygous animals over 3 months of age can be identified by measuring erythrocyte PFK activity. Heterozygous carrier dogs have approximately half of the normal enzyme activities in erythrocytes, but some overlap in activity may occur with normal animals.[54] Fortunately, a PCR-based DNA test can clearly differentiate normal, carrier, and affected dogs regardless of age.[31,63.]

Total body iron is increased in PFK-deficient dogs, as indicated by increased serum ferritin concentration and hepatic hemosiderosis,[49] but the myelofibrosis, myelosclerosis, and liver failure seen in PK-deficient dogs have not been recognized in PFK-deficient dogs. Although PFK-deficient dogs can die during a hemolytic crisis, affected dogs can have a normal life span if properly managed. Owners should avoid placing affected dogs in stressful situations or subjecting them to strenuous exercise, excitement, or high environmental temperatures that might result in hyperventilation.

DIAGNOSTIC TESTS

Blood samples collected in EDTA (1 to 2 mL of whole blood) are suitable for both spectrophotometric (usually kinetic) enzyme assays and DNA-based tests. Cheek swabs (2 or 3 buccal swabs) may also be used for DNA-based assays.[31] Samples for DNA-based assays do not require refrigeration or overnight shipping and can be shipped via regular mail.

DNA-based assays can differentiate between heterozygous and homozygous animals and are available for both PK and PFK deficiencies; however, all animals deficient in a particular enzyme do not necessarily have the same genetic defect. Therefore, different DNA–based assays may be needed to diagnose a specific enzyme deficiency in different breeds.[31] Breed and mutation specific DNA–based assays are required to diagnose PK deficiency in Basenji, beagle, and West Highland white and Cairn terrier dogs. In contrast, a single DNA–based assay is available to identify the common PK mutation in Abyssinians, Somali, and domestic short-hair cats and in identifying the common PFK mutation in English Springer spaniels, cocker spaniels, whippets, and mixed-breed dogs. Wachtelhund dogs have a unique PFK mutation that has yet to be identified. Without a specific genetic test, diagnosis of PFK deficiency in this breed requires measuring PFK enzymatic activity.[41]

Enzyme assays are performed in a limited number of research laboratories; thus, arrangements must generally be made with a laboratory before samples are collected to ensure that the laboratory can perform the assay in the required time. Blood samples for enzyme assays should be kept cool (not frozen) and shipped overnight so the assay(s) can be performed within one day. Commercial controls are not available for erythrocyte enzyme assays. Therefore, at least one control blood sample from a healthy animal of the same species should be collected the same day and shipped with the blood sample from the patient.[64] With the exception of PK deficiency in dogs (see the discussion in "Pyruvate Kinase Deficiency in Dogs and Cats"), homozygous-deficient animals can be recognized using spectrophotometric enzyme assays.[65] There is generally some overlap between heterozygous-deficient animals and normal animals; consequently, the identification of carrier animals by enzyme assays is less certain than DNA-based tests.

SUMMARY

Erythrocyte enzyme deficiencies do not usually shorten life expectancy except for PK deficiency in dogs and the potential for PFK-deficient dogs to die during hemolytic crises. In addition, erythrocyte enzyme deficiencies are uncommon or rare, so they are generally not seriously considered in the differential diagnosis of anemia until common causes of anemia have been excluded. However, unique clinical and/or laboratory findings like sporadic hemoglobinuria in English Springer spaniels (PFK deficiency) may quickly point to the possibility of an inherited erythrocyte enzyme defect. The ability to diagnose deficient or carrier animals allows for the possibility of eliminating these undesirable traits in future breeding. Continued research is needed to document additional enzyme deficiencies that likely occur and to develop additional DNA-based assays that are especially important in the recognition of heterozygous or carrier animals that have no clinical signs.

ACKNOWLEDGMENTS

The authors thank the many collaborators, practicing veterinarians, and technologists who were instrumental in generating the research findings summarized in this report. Special thanks are given to Dr Urs Giger for collaborative studies in PFK and

PK deficiencies and to Melanie Pate for her technical support in studying all of the defects discussed.

REFERENCES

1. Harvey JW. The erythrocyte: physiology, metabolism and biochemical disorders. In: Kaneko JJ, Harvey JW, Bruss ML, editors. Clinical biochemistry of domestic animals. 6th edition. San Diego (CA): Academic Press; 2008. p. 173–240.
2. Giger U, Noble NA. Determination of erythrocyte pyruvate kinase deficiency in Basenjis with chronic hemolytic anemia. J Am Vet Med Assoc 1991;198:1755–61.
3. Searcy GP, Miller DR, Tasker JB. Congenital hemolytic anemia in the Basenji dog duo to erythrocyte pyruvate kinase deficiency. Can J Comp Med 1971;35:67–70.
4. Searcy GP, Tasker JB, Miller DR. Animal model: pyruvate kinase deficiency in dogs. Am J Physiol 1979;94:689–92.
5. Giger U, Mason GD, Wang P. Inherited erythrocyte pyruvate kinase deficiency in a beagle dog. Vet Clin Pathol 1991;20:83–6.
6. Harvey JW, Kaneko JJ, Hudson EB. Erythrocyte pyruvate kinase deficiency in a beagle dog. Vet Clin Pathol 1977;6:13–7.
7. Prasse KW, Crouser D, Beutler E, et al. Pyruvate kinase deficiency anemia with terminal myelofibrosis and osteosclerosis in a beagle. J Am Vet Med Assoc 1975;166: 1170–5.
8. Chapman BL, Giger U. Inherited erythrocyte pyruvate kinase deficiency in the West Highland white terrier. J Small Anim Pract 1990;31:610–6.
9. Schaer M, Harvey JW, Calderwood Mays MB, et al. Pyruvate kinase deficiency causing hemolytic anemia with secondary hemochromatosis in a Cairn terrier dog. J Am Anim Hosp Assoc 1992;28:233–9.
10. Giger U. Hereditary erythrocyte enzyme abnormalities. In: Weiss DJ, Wardrop KJ, editors. Schalm's veterinary hematology. 6th edition. Ames (IA): Wiley-Blackwell; 2010. p. 179–86.
11. Harvey JW. Congenital erythrocyte enzyme deficiencies. Vet Clin North Am Small Anim Pract 1996;26:1003–11.
12. Dhindsa DS, Black JA, Koler RD, et al. Respiratory characteristics of blood from basenji dogs with classical erythrocyte pyruvate kinase deficiency. Respir Physiol 1976;26:65–75.
13. Whitney KM, Lothrop CD Jr. Genetic test for pyruvate kinase deficiency of Basenjis. J Am Vet Med Assoc 1995;207:918–21.
14. Chandler FW, Prasse KW, Callaway CS. Surface ultrastructure of pyruvate kinase-deficient erythrocytes in the basenji dog. Am J Vet Res 1975;36:1477–80.
15. Becker KJ, Geyer H, Eigenbrodt E, et al. Purification of pyruvate kinase isoenzymes type M_1 and M_2 from dog (Canis familiaris) and comparison of their properties with those from chicken and rat. Comp Biochem Physiol B 1986;83B:823–9.
16. Black JA, Rittenberg MB, Standerfer RJ, et al. Hereditary persistence of fetal erythrocyte pyruvate kinase in the basenji dog. Prog Clin Biol Res 1978;21:275–90.
17. Whitney KM, Goodman SA, Bailey EM, et al. The molecular basis of canine pyruvate kinase deficiency. Exp Hematol 1994;22:866–74.
18. Smith JE, Agar NS. The effect of phlebotomy on canine erythrocyte metabolism. Res Vet Sci 1975;18:231–6.
19. Brun A, Gaudernack G, Sandberg S. A new method for isolation of reticulocytes: positive selection of human reticulocytes by immunomagnetic separation. Blood 1990;76:2397–403.

20. Inaba M, Maede Y. Inherited persistence of immature type pyruvate kinase and hexokinase isozymes in dog erythrocytes. Comp Biochem Physiol B 1989;92B: 151–6.
21. Brown RV, Teng YS. Studies of inherited pyruvate kinase deficiency in the basenji. J Am Anim Hosp Assoc 1975;11:362–5.
22. Standerfer RJ, Templeton JW, Black JA. Anomalous pyruvate kinase deficiency in the basenji dog. Am J Vet Res 1974;35:1541–3.
23. Harvey JW, Peteya DJ, Kociba GJ. Utilization of an enzyme heat stability test and erythrocyte glycolytic intermediate assays in the diagnosis of canine pyruvate kinase deficiency. Vet Clin Pathol 1990;19:55–8.
24. Nakashima K, Miwa S, Shinohara K, et al. Electrophoretic, immunologic and kinetic characterization of erythrocyte pyruvate kinase in the basenji dog with pyruvate kinase deficiency. Tohoku J Exp Med 1975;117:179–85.
25. Stewart WB, Vassar PS, Stone RS. Iron absorption in dogs during anemia due to acetylphenylhydrazine. J Clin Invest 1953;32:1225–8.
26. Weiden PL, Hackman RC, Deeg J, et al. Long-term survival and reversal of iron overload after marrow transplantation in dogs with congenital hemolytic anemia. Blood 1981;57:66–70.
27. Zaucha JA, Yu C, Lothrop CDJ, et al. Severe canine hereditary hemolytic anemia treated by nonmyeloablative marrow transplantation. Biol Blood Marrow Transplant 2001;7:14–24.
28. Boivin P, Galand C. Iron overload in congenital haemolytic anaemia due to pyruvate kinase deficiency: a major late complication. Presse Med 1990;19:1087–90.
29. Bader R, Bode G, Rebel W, et al. Stimulation of bone marrow by administration of excessive doses of recombinant human erythropoietin. Pathol Res Pract 1992;188: 676–9.
30. Skelly BJ, Wallace M, Rajpurohit YR, et al. Identification of a 6 base pair insertion in West Highland white terriers with erythrocyte pyruvate kinase deficiency. Am J Vet Res 1999;60:1169–72.
31. Giger U. PennGen. Available at http://research.vet.upenn.edu/penngen. Accessed June 22, 2011.
32. Ford S, Giger U, Duesberg C, et al. Inherited erythrocyte pyruvate kinase (PK) deficiency causing hemolytic anemia in an Abyssinian cat abstract. J Vet Intern Med 1992;6:123.
33. Giger U, Rajpurohit Y, Wang P, et al. Molecular basis of erythrocyte pyruvate kinase (R-PK) deficiency in cats abstract. Blood 1997;90(Suppl 1):5b.
34. Mansfield CS, Clark P. Pyruvate kinase deficiency in a Somali cat in Australia. Aust Vet J 2005; 83:483–5.
35. Kohn B, Fumi C, Seng A, et al. Anemia due to erythrocytic pyruvate kinase deficiency and its incidence in Somali and Abyssinian cats in Germany. Kleintierpraxis 2005;50: 305–12.
36. Vora S, Giger U, Turchen S, et al. Characterization of the enzymatic lesion in inherited phosphofructokinase deficiency in the dog: an animal analogue of human glycogen storage disease type VII. Proc Natl Acad Sci U S A 1985;82:8109–13.
37. Mhaskar Y, Harvey JW, Dunaway GA. Developmental changes of 6-phosphofructo-1-kinase subunit levels in erythrocytes from normal dogs and dogs affected by glycogen storage disease type VII. Comp Biochem Physiol B 1992;101B:303–7.
38. Giger U, Harvey JW, Yamaguchi RA, et al. Inherited phosphofructokinase deficiency in dogs with hyperventilation-induced hemolysis: increased in vitro and in vivo alkaline fragility of erythrocytes. Blood 1985;65:345–51.

39. Giger U, Harvey JW. Hemolysis caused by phosphofructokinase deficiency in English springer spaniels: seven cases (1983–1986). J Am Vet Med Assoc 1987;191:453–9.

40. Giger U, Smith BF, Woods CB, et al. Inherited phosphofructokinase deficiency in an American cocker spaniel. J Am Vet Med Assoc 1992;201:1569–71.

41. Hillström A, Tvedten H, Rowe A, et al. Hereditary phosphofructokinase deficiency in Wachtelhunds. J Am Anim Hosp Assoc 2011;47:145–50.

42. Gerber K, Harvey JW, D'Agorne S, et al. Hemolysis, myopathy, and cardiac disease associated with hereditary phosphofructokinase deficiency in two Whippets. Vet Clin Path 2009;38:46–51.

43. Mhaskar Y, Giger U, Dunaway GA. Presence of a truncated M-type subunit and altered kinetic properties of 6-phosphofructo-1-kinase isozymes in the brain of a dog affected by glycogen storage disease type VII. Enzyme 1991;45:137–44.

44. Smith BF, Henthorn PS, Rajpurohit Y, et al. A cDNA encoding canine muscle-type phosphofructokinase. Gene 1996;168:275–6.

45. Harvey JW, Pate MG, Mhaskar Y, et al. Characterization of phosphofructokinase-deficient canine erythrocytes. J Inherit Metab Dis 1992;15:747–59.

46. Hladky SB, Rink TJ. pH equilibrium across the red cell membrane. In: Lew VL, Ellory JC, editors. Membrane transport in red cells. New York: Academic Press; 1977. p. 115–35.

47. Giger U, Reilly MP, Asakura T, et al. Autosomal recessive inherited phosphofructokinase deficiency in English springer spaniels. Anim Genet 1986;17:15–23.

48. Giger U. Survival of phosphofructokinase-deficient erythrocytes in a canine model abstract. Blood 1987;70(Suppl):52a.

49. Harvey JW, Smith JE. Haematology and clinical chemistry of English springer spaniel dogs with phosphofructokinase deficiency. Comp Haematol Int 1994;4:70–4.

50. De Schepper J. Degradation of haemoglobin to bilirubin in the kidney of the dog. Tijdschr Diergeneeskd 1974;99:699–707.

51. Iampietro PF, Burr MJ, Fiorica V, et al. pH-dependent lysis of canine erythrocytes. J Appl Physiol 1967;23:505–10.

52. Waddell WJ. Lysis of dog erythrocytes in mildly alkaline isotonic media. Am J Physiol 1956;186:339–42.

53. Harvey JW, Sussman WA, Pate MG. Effect of 2,3-diphosphoglycerate concentration on the alkaline fragility of phosphofructokinase-deficient canine erythrocytes. Comp Biochem Physiol B 1988;89B:105–7.

54. Harvey JW, Reddy GR. Postnatal hematologic development in phosphofructokinase-deficient dogs. Blood 1989;74:2556–61.

55. Giger U, Kelly AM, Teno PS. Biochemical studies of canine muscle phosphofructokinase deficiency. Enzyme 1988;40:25–9.

56. Harvey JW, Gropp KE, Bellah JR. Biochemical findings in phosphofructokinase-deficient canine skeletal muscle. In: Ubaldi A, editor. State of art in animal clinical biochemistry. Parma (Italy): Boehringer Mannheim; 1992. p. 79.

57. Brechue WF, Gropp KE, Ameredes BT, et al. Metabolic and work capacity of skeletal muscle of PFK-deficient dogs studied in situ. J Appl Physiol 1994;77:2456–67.

58. Giger U, Argov Z, Schnall M, et al. Metabolic myopathy in canine muscle-type phosphofructokinase deficiency. Muscle Nerve 1988;11:1260–5.

59. McCully K, Chance B, Giger U. In vivo determination of altered hemoglobin saturation in dogs with M-type phosphofructokinase deficiency. Muscle Nerve 1999;22:621–7.

60. Snow DH, Billeter R, Mascarello F, et al. No classical type IIB fibres in dog skeletal muscle. Histochemistry 1982;75:53–65.

61. Harvey JW, Calderwood Mays MB, Gropp KE, et al. Polysaccharide storage myopathy in canine phosphofructokinase deficiency (type VII glycogen storage disease). Vet Pathol 1990;27:1–8.
62. Gropp KE. Morphology, morphometry, and development of skeletal muscle in muscle-type phosphofructokinase deficient dogs [PhD thesis]. Gainesville: University of Florida; 1991.
63. Giger U, Smith BF, Rajpurohit Y. PCR-based screening test for phosphofructokinase (PFK) deficiency: a common inherited disease in English springer spaniels abstract. J Vet Intern Med 1995;9:187.
64. Christopher MM, Harvey JW. Specialized hematology tests. Semin Vet Med Surg Small Anim 1992;7:301–10.
65. Beutler E. Red cell metabolism: A manual of biochemical methods. Orlando (FL): Grune & Stratton; 1984. p. 42–82.

Role of Hepcidin in Iron Metabolism and Potential Clinical Applications

Carolyn N. Grimes, DVM[a], Luca Giori, DVM[b],
Michael M. Fry, DVM, MS[a],*

KEYWORDS

• Erythrocyte • Hematology • Hepcidin • Iron • Liver

Iron is vital in a variety of homeostatic processes. Although best known for its roles in oxygen storage and transport (ie, in hemoglobin and myoglobin), iron is a necessary component of many molecules involved in other critical metabolic processes.[1,2]

Unless given parenterally or in the form of a blood transfusion, iron enters the body exclusively through the diet. Dietary iron occurs in heme and nonheme forms, which come predominantly from animal and plant sources, respectively. Digestive processes liberate iron from dietary sources and make it available for absorption via specific apical membrane transport proteins on enterocytes. Movement of iron from the enterocyte into the plasma occurs via the basolateral membrane transport protein, ferroportin. Once in plasma, iron binds to the transport protein, transferrin, for distribution to various tissues.[1,3]

A small amount of iron is lost daily from the healthy animal through sweat, blood, and sloughed or desquamated cells of the integument, intestine, and urinary tract. Additionally, menstruating primates and egg-laying birds may experience moderate iron losses in association with reproductive processes.[4] Iron is not, however, actively excreted from the body; total body iron is controlled via regulation of intestinal absorption. This is an important concept, as the body cannot upregulate iron excretion in circumstances of iron overload.[5]

The majority of total body iron is in erythrocytes; in the healthy animal, 60%-70% of total body iron exists in the form of hemoglobin. Erythroid precursors are the primary site of iron utilization. Because they synthesize hemoglobin, they have, by far, the highest iron requirements of any cell type.[1,5] Storage iron exists principally in

The authors have nothing to disclose.

[a] Department of Biomedical and Diagnostic Sciences, College of Veterinary Medicine, University of Tennessee, 2407 River Drive, Knoxville, TN 37996-4542, USA
[b] Department of Veterinary Pathology, Hygiene and Health, Università degli Studi di Milano, Via Celoria 10, Milano 20133, Italy
* Corresponding author.
E-mail address: mfry@utk.edu

macrophages and hepatocytes in the form of ferritin; approximately 20%–30% of total iron is stored this way in various tissues, primarily the liver, spleen, and bone marrow.[1,6] Hepatocytes take up iron from the plasma via a membrane receptor (transferrin receptor 1 [TfR1]). Hepatocytes not only store iron but also synthesize hepcidin, transferrin, and other proteins important in iron homeostasis.[7,8] In addition to storing iron, macrophages play a critical role in iron recycling that occurs as part of normal clearance of erythrocytes. Because only small amounts of iron are obtained from the diet, iron recycling in macrophages is largely responsible for maintaining adequate plasma iron concentrations.[5] As in hepatocytes, iron uptake by erythroid precursors is facilitated by TfR1.[1,9]

Regulation of iron metabolism occurs at cellular and systemic levels. Intracellular iron content[1,3,10] and interaction of iron with one or more iron responsive elements (IREs) present in mRNA[3,11] influence synthesis of many proteins involved in iron metabolism (transferrin, TfR1, ferritin, ferroportin, and others). Cytoplasmic iron sensors called iron regulatory proteins (IRPs) bind IREs when iron is scarce, and, depending on the nature of the IRP–IRE interaction, protein synthesis may be inhibited or enhanced.[1,3,12]

Systemic control of iron metabolism depends largely on hepcidin, a hormone that decreases bioavailability of iron by limiting absorption from the diet and mobilization of intracellular iron stores. Hepcidin is discussed more in subsequent sections.

Regulation or dysregulation of iron metabolism is important in the pathophysiology of many disorders, including iron deficiency, anemia of inflammation (formerly known as anemia of chronic disease), portosystemic shunt, copper deficiency, and iron excess (in association with iron toxicity, dietary iron overload, serial blood transfusions, hemolytic anemia, primary and secondary hemochromatosis, and hemosiderosis).[2]

HEPCIDIN: NORMAL BIOLOGY
Structure, Synthesis, and Excretion

In 2000 and 2001, several independent research groups reported the discovery of a novel peptide, first termed liver-expressed antimicrobial peptide-1 (LEAP-1) and subsequently termed hepcidin (because it is highly expressed in the liver and has weak antimicrobial activity in vitro).[13–15] This molecule was first recognized as a member of the defensin family of antimicrobial peptides, and only later identified as a key hormonal regulator of iron.

The biologically active form of hepcidin is a 25-amino-acid peptide. Hepcidin is synthesized as a larger precursor molecule and then processed to its active form by proteolytic cleavage, forming a hairpin structure (an amphipathic beta sheet) with 4 highly conserved disulfide bonds.[16] Hepcidin is highly conserved across species.[17,18]

Hepatocytes are the primary sites of hepcidin synthesis and, in physiologic conditions, hepatic hepcidin expression is regulated by a cohort of proteins (hereditary hemochromatosis protein [HFE], transferrin receptor 2 [TfR2], hemojuvelin [HJV], bone morphogenetic protein 6 [BMP6], and others). As discussed later, these proteins upregulate or downregulate hepcidin expression depending on intracellular and extracellular iron concentrations, erythroid factors, and inflammatory cytokines.[19,20] Hepcidin circulates in plasma bound to alpha$_2$-macroglobulin.[21] Evidence suggests that other cells may express hepcidin mRNA but at a much lower level than hepatoctyes; the biologic significance of extrahepatic hepcidin production remains unclear.[6]

Plasma hepcidin is freely filtered by the glomerulus and undergoes rapid urinary excretion in animals with normal renal function. A fraction of hepcidin is also cleared by codegradation with ferroportin.[5]

Biological Activity

The primary (known) role of hepcidin is to decrease the amount of iron in the plasma. Hepcidin expression is regulated by intracellular and extracellular iron stores, erythropoietic demand, and inflammation (see later). Hepcidin decreases iron flow into the plasma by restricting intestinal iron absorption and the release of iron already stored in macrophages and hepatocytes. It accomplishes these effects by interacting with the iron efflux protein, ferroportin, which is the primary known ligand for hepcidin.[5,6,19,22] Ferroportin is the most important molecule in the regulation of iron transfer from cells into the plasma—in fact, in vivo, iron transfer from cells into plasma is completely dependent on ferroportin.[23] Ferroportin is a surface membrane protein present on macrophages, hepatocytes, and the basolateral aspect of duodenal enterocytes, where it is the conduit for iron export. Circulating hepcidin binds to membrane ferroportin, triggering the internalization and subsequent degradation of ferroportin, thus trapping iron within the cells and preventing its efflux into the plasma.[5,6,19,22]

Regulation of Expression and Serum Concentration

Systemic and intracellular iron concentrations

Hepcidin production is transcriptionally regulated in the hepatocyte. Serum iron (bound to transferrin) and intracellular iron stores influence intracellular signaling molecules that control hepcidin transcription. The BMP signaling cascade is the most critical of these processes. Upregulation of the BMP signaling pathway results in increased hepcidin expression. Transferrin receptors (TfR1 and TfR2) on the hepatocyte membrane serve as physiologic sensors of changes in extracellular (ie, serum) iron. Increased serum iron concentration leads to increased transferrin binding to TfR1 and TfR2 and subsequent upregulation of the BMP pathway, resulting in increased hepcidin expression. Similarly, intrahepatocytic iron stores cause increased production of BMP6, a molecule that activates the BMP receptor, upregulating the BMP pathway.[5,19]

Erythropoietic signals

Expansion of erythropoietic precursors is associated with a decrease in hepcidin production.[24] This relationship makes sense, since erythroid precursors are the primary site of iron utilization in the body. Effective erythropoietic activity thus relies on adequate iron availability. Although the exact mechanism of decreased hepcidin synthesis associated with erythropoiesis is not yet known, it appears to be more directly related to erythropoiesis (ie, bone marrow activity), rather than erythropoiesis-inducing factors, such as hypoxia or erythropoietin.[5,19]

Inflammation

Long before the discovery of hepcidin, iron sequestration in inflammatory conditions was recognized as a possible evolutionary adaptation to limit microbial access to iron.[25,26] More recently, study of hepcidin has led to breakthroughs in the understanding of the mechanisms of anemia of inflammation. Hepcidin is an acute phase protein,[27] and both acute and chronic systemic inflammatory disorders are associated with increased serum hepcidin concentration.[25,28] Interleukins 1 and 6 (IL-1 and IL-6) are inflammatory cytokines that upregulate hepcidin transcription[5,29]; lipopolysaccharide (LPS) likewise induces hepcidin production[19,30]; and other inflammatory cytokines and molecules may also have similar effects. The upregulation of hepcidin associated with inflammation results in hypoferremia and, potentially, iron-restricted erythropoiesis and anemia. The association between inflammatory disease, hepcidin expression, and anemia has been extensively described elsewhere[25,26] and is discussed in more detail later in this chapter.

Impaired renal clearance
Because of its small size, hepcidin passes freely through the glomerulus into the urinary filtrate in animals with normal renal function. As with other filtered analytes, changes in the glomerular filtration rate (GFR) may affect serum concentrations of hepcidin. Most hepcidin in the urinary filtrate is resorbed and subsequently broken down by proximal tubular epitheliocytes; a small fraction remains intact and passes into the urine.[6]

ROLE OF HEPCIDIN IN VARIOUS DISORDERS
Disorders Associated with Decreased Hepcidin Activity

Hereditary hemochromatosis
In hemochromatoses, increased intestinal iron absorption results in iron accumulation in tissues and resultant organ (often liver) damage. In most forms of the disease, mutations in the HJV or hepcidin (HFE) gene result in failure of hepatocytes to produce sufficient hepcidin. Patients thus have decreased serum hepcidin concentration and increased circulating iron and tissue iron stores.[6] Hereditary hemochromatosis is rare in domestic animals, although mouse models exist.[6,31] Hemochromatosis has been identified in 6 related Salers cattle, in which it is presumed to be inherited.[31] Additionally, mynah birds demonstrate features of hemochromatosis that resemble hereditary hemochromatosis in humans (possibly an evolutionary adaptation to low iron availability in their natural habitat).[32]

Anemias of ineffective erythropoiesis
Expansion of erythroid precursors in the bone marrow stimulated by erythropoietin (EPO) is associated with decreased serum hepcidin levels.[24] Human patients with β-thalassemia and some forms of congenital dyserythropoiesis that are characterized by anemia despite marked erythroid hyperplasia (ineffective erythropoiesis) have low serum hepcidin concentration, which leads to increased intestinal iron absorption and, potentially, parenchymal iron overload and increased serum ferritin.[6,19] β-Thalassemia has not been reported in domestic animals.[33] Interestingly, some forms of congenital dyserythropoiesis recognized in animals have been associated with hyperferremia[34]; to the authors' knowledge, the role of hepcidin in those cases has not been investigated.

Hypotransferrinemia
Humans and mouse models with primary hypotransferrinemia develop microcytic, hypochromic (iron deficiency) anemia despite parenchymal iron overload and decreased serum hepcidin concentrations. Suspected mechanisms for these abnormalities include decreased effects of transferrin on hepcidin expression and decreased hepcidin expression associated with EPO-stimulated bone marrow.[19] A rare form of hereditary hemochromatosis in humans is due to autosomal recessive mutations in TfR2. This mutation in TfR2 precludes cellular binding of iron-bound transferrin, which results in downregulation of hepcidin expression and subsequent iron overload.[6]

Iron deficiency anemia
In iron deficiency, as may occur due to chronic blood loss or malnutrition, decreased iron availability (detected as decreased iron-bound transferrin and decreased intracellular iron stores) effectively downregulates the BMP signaling cascade (previously discussed), decreasing hepcidin expression.[19]

Chronic liver disease

Some forms of chronic liver disease in humans (alcoholic liver disease and hepatitis C, in particular) are associated with decreased production of hepcidin. This process is suspected to be multifactorial. Reactive oxygen species induced by alcohol and hepatitis C, among other factors, have been shown to directly reduce hepcidin transcription.[35,36] Additionally, failure of hepatocytes to synthesize hepcidin in end-stage liver disease is suspected to contribute to low hepcidin concentrations in these patients.[35]

Disorders Associated with Hepcidin Resistance

Ferroportin mutations

A rare disorder in humans associated with hepcidin resistance is due to autosomal dominant ferroportin mutations that interfere with ferroportin function. One such mutation interferes with the ability of ferroportin to bind hepcidin, thus preventing hepcidin-induced ferroportin internalization. Patients with this mutation develop parenchymal iron overload despite high (or high normal) serum hepcidin concentrations.[37,38] Other mutations may interfere with ferroportin internalization and degradation.[19]

Disorders Associated with Increased Hepcidin Activity

Anemia of inflammation

As previously discussed, inflammatory cytokines (in particular, IL-1 and IL-6) and other molecules (e.g., LPS) cause upregulation of hepcidin transcription.[5] This results in increased circulating concentration of hepcidin and subsequent hypoferremia in inflammatory disorders. There is also evidence that IL-1, IL-6, IL-10, and tumor necrosis factor (TNF)-α upregulate ferritin expression, resulting in increased intracellular retention of iron. IL-10 has been shown to increase transferrin receptor expression (causing increased cellular iron uptake)[39]; however, transferrin is also a negative acute phase protein and may decrease in inflammation.[1] The combined effect of these processes is increased iron retention and decreased circulating iron availability (hypoferremia), causing a functional iron deficiency (ie, an iron-*restricted*, but not iron-*depleted*, state), in which iron is not available for erythropoiesis. This is thought to have evolved as a defense mechanism whereby iron is less available to pathogenic microbes (interestingly, hepcidin also appears to demonstrate moderate antimicrobial activity in vitro but only at very high concentrations, making its significance in this capacity in vivo unclear).[39]

The described nonregenerative anemia and hypoferremia resulting from cytokine-induced iron sequestration is sometimes referred to as "anemia of chronic disease." It is important to note that these pathophysiologic changes may be associated with disorders that are either acute or chronic in nature and that the resultant laboratory abnormalities are not necessarily characteristic of all chronic diseases. Therefore, some consider the term "anemia of inflammation" to be more accurate and appropriate.[19]

Iron refractory iron deficiency anemia

Matriptase-2 (*TMPRSS6*) is a membrane protease (expressed primarily in the liver) that cleaves membrane HJV and, therefore, functions as a negative regulator of hepcidin.[40] An autosomal recessive disorder in humans caused by mutations in *TMPRSS6* (familial iron refractory iron deficiency anemia) thus causes excess serum hepcidin resulting in severe hypoferremia and resultant anemia that is resistant to iron supplementation therapy.[41,42] Functional hepatic adenomas that overexpress hepcidin have also been identified in humans and cause similar hematologic and clinical abnormalities.[42] To the authors' knowledge, analogous disease processes have not been reported in veterinary species.

Renal disease

In the past, impaired erythropoietin production was assumed to be the cause of anemia related to chronic kidney disease. However, *increased* serum erythropoietin concentrations and concurrent increased serum hepcidin concentrations in some human patients with chronic kidney disease suggest otherwise.[6,43] Hepcidin is freely filtered at the level of the glomerulus and rapidly cleared from the plasma. Thus, serum hepcidin concentrations increase when GFR decreases, as in renal insufficiency.[43] It is therefore plausible that increased serum hepcidin may be an important cause of nonregenerative anemia in patients with chronic kidney disease. Additionally, hypercytokinemia associated with the underlying disease process may contribute to increased serum hepcidin concentration in some cases.[6]

HEPCIDIN STUDIES IN ANIMALS

The recent discovery and characterization of hepcidin have led to renewed interest in iron-related research and the development and use of animal models in this field. Most hepcidin-related animal research has been basic research involving laboratory animals, especially mice. Following the identification of the gene encoding a protein homologous to human hepcidin in mice,[15] hepcidin has been identified and sequenced in rats,[44] other mice,[45] various fish,[46–51] dogs,[17] swine,[52] pigeons,[53] cattle,[30] cat,[54] buffalo,[55] nonhuman primates,[56] horses,[57] and sheep.[30]

Phylogenetic analysis indicates that hepcidin is highly conserved among animals and humans in its DNA sequence and secondary structure. Canine hepcidin has greater homology with human hepcidin than does mouse or rat hepcidin.[17] Based on this, the dog has been suggested as a promising animal model for research of hepcidin in human health and disease.

Clinically oriented reports on hepcidin in animals other than rodents or nonhuman primates include investigations in dogs, calves, and sheep. Dogs with experimentally induced nutritional iron deficiency anemia had markedly decreased hepatic hepcidin gene expression and increased hepatic transferrin receptor gene expression.[58] Calves fed supplementary iron had increased hepatic hepcidin gene expression and decreased duodenal expression of the ferroportin protein.[59] Sheep with experimentally induced inflammation had increased hepatic mRNA expression and developed hypoferremia.[30] These findings are consistent with known biology of hepcidin in humans and laboratory animals and suggest that the body of knowledge about hepcidin in those species is likely to be applicable to domestic animal species in general. Translation of basic research findings into diagnostic and therapeutic applications in people has already begun, and a similar pattern seems likely to occur in veterinary medicine.

LABORATORY EVALUATION OF HEPCIDIN

Evaluation of iron status typically relies on commonly available blood tests. The most frequently used tests are conventional indices (mean cell volume [MCV], mean cell hemoglobin concentration [MCHC]) that are part of the complete blood count, and serum tests that are often run as a panel (serum iron concentration, total iron binding capacity, % transferrin saturation, and ferritin concentration) at some reference laboratories. Reticulocyte indices (reticulocyte hemoglobin [CHr], reticulocyte mean cell volume [MCVr], others), which are better indicators of current iron availability at the level of erythropoiesis than are MCV or MCHC,[60] are now available at many veterinary reference laboratories. Many of the other serum markers of iron status that are available for use in people—for example, soluble erythrocyte zinc protoporphyrin concentration, soluble transferrin receptor concentration, and others—are not presently available for use in domestic animals. *An explanation of the mechanics, utility, and limitations of assays for clinical evaluation of iron status Is beyond the scope of this discussion and may be found elsewhere.*[1,2,39,61,62] However, the commonly available tests often do not provide sufficient information for differentiation among various iron-related metabolopathies. Measurement of serum hepcidin concentration may prove quite useful to this end and is an area of active investigation. At present, there is no consensus on the best assay method for hepcidin. Diagnostic assays are not routinely available for use in people, but several immunoassays for measuring serum hepcidin concentration have been developed and evaluated.[63–66] One or more of these seems likely to emerge as the method(s) of choice for clinical application.

Challenges associated with laboratory evaluation of hepcidin include limited antigenicity because of the small size of the protein and high homology between species, which makes it difficult to develop useful antibodies[67]; low concentration in and rapid clearance from the plasma[67]; and normal biological (eg, diurnal) variation.[68] Some investigations have focused on measuring hepcidin concentration in urine; however, these typically require complex and time-consuming laboratory methods,[67] and, in general, urine assays are not as suitable for routine diagnostic testing as serum assays.[67,69] Other studies have used an enzyme-linked immunosorbent assay (ELISA) that measures the serum concentration of prohepcidin, which is the larger precursor of the 25-amino-acid biologically active peptide.[70,71] Since prohepcidin appears to be an unstable analyte in serum and its levels do not correlate with urinary and serum hepcidin, the relevance of these data is controversial.

Methods for measuring hepcidin concentration in serum include assays based on mass spectrometry[72–76] and immunoassays.[63,64,66] The former can distinguish between the biologically active form of hepcidin and other isoforms (hepcidin-22 and -20) that have no known biological function but are impractical for routine diagnostic testing. Immunoassays are more suitable for clinical laboratory applications but only measure total hepcidin concentrations. As mentioned, several competitive ELISA methods have been described for measuring hepcidin concentration in human serum; one of these competitive ELISAs was the basis for a recent large study that generated age- and sex-specific reference values for serum hepcidin concentration in people.[65]

HEPCIDIN: CLINICAL APPLICATIONS
Diagnostic Applications

Although hepcidin assays are not currently being used routinely in clinical medicine, the utility of such assays seems promising. Hepcidin assays may prove complementary to or a useful alternative to ferritin and other assays in the diagnosis of iron-related disorders. Additionally, studies evaluating hepcidin concentrations in various clinical situations imply that these assays may help guide certain therapeutic decisions and answer some prognostic questions.

Although both ferritin and hepcidin have similar responses to inflammation and iron availability,[63] adding hepcidin assays to the arsenal of diagnostics used in the evaluation of iron status may be beneficial. First, hepcidin is an acute phase protein and changes in serum hepcidin concentration take place in a matter of hours, whereas changes in ferritin are slower,[28] making hepcidin more of a "real-time" marker of iron status. This may provide useful information about iron deficiency before other laboratory abnormalities can be identified.

Second, although ferritin concentration is useful in the diagnosis of many iron-related disorders, changes in hepcidin concentration may be the *cause* of some of these disorders, and unexpected patterns of ferritin/hepcidin change may be characteristic of certain disorders (see previous discussion of the role of hepcidin in various disorders).

Third, evaluation of hepcidin may help differentiate among causes of anemia. Of particular importance, hepcidin concentrations may help distinguish between anemia of inflammation and iron deficiency anemia (the 2 most common causes of anemia in humans). Anemia caused by true iron deficiency is likely to be associated with decreased hepcidin concentration and decreased iron stores (eg, ferritin), whereas anemia of inflammation (which is considered a "functional" iron deficiency) is associated with increased levels of hepcidin, despite adequate tissue iron stores.[6,77] Additionally, hepcidin levels may be useful in determining the cause of anemia associated with chronic kidney disease in some patients.[6,78]

Finally, evaluation of hepcidin offers promise in guiding therapeutic decisions related to treatment of anemias with iron supplementation, erythropoietin, anticytokine therapies, and hemodialysis.[19] In particular, knowledge of hepcidin concentrations may help clinicians predict whether patients with anemia and iron deficiency will be refractory to iron supplementation[63] and may help guide treatment decisions in patients with chronic renal disease.[6,78,79]

Therapeutic Applications

Hepcidin agonists are being investigated for potential use in the treatment and prevention of iron overload in diseases associated with hepcidin deficiency.[6,19] Overexpression of *Hamp1* (a gene encoding hepcidin) inhibited iron accumulation in mouse models of hereditary hemochromatosis and β-thalassemia.[80,81] Additionally, small molecules to augment hepcidin synthesis or mimic its effects on ferroportin are being considered in the treatment of various iron-overload disorders.[5]

Conversely, agents that decrease hepcidin production, sequester or neutralize hepcidin, interfere with hepcidin binding by ferroportin, or inhibit ferroportin internalization may be useful in the treatment of iron-restricted anemias (e.g., anemia of inflammation, iron refractory iron deficiency anemia).[6] Of particular interest is the potential role of hepcidin antagonism in the treatment of anemia of inflammation: hepcidin-neutralizing antibodies and hepcidin "small interfering RNAs" augmented erythropoietin therapy in the treatment of anemia in a mouse model of anemia of inflammation.[82] Also, inhibition of IL-6 (with anti–IL-6 antibodies) in monkeys with anemia of inflammation showed decreased hepcidin expression and improvement of anemia.[83] Although these and other potential therapies are promising, they are not necessarily without risk. Compromising the physiologic role of hepcidin could potentially promote infections or cause other adverse effects.[79] Such aspects of hepcidin-modulating therapeutics comprise a current area of active investigation.

SUMMARY

The relatively recent discovery of hepcidin has stimulated renewed research interest in iron metabolism and iron-related disorders, emphasizing the importance of this hormone in many normal and pathologic processes. Important questions still remain to be answered; however, research to date offers promising diagnostic and therapeutic implications for both humans and veterinary species.

REFERENCES

1. Harvey JW. Iron metabolism and its disorders. In: Kaneko J, Harvey J, Bruss ML, editors. Clinical biochemistry of domestic animals. 6th edition. Burlington (MA): Elsevier; 2008. p. 259–86.
2. Weiss DJ. Iron and copper deficiencies and disorders of iron metabolism. In: Weiss D, Wardrop K, editors. Schalm's veterinary hematology. 6th edition. Ames (IA): Blackwell Publishing; 2010. p. 167–71.
3. Andrews NC. Forging a field: the golden age of iron biology. Blood 2008;112:219–30.
4. Finch CA, Ragan HA, Dyer IA, et al. Body iron loss in animals. Proc Soc Exp Biol Med 1978;159:335–8.
5. Hentze MW, Muckenthaler MU, Galy B, et al. Two to tango: regulation of mammalian iron metabolism. Cell 2010;142:24–38.
6. Ganz T, Nemeth E. Hepcidin and disorders of iron metabolism. Annu Rev Med 2011;62:347–60.
7. Anderson GJ, Frazer DM. Hepatic iron metabolism. Semin Liver Dis 2005;25:420–32.
8. Rivera S, Liu L, Nemeth E, et al. Hepcidin excess induces the sequestration of iron and exacerbates tumor-associated anemia. Blood 2005;105:1797–802.
9. Mackenzie B, Garrick MD. Iron imports. II. Iron uptake at the apical membrane in the intestine. Am J Physiol Gastrointest Liver Physiol 2005;289:G981–6.
10. Piccinelli P, Samuelsson T. Evolution of the iron-responsive element. RNA 2007;13: 952–66.
11. Thomson AM, Rogers JT, Leedman PJ. Iron-regulatory proteins, iron-responsive elements and ferritin mRNA translation. Int J Biochem Cell Biol. 1999;31:1139–52.
12. Rouault TA. The role of iron regulatory proteins in mammalian iron homeostasis and disease. Nat Chem Biol 2006;2:406–14.
13. Adermann K, Krause A, Neitz S, et al. LEAP-1, a novel highly disulfide-bonded human peptide, exhibits antimicrobial activity. FEBS Lett 2000;480(2-3):147–50.
14. Ganz T, Park CH, Valore EV, et al. Hepcidin, a urinary antimicrobial peptide synthesized in the liver. J Biol Chem 2001;276:7806–10.
15. Pigeon C, Ilyin G, Courselaud B, et al. A new mouse liver-specific gene, encoding a protein homologous to human antimicrobial peptide hepcidin, is overexpressed during iron overload. J Biol Chem 2001;276:7811–9.
16. Jordan JB, Poppe L, Haniu M, et al. Hepcidin revisited, disulfide connectivity, dynamics, and structure. J Biol Chem 2009;284:24155–67.
17. Fry MM, Liggett JL, Baek SJ. Molecular cloning and expression of canine hepcidin. Vet Clin Pathol 2004;33:223–7.
18. Verga Falzacappa MV, Muckenthaler MU. Hepcidin: iron-hormone and anti-microbial peptide. Gene 2005;364:37–44.
19. Ganz T. Hepcidin and iron regulation, 10 years later. Blood 2011;117:4425–33.
20. Zhang AS, Enns CA. Molecular mechanisms of normal iron homeostasis. Hematol Am Soc Hematol Educ Progr 2009:207–14.
21. Peslova G, Petrak J, Kuzelova K, et al. Hepcidin, the hormone of iron metabolism, is bound specifically to alpha-2-macroglobulin in blood. Blood 2009;113:6225–36.
22. Nemeth E, Tuttle MS, Powelson J, et al. Hepcidin regulates cellular iron efflux by binding to ferroportin and inducing its internalization. Science 2004;306(5704): 2090–3.
23. Donovan A, Lima CA, Pinkus JL, et al. The iron exporter ferroportin/Slc40a1 is essential for iron homeostasis. Cell Metab 2005;1:191–200.
24. Pak M, Lopez MA, Gabayan V, et al. Suppression of hepcidin during anemia requires erythropoietic activity. Blood 2006;108:3730–5.

25. Theurl I, Aigner E, Theurl M, et al. Regulation of iron homeostasis in anemia of chronic disease and iron deficiency anemia: diagnostic and therapeutic implications. Blood 2009;113:5277–86.

26. Ganz T, Nemeth E. Iron sequestration and anemia of inflammation. Semin Hematol 2009;46:387–93.

27. Nemeth E, Valore EV, Territo M, et al. Hepcidin, a putative mediator of anemia of inflammation, is a type II acute-phase protein. Blood 2003;101:2461–3.

28. Kemna E, Pickkers P, Nemeth E, et al. Time-course analysis of hepcidin, serum iron, and plasma cytokine levels in humans injected with LPS. Blood 2005;106:1864–6.

29. Lee P, Peng H, Gelbart T, et al. Regulation of hepcidin transcription by interleukin-1 and interleukin-6. Proc Natl Acad Sci U S A 2005;102:1906–10.

30. Badial PR, Oliveira Filho JP, Cunha PH, et al. Identification, characterization and expression analysis of hepcidin gene in sheep. Res Vet Sci 2011;90:443–50.

31. O'Toole D, Kelly EJ, McAllister MM, et al. Hepatic failure and hemochromatosis of Salers and Salers-cross cattle. Vet Pathol 2001;38:372–89.

32. Mete A, Hendriks HG, Klaren PH, et al. Iron metabolism in mynah birds (Gracula religiosa) resembles human hereditary haemochromatosis. Avian Pathol 2003;32:625–32.

33. Giger U. Hereditary erythrocyte enzyme abnormalities. In: Weiss D, Wardrop K, editors. Schalm's veterinary hematology. 6th edition. Ames (IA): Blackwell; 2010. p. 179–86.

34. Steffen DJ, Elliott GS, Leipold HW, et al. Congenital dyserythropoiesis and progressive alopecia in Polled Hereford calves: hematologic, biochemical, bone marrow cytologic, electrophoretic, and flow cytometric findings. J Vet Diagn Invest 1992;4:31–7.

35. Fargion S, Valenti L, Fracanzani AL. Beyond hereditary hemochromatosis: new insights into the relationship between iron overload and chronic liver diseases. Dig Liver Dis 2011;43:89–95.

36. Fujita N, Sugimoto R, Takeo M, et al. Hepcidin expression in the liver: relatively low level in patients with chronic hepatitis C. Mol Med 2007;13:97–104.

37. Fernandes A, Preza GC, Phung Y, et al. The molecular basis of hepcidin-resistant hereditary hemochromatosis. Blood 2009;114:437–43.

38. Sham RL, Phatak PD, Nemeth E, et al. Hereditary hemochromatosis due to resistance to hepcidin: high hepcidin concentrations in a family with C326S ferroportin mutation. Blood 2009;114:493–4.

39. McCown JL, Specht AJ. Iron homeostasis and disorders in dogs and cats: a review. J Am Anim Hosp Assoc 2011;47:151–60.

40. Silvestri L, Pagani A, Nai A, et al. The serine protease matriptase-2 (TMPRSS6) inhibits hepcidin activation by cleaving membrane hemojuvelin. Cell Metab 2008;8:502–11.

41. Finberg KE, Heeney MM, Campagna DR, et al. Mutations in TMPRSS6 cause iron-refractory iron deficiency anemia (IRIDA). Nat Genet 2008;40:569–71.

42. Weinstein DA, Roy CN, Fleming MD, et al. Inappropriate expression of hepcidin is associated with iron refractory anemia: implications for the anemia of chronic disease. Blood 2002;100:3776–81.

43. Zaritsky J, Young B, Wang HJ, et al. Hepcidin—a potential novel biomarker for iron status in chronic kidney disease. Clin J Am Soc Nephrol 2009;4:1051–6.

44. Schwarz P, Strnad P, Singer N, et al. Identification, sequencing, and cellular localization of hepcidin in guinea pig (Cavia porcellus). J Endocrinol 2009;202:389–96.

45. Ilyin G, Courselaud B, Troadec MB, et al. Comparative analysis of mouse hepcidin 1 and 2 genes: evidence for different patterns of expression and co-inducibility during iron overload. FEBS Lett 2003;542(1–3):22–6.

46. Shike H, Shimizu C, Lauth X, et al. Organization and expression analysis of the zebrafish hepcidin gene, an antimicrobial peptide gene conserved among vertebrates. Dev Comp Immunol 2004;28(7-8):747–54.
47. Chen SL, Xu MY, Ji XS, et al. Cloning, characterization, and expression analysis of hepcidin gene from red sea bream (Chrysophrys major). Antimicrob Agents Chemother 2005;49:1608–12.
48. Douglas SE, Gallant JW, Liebscher RS, et al. Identification and expression analysis of hepcidin-like antimicrobial peptides in bony fish. Dev Comp Immunol 2003;27(6-7): 589–601.
49. Lauth X, Babon JJ, Stannard JA, et al. Bass hepcidin synthesis, solution structure, antimicrobial activities and synergism, and in vivo hepatic response to bacterial infections. J Biol Chem 2005;280:9272–82.
50. Wang KJ, Cai JJ, Cai L, et al. Cloning and expression of a hepcidin gene from a marine fish (Pseudosciaena crocea) and the antimicrobial activity of its synthetic peptide. Peptides 2009;30:638–46.
51. Zhang YA, Zou J, Chang CI, et al. Discovery and characterization of two types of liver-expressed antimicrobial peptide 2 (LEAP-2) genes in rainbow trout. Vet Immunol Immunopathol 2004;101:259–69.
52. Sang Y, Ramanathan B, Minton JE, et al. Porcine liver-expressed antimicrobial peptides, hepcidin and LEAP-2: cloning and induction by bacterial infection. Dev Comp Immunol 2006;30:357–66.
53. Fu YM, Li SP, Wu YF, et al. Identification and expression analysis of hepcidin-like cDNAs from pigeon (Columba livia). Mol Cell Biochem 2007;305:191–7.
54. Hilton KB, Lambert LA. Molecular evolution and characterization of hepcidin gene products in vertebrates. Gene 2008;415:40–8.
55. Khangembam VC, Kumar A. Buffalo hepcidin: characterization of cDNA and study of antimicrobial property. Vet Res Commun 2011;35:79–87.
56. Segat L, Pontillo A, Milanese M, et al. Evolution of the hepcidin gene in primates. BMC Genom 2008;9:120.
57. Oliveira Filho JP, Badial PR, Cunha PH, et al. Cloning, sequencing and expression analysis of the equine hepcidin gene by real-time PCR. Vet Immunol Immunopathol 2010;135:34–42.
58. Fry MM, Kirk CA, Liggett JL, et al. Changes in hepatic gene expression in dogs with experimentally induced nutritional iron deficiency. Vet Clin Pathol 2009;38:13–9.
59. Hansen SL, Ashwell MS, Moeser AJ, et al. High dietary iron reduces transporters involved in iron and manganese metabolism and increases intestinal permeability in calves. J Dairy Sci 2010;93:656–65.
60. Fry MM, Kirk CA. Reticulocyte indices in a canine model of nutritional iron deficiency. Vet Clin Pathol 2006;35:172–81.
61. Koulaouzidis A, Said E, Cottier R, et al. Soluble transferrin receptors and iron deficiency, a step beyond ferritin. A systematic review. J Gastrointestin Liver Dis 2009;18:345–52.
62. Thomas C, Kirschbaum A, Boehm D, Thomas L. The diagnostic plot: a concept for identifying different states of iron deficiency and monitoring the response to epoetin therapy. Med Oncol 2006;23:23–36.
63. Ganz T, Olbina G, Girelli D, et al. Immunoassay for human serum hepcidin. Blood 2008;112:4292–7.
64. Koliaraki V, Marinou M, Vassilakopoulos TP, et al. A novel immunological assay for hepcidin quantification in human serum. PLoS One 2009;4:e4581.
65. Galesloot TE, Vermeulen SH, Geurts-Moespot AJ, et al. Serum hepcidin: reference ranges and biochemical correlates in the general population. Blood 2011;117:e218–25.

66. Fry MM, Kania SA, Flatland B, et al. Development of a canine hepcidin serum immunoassay. Paper presented at: American Society for Veterinary Clinical Pathology 44th Annual Meeting. Monterey (CA), 2009.

67. Malyszko J. Hepcidin assays: ironing out some details. Clin J Am Soc Nephrol 2009;4:1015–6.

68. Kroot JJ, Hendriks JC, Laarakkers CM, et al. (Pre)analytical imprecision, between-subject variability, and daily variations in serum and urine hepcidin: implications for clinical studies. Anal Biochem 2009;389:124–9.

69. Schaub S, Wilkins J, Weiler T, et al. Urine protein profiling with surface-enhanced laser-desorption/ionization time-of-flight mass spectrometry. Kidney Int 2004;65: 323–32.

70. Roe MA, Spinks C, Heath AL, et al. Serum prohepcidin concentration: no association with iron absorption in healthy men; and no relationship with iron status in men carrying HFE mutations, hereditary haemochromatosis patients undergoing phlebotomy treatment, or pregnant women. Br J Nutr 2007;97:544–9.

71. Sasu BJ, Li H, Rose MJ, et al. Serum hepcidin but not prohepcidin may be an effective marker for anemia of inflammation (AI). Blood Cells Mol Dis 2010;45:238–45.

72. Li H, Rose MJ, Tran L, et al. Development of a method for the sensitive and quantitative determination of hepcidin in human serum using LC-MS/MS. J Pharmacol Toxicol Methods 2009;59:171–80.

73. Kemna E, Tjalsma H, Laarakkers C, et al. Novel urine hepcidin assay by mass spectrometry. Blood 2005;106:3268–70.

74. Kemna EH, Tjalsma H, Podust VN, et al. Mass spectrometry-based hepcidin measurements in serum and urine: analytical aspects and clinical implications. Clin Chem 2007;53:620–8.

75. Campostrini N, Castagna A, Zaninotto F, et al. Evaluation of hepcidin isoforms in hemodialysis patients by a proteomic approach based on SELDI-TOF MS. J Biomed Biotechnol 2010;2010:329646.

76. Castagna A, Campostrini N, Zaninotto F, et al. Hepcidin assay in serum by SELDI-TOF-MS and other approaches. J Prot 2010;73:527–36.

77. Thomas C, Kobold U, Balan S, et al. Serum hepcidin-25 may replace the ferritin index in the Thomas plot in assessing iron status in anemic patients. Int J Lab Hematol 2011;33(2):187–93.

78. Macdougall IC, Malyszko J, Hider RC, et al. Current status of the measurement of blood hepcidin levels in chronic kidney disease. Clin J Am Soc Nephrol 2010;5(9): 1681–9.

79. Coyne DW. Hepcidin: clinical utility as a diagnostic tool and therapeutic target. Kidney Int 2011;80:240–4.

80. Nicolas G, Viatte L, Lou DQ, et al. Constitutive hepcidin expression prevents iron overload in a mouse model of hemochromatosis. Nat Genet 2003;34:97–101.

81. Gardenghi S, Ramos P, Marongiu MF, et al. Hepcidin as a therapeutic tool to limit iron overload and improve anemia in beta-thalassemic mice. J Clin Invest 2010;120: 4466–77.

82. Sasu BJ, Cooke KS, Arvedson TL, et al. Antihepcidin antibody treatment modulates iron metabolism and is effective in a mouse model of inflammation-induced anemia. Blood 2010;115:3616–24.

83. Hashizume M, Uchiyama Y, Horai N, et al. Tocilizumab, a humanized anti-interleukin-6 receptor antibody, improved anemia in monkey arthritis by suppressing IL-6-induced hepcidin production. Rheumatol Int 2010;30:917–23.

Molecular Diagnostics of Hematologic Malignancies in Small Animals

Anne C. Avery, VMD, PhD

KEYWORDS

- Lymphoma • Canine • Clonality • Mast cell tumors
- Feline • c-kit

Over the past 20 years, human pathologists and oncologists have become increasingly reliant on genetic testing to diagnose, prognosticate and choose treatment for almost every kind of cancer. We are beginning to adopt such testing in veterinary medicine and, as a result, can often offer clients more cost-effective and less invasive diagnostics, and more reliable prognostic information.

Our ability to inexpensively identify various types of genetic changes associated with cancer not only adds to our diagnostic armament but also expands the kinds of questions we can ask in both the laboratory and clinically. For example, molecular testing allows us to distinguish a reactive population of lymphocytes from a neoplastic one and also allows us to determine if this patient's lymphoma is the same one he was treated for 1 year ago or if it is a newly arising tumor. The number of tumor cells in the peripheral blood of lymphoma patients can be precisely quantified and followed throughout treatment. Detection of a mutation in the c-kit gene in canine mast cell tumors gives us prognostic information, and in addition helps clinicians choose the type of chemotherapy that will be most efficacious in that patient. Most polymerase chain reaction (PCR)-based tests are relatively inexpensive and may help save owners money in the long run.

Molecular based diagnostic tests in hematologic malignancy can be placed into 3 broad categories: (1) detection of individual mutations in oncogenes, (2) detection of clonality in lymphoma and leukemia by taking advantage of their unique antigen receptor genes (immunoglobulin and T-cell receptor genes, and (3) detection of chromosomal translocations, deletions, and duplications. Clonality testing and detection of the c-kit oncogene in mast cell tumors are both now in routine use and widely available to practitioners. The uses and limitations of both of these assays will

The author has nothing to disclose.

Clinical Immunology Laboratory, Department of Microbiology, Immunology and Pathology, College of Veterinary Medicine and Biomedical Sciences, Colorado State University, 200 West Lake Street, Fort Collins, CO 80523, USA

E-mail address: Anne.Avery@colostate.edu

Vet Clin Small Anim 42 (2012) 97–110
doi:10.1016/j.cvsm.2011.11.001
0195-5616/12/$ – see front matter © 2012 Published by Elsevier Inc.

be discussed here. Many of the general principles would apply to any type of genetic testing that eventually becomes available.

DETECTION OF MUTATIONS IN INDIVIDUAL ONCOGENES

In 1999, 2 reports described the presence of mutations in the gene c-kit in canine mast cell tumors.[1,2] c-kit is a receptor tyrosine kinase for stem cell factor (SCF), which stimulates mast cell growth. Both reports described small duplications of DNA within the c-kit gene called internal tandem duplications (ITDs). These mutations were found within exons 11 and 12 of the c-kit gene (**Fig. 1**, referred to hereafter as the exon 11

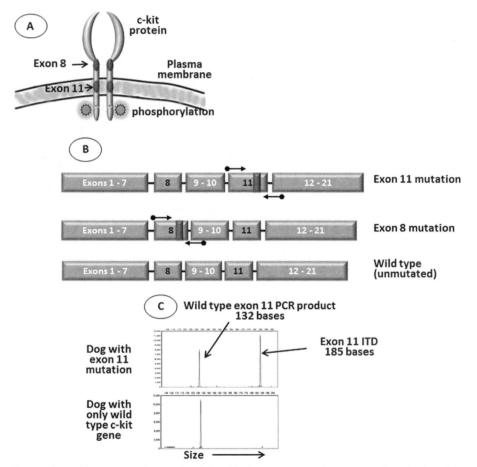

Fig. 1. The c-kit gene and protein. (*A*) C-kit is a transmembrane protein which, when activated by SCF, is phosphorylated on the cytoplasmic tail. Internal tandem duplications (ITDs) are seen in the region of the protein encoded by exon 8 (extracellular) and exon 11 (transmembrane). (*B*) c-kit mutations are found in exons 8, 9, 11, and 17, but currently available assays only detect ITDs in exon 8 (always a 12-base insertion), and exon 11 (a variety of different insertions). The arrows illustrate the location of the PCR primers used to detect the two different mutations (not drawn to scale). (*C*) Amplification of exon 11 by PCR reveals a wild-type product (132 bases) in all cases and a larger product in dogs with an exon 11 ITD. Similar results would be seen with exon 8 primers (not shown).

mutation). When SCF binds to unmutated c-kit, the cytoplasmic portion of the receptor undergoes autophosphorylation. In the presence of the exon 11 ITD, the receptor is constitutively phosphorylated, regardless of whether SCF is present (see **Fig. 1**). c-kit phosphorylation activates signaling pathways that stimulate mast cell growth. Therefore, the presence of this mutation is directly responsible for the uncontrolled proliferation of mast cells. The finding that some mast cell tumors are caused by constitutive activation through a receptor tyrosine kinase lead investigators to hypothesize that tyrosine kinase inhibitors would be useful therapies against this disease.

A comprehensive analysis of mutations in 50 canine mast cell tumors demonstrated that while the exon 11 ITDs were the most common (half of the cases), other c-kit mutations could also cause constitutive activation of the c-kit gene.[3] This included 8 examples of an identical 12–base pair ITD in exon 8 (16% of all mutations detected), as well as 8 examples of a single base change in exon 9 (16% of all mutations detected). Each of these was shown to cause constitutive phosphorylation of c-kit, suggesting that each might be rational targets of tyrosine kinase inhibitors. There were additional single base changes and rare deletions and insertions detected in exon 11 and 1 in exon 17 that did not undergo functional analysis. Together these 50 c-kit mutations represented 26% of the 191 mast cells tested. The patient population was dogs with a grade II or III mast cell tumor that had failed surgical resection or was unresectable. The prevalence of c-kit mutations in the population of mast cell tumors as a whole is probably lower.

Technical Aspects of c-kit Mutation Analysis

The discovery of dysregulated tyrosine kinase activity in the c-kit receptor led to the investigation of tyrosine kinase inhibitors as therapy and the eventual development of tyrosine kinase inhibitors such as Palladia (toceranib phosphate, Pfizer Animal Health) for use in this disease. Detection of c-kit mutations has therefore become a routine part of mast cell tumor diagnostics, because the presence of these mutations can guide therapy choices. Several laboratories now offer c-kit mutation analysis, most commonly for the exon 11 ITD. The assay is carried out by isolating DNA from cytology specimens or formalin-fixed, paraffin-embedded biopsy samples. The portion of the gene that most commonly carries the mutation is amplified by PCR using primers bracketing the region, and the products are separated by gel electrophoresis (see **Fig. 1**). All samples should show amplification of the wild-type, unmutated gene, since only 1 chromosome is likely to be affected by the mutation. In addition, there will invariably be nontumor tissue in the sample, which will have only the wild-type gene. This amplification can serve as the positive control, revealing adequate quantities of good-quality DNA. If the mutation is present, there will be a second, larger product visible as well (see **Fig. 1**). The size of the exon 11 ITD differs within each novel mast cell tumor.

Additional testing for the exon 8 ITD is offered by some laboratories. The principle is the same as detection of exon 11 mutations, but this mutation may be more difficult to detect using standard agarose gel separation methods, since the insertion is 12 bases. Single base resolution is possible using DNA sequencing instrumentation,[4] and this method may be more appropriate for exon 8 analysis.

The methodology for these assays, however, will not detect single base pair changes, such as have been reported in exon 9.[3,5] Therefore, the absence of a positive result in the commonly offered c-kit mutation assays for exon 8 and 11 does not mean that an activating mutation is not present. Assays for exon 9 have been developed (A. Avery and R. Burnett, unpublished observations, 2011), but this mutation appears to have low prevalence in the population and exon 9 testing is not routinely carried out.

The detection methods currently offered require that approximately 10% of the cells in the sample be mast cells[3] (A. Avery and R. Burnett, unpublished observations, 2011). This is because the mutated c-kit gene gives rise to a larger PCR product than does the wild-type gene. These products compete with one another during the amplification process, and amplification of the smaller, wild-type product is more efficient. Therefore, when the number of mast cells is low, a mutation may be missed. For this reason the standard assay is not likely to be useful for detecting metastasized mast cells in draining lymph nodes or for minimum residual disease detection. Tumor-specific primers, based on the specific mutation present, could be constructed for this purpose since such reagents are significantly more sensitive.

c-kit Mutations and Prognosis Using Conventional Therapy

The presence of a mutation in exon 11 of c-kit has been associated with poor prognosis in 2 studies conducted by the same group. Webster and coworkers[6] demonstrated that in cases treated by surgical excision alone (no chemotherapy), the presence of a mutation in exon 11 was highly correlated with a poor outcome. Subsequently, the same group evaluated the response to vinblastine and prednisone in 28 dogs and found that dogs with an exon 11 mutation had a disease-free interval of 6.5 months compared to those without this mutation (11 months).[7] Immunohisto-chemical staining for c-kit and histologic grade were also independently prognostic in this study. On the other hand, a large study[8] found a trend toward a worse outcome when a mutation was present, but this trend did not reach significance. There was no control for treatment, however, so an effect of the mutation may have been missed.

c-kit Mutation Status and Response to Receptor Tyrosine Kinase Inhibitors

These reports compared the response of mast cell tumors to conventional chemo-therapy (vinblastine and prednisone) with no therapy at all. Receptor tyrosine kinase inhibitors, such as Palladia, specifically target the c-kit receptor and therefore were predicted to be most effective in mast cell tumors with a constitutively activated c-kit gene. Consistent with this notion, Hahn and colleagues[9] found that in 202 dogs with recurrent or nonresectable grade II or III mast cell tumors, first-line treatment with the tyrosine kinase inhibitor masitinib was more effective than placebo regardless of whether a c-kit mutation was present. Dogs that had received other therapy prior to masitinib, however, only responded if the c-kit mutation was present. This study included all c-kit mutations, not just those found in exon 11. In another study,[10] dogs with recurrent mast cell disease responded better to the tyrosine kinase inhibitor Palladia if they carried the exon 11 c-kit mutation than if they did not. The effect of activating c-kit mutations on a patient's response to tyrosine kinase inhibitors compared with conventional chemotherapy has not yet been reported.

Detection of c-kit mutations in mast cell tumors is now routinely used for prognosis and guiding treatment. Most commonly, mutation status is determined together with immunohistochemical staining to examine proliferation markers and the cellular location of c-kit. These factors help establish prognosis and the need for additional therapy.[11,12] At least one clinical study[5] demonstrated that dogs with a single base pair change in exon 9 of c-kit responded very favorably to imatinib, although testing for this mutation is not currently offered.

c-kit Mutations Can Be Used as a Tumor Fingerprint

Patients often suffer from recurrent mast cell tumors, but it is not clear if these are derived from a single clone. Zavodska and coworkers[13] addressed this question in 2 patients by exploiting the fact that exon 11 mutations differ from tumor to tumor, thus providing a unique fingerprint to a tumor that carries it. They described 2 patients with mast cell tumors that recurred over a period of 3 years. One of these patients had 1 mast cell tumor occur each year for 3 years, with no therapy between the appearances of each tumor, and the tumor recurring in a different location each time. Since the tumor harbored a c-kit mutation, this allowed the investigators to demonstrate that the same mutation was present in each of the 3 tumors, indicating that the tumors were all derived from the same clone. Therefore, the neoplastic mast cells were never eradicated. A second case also involved a dog with multiple mast cells, which had a cytologically more aggressive appearance (grade III). Again, each of the individual tumors had the same tandem duplication, indicating they all arose from the same neoplastic clone. This approach could be extended by creating tumor-specific PCR primers based on the mutated sequence. Such primers would be far more sensitive than the standard assay and could detect distant metastases and the presence of neoplastic cells in the blood and can even be used to quantify tumor cells.

c-kit Mutations in Cats

Feline mast cell tumors also have c-kit mutations. The overall rate of mutation, based on 62 tumors, was 68%, higher than that seen in dogs.[14] The majority of these mutations involved an ITD of exon 8, similar to that seen in dogs, although a number of other mutations were also identified. Seven of 8 cats with c-kit mutations had objective clinical responses to the tyrosine kinase inhibitor imatinib, but there have not yet been controlled trials to determine if the presence of a c-kit mutation results in better clinical responses with tyrosine kinase inhibitors. Although c-kit testing in cats is not currently offered commercially, an assay to detect the majority of exon 8 mutations would be straightforward.

c-kit in Gastrointestinal Stromal Cell Tumors

c-kit is expressed in many different types of tumors. In particular, activating mutations in exon 11 of c-kit have been found in approximately 70% of human gastrointestinal stromal cell tumors (GISTs), and these cases respond well to tyrosine kinase inhibitors compared with the response by mutation-negative tumors. To date, the relevant region of c-kit has been sequenced in 21 cases of canine GIST, and mutations found in 8 (38%) of these.[15,16] Seven of the 8 involved a 3– or 6–base pair deletion and would therefore be detectable by some laboratories offering c-kit mutation analysis, depending on their level of resolution of the amplified gene product. It is important to note, however, that it has not yet been established that GISTs in dogs will response to tyrosine kinase inhibitors such as Palladia, or if the mutation has any prognostic significance.

CLONALITY ASSAYS
Principals of Clonality Assays

A clonality assay demonstrates that a group of cells is derived from a single clone. The term is usually used to refer to detection of the unique genes found in each individual B or T cell—immunoglobulin genes in B cells and T-cell receptor genes in T cells. The portion of these genes that encodes the antigen binding region is the portion that varies between cells, in both size and sequence. Once a B or T cell is mature and divides in response to antigenic stimulation, the immunoglobulin and T-cell receptor genes are passed on to the daughter cells.[17,18]

In the course of a normal immune response to a pathogen, B and T cells are activated, expand, and eventually die leaving behind a small number of residual memory cells. On the other hand, when a cell becomes neoplastic, it is no longer responds to growth controls and can expand significantly more than the cells during an immune response. Therefore, if one can establish that the majority of cells in a particular collection of lymphocytes have the same immunoglobulin or T-cell receptor gene, it is most likely that these cells are neoplastic rather than reactive.[19]

When immunoglobulin and T-cell receptor genes rearrange during the course of B-cell and T-cell development, respectively, the length and sequence of the resultant gene differ from cell to cell. There are many reasons for this, including the fact that nucleotides are added between V, D, and J segments as they rearrange into a contiguous formation. The clonality assay takes advantage of this fact. In a sample consisting of many different lymphocytes, as in a reactive process (the lymph nodes of a dog with chronic pyoderma or poor dental hygiene, for example), there will be multiple different-sized T-cell receptor and immunoglobulin genes (**Fig. 2**). On the other hand, in a sample consisting of neoplastic lymphocytes, the immunoglobulin gene or the T-cell receptor gene (depending on whether it is a B-cell or a T-cell lymphoma) will be a single size.

Technical Aspects of Clonality Assays

Clonality assays are accomplished by isolating DNA from cells suspected to be neoplastic and then, using PCR primers directed at the conserved regions of T-cell receptor or immunoglobulin genes that flank the hypervariable regions of these genes, amplifying the variable regions. The PCR products are separated by size using a variety of possible methods. The presence of a single-sized PCR product is indicative of clonality, whereas the presence of multiple PCR products supports a reactive process (see **Fig. 2**). This assay has now been reported by a number of laboratories[20–23] and used to answer a variety of clinical questions.[24–26] We have termed this assay the PARR assay (PCR for Antigen Receptor Rearrangements) in order to distinguish it from other types of clonality assays.[21] It should be noted, however, that this term is not used in the human literature.

The PARR assay differs from more commonly performed PCR assays—for example, those that are used to detect DNA from infectious agents where the result is read as "positive" or "negative"—in that the quality of the results relies very heavily on the source of the DNA (formalin-fixed paraffin-embedded tissue vs frozen or fresh samples), the primers used, the PCR cycling protocol, and particularly on the resolution of the PCR product separation technique. Because each of these factors will differ between laboratories, it is essential that a laboratory carrying out clonality analysis provide an assessment of the sensitivity and specificity of their assay. PCR products may look clonal if the products are not separated with sufficient resolution, if there was too little DNA, or if the DNA was poor quality. Thus the finding of a clonal product needs to be accompanied with information on how many non-neoplastic samples the laboratory has analyzed, and how many of these would be called clonal under that laboratory's conditions. Ideally, separation techniques that give single base resolution, such as capillary electrophoresis, should be used, but at minimum resolution of three base pairs is necessary. Agarose gels, commonly used for most conventional end point PCR assays, do not afford this kind of resolution.

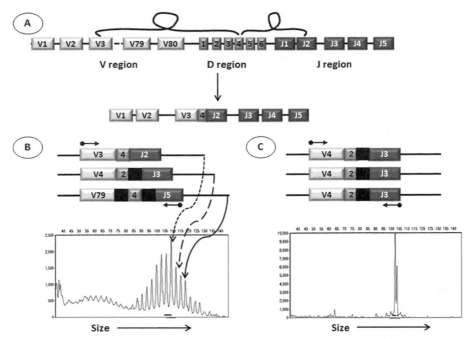

Fig. 2. Rearrangement of immunoglobulin genes. (*A*) There are approximately 80 V region genes, 6 D region genes, and 5 J region genes (Bao and colleagues[42] and A. Avery, unpublished observations, 2011) in dogs (this figure does not represent the actual numerical order of the genes). A single V, D, and J are brought together at random to create a single VDJ gene segment that encodes the antigen binding portion an antibody, and the intervening sequence is removed. (*B*) In the process of bringing together V, D, and J genes, a variable number of nucleotides (depicted in *black*) are added between V and D and between D and J. As a result, each individual B cell will have a VDJ gene segment with a unique length. When DNA from a heterogeneous population of B cells is isolated and amplified with primers bracketing the VDJ gene segment (*small arrows*), the PCR products will be different lengths. The bottom panel shows the PCR products separated by size using capillary gel electrophoresis and illustrates multiple different-sized PCR products. (*C*) When a population of B cells is composed of cells derived from a single clone, all the VDJ gene segments will be identically sized. PCR amplification of the VDJ gene segment will yield a single-sized product as shown in the bottom panel. All the principles illustrated here apply to T-cell receptor genes. For the clonality assay, the T-cell receptor gamma chain is amplified, although in theory T-cell receptor beta could also be used.

Limitations of the PARR Assay

Sensitivity

There are two types of sensitivity limitations in the PARR assay. First is the ability of the PCR primers used in these assays to detect all possible V and J regions that are used in the generation of immunoglobulin and T-cell receptor gene. Depending on the primers and conditions used and the nature of the tumor, the sensitivity of the assay for detecting clonal populations of B or T cells in confirmed cases of lymphoma or leukemia ranges from 63% to 100%.[21,27,28] Failure to detect a clonal product in a case of unequivocally diagnosed lymphoma may be due to utilization of rare V or J genes, polymorphism within the species in V and J genes, or, in the case of immunoglobulin genes, somatic hypermutation of those genes in the site where the primers bind. Since the original descriptions of the clonality assay,[20,21] the complete canine genome has become available and is well annotated. This resource has allowed investigators to develop primers that will detect a higher percentage of T-cell receptor and immunoglobulin genes and, when widely used, should increase the sensitivity of the PARR assay.[22,23]

The second type of sensitivity limitation is in how many individual tumor cells can be detected within a background of normal cells. As with all aspects of the assay, this limit will probably differ between laboratories, but in the original description of the assay it was estimated that approximately 1 tumor cell in 100 normal cells could be detected.[21] The use of tumor specific primers can detect a significantly smaller proportion of neoplastic cells $(1:10^4)$,[26] but this kind of assay is not in routine clinical use.

Determining phenotype

B-cell lymphomas have clonal immunoglobulin gene rearrangements but should not have clonal T-cell receptor rearrangements, and vice versa. Thus in theory, the clonality assay can be used to determine the phenotype of a lymphoma. The original descriptions of this assay reported high fidelity of the assay to lineage—for cases of confirmed lymphoma, the type of rearrangement was consistent with the immuno-phenotype in all cases (n = 42) except for 1 case in which both immunoglobulin and T-cell receptor rearrangements were identified.[21] Subsequently, several reports have suggested that a higher percentage of cases will have clonal rearrangements of both immunoglobulin and T-cell receptor genes in both dogs[28] and cats.[29] Each of these studies had different case selection criteria (Valli and colleagues specifically looked at indolent lymphomas, whereas the original report included any immunophenotyped case of lymphoma), which may explain the differing results. Nonetheless, although flow cytometry, immunocytochemistry, and immunohistochemistry are the tests of choice for determining the phenotype of a lymphoma, in most cases of lymphoma and lymphocytic leukemia, the lineage can be deduced from the PARR assay. It is important to note, however, the simply identifying a lymphoma as B or T cell in origin can be prognostically misleading. While there is a great deal of data supporting the idea that B-cell lymphomas overall have a poorer prognosis than T-cell lympho-mas,[30,31] there are many exceptions. Ponce and coworkers[32] demonstrated that Burkitt lymphoma (a B-cell origin tumor) had the gravest prognosis of all the histologic subtypes, B or T cell, and small clear-cell T lymphoma had the best. Furthermore, Rao and colleagues described a subset of B-cell lymphomas characterized by flow cytometry with a median survival of 136 days, closer to that typically reported for T-cell lymphomas.[33] Therefore, if the goal of phenotyping is to establish prognosis, histology or flow cytometry is preferable to clonality testing.

The PARR assay should not be used to establish whether a tumor is lymphoid or myeloid in origin in cytologically ambiguous cases. Burnett and coworkers[21] reported an acute myeloid leukemia with a clonally rearranged immunoglobulin gene, and similar findings have been reported in human myelogenous leuke-mias.[34] Thus, while the presence or absence of a clonally rearranged immuno-globulin or T-cell receptor gene can contributed to lineage determination, it should not be the sole determinant.

Uses of the PARR Assay

The PARR assay is most commonly used to aid in distinguishing reactive (polyclonal) from neoplastic (monoclonal) lymphocytes when these distinctions are difficult to make with other means. For example, while cytologic examination of lymph node aspirates can often be diagnostic for lymphoma, in cases where the majority of cells are small and mature, it is difficult to make the diagnosis of lymphoma definitively. Additional diagnostics in such cases can include histology, flow cytometry, or clonality assays. Unfortunately, to date there has been no systematic effort to compare the diagnostic utility of each of these methods, and the choice of which will be guided by the question being asked, owner finances, and the availability of sample. PARR is useful because the amount of sample required is small and the assay can be carried out on almost any tissue. On the other hand, as noted earlier, flow cytometry and histopathology can give more prognostic information than can PARR.

One example of the utility of PARR assays is in the diagnosis of indolent lymphoma. Indolent lymphomas that have been described in dogs include marginal zone lymphoma, mantle cell lymphoma and follicular lymphoma (B-cell origin) and T zone lymphomas (T-cell origin).[28] These tumors can be difficult to diagnose by histology because they can retain follicular architecture and, especially in the early stages, can be mistaken for hyperplastic lymph nodes. Valli and colleagues used the presence of a clonal lymphocyte population assessment to reclassify several cases of indolent lymphoma that had originally been diagnosed as hyperplastic but contained clonally rearranged antigen receptor genes. In this study, detection of immunoglobulin rearrangements in cases of histologically diagnosed B-cell indolent lymphoma ranged from 80% to 100% (depending on the histologic subtype) and 63% of indolent T-cell lymphomas. It is important to note that neither diagnostic procedure (histology or clonality) is 100% specific or sensitive, so the final clinical diagnosis in such ambiguous cases would require systematic clinical follow up. Nonetheless, this study suggests that indolent lymphoma is likely underdiagnosed, and clonality assays may help to correct this. It would be useful to see a wider survey of cases diagnosed with lymphoid hyperplasia, coupled with clinical follow-up information, to determine to what degree indolent lymphoma may be underdiagnosed.

Clonality has also been used to demonstrate that the entity known as cutaneous lymphocytosis in dogs is likely an indolent cutaneous lymphoma.[35] This study described 8 dogs presenting with cutaneous lesions that were composed of well-differentiated T cells and a histologically benign appearance. Nonetheless, in 7 of the 8 dogs, the lymphocyte population was shown to be clonal using PCR for T-cell receptor genes. Clinical follow-up of these cases showed that the disease did not regress in any of the patients, and progressed in several leading to euthanasia. Thus, the clinical progression in these cases supported the clonality results, and illustrates the utility of this kind of analysis.

PARR can be used to determine the relatedness of lymphocyte populations
Other than being used to distinguish reactive from neoplastic lymphocyte expansions, the PARR assay has been used in human medicine to detect lymphocytes that will eventually become lymphoma in pre-neoplastic tissues. The best example of such a study was the demonstration that the lymphoid hyperplasia seen in early *Helicobacter pylori* infection contains the B cells that eventually become neoplastic in MALT-lymphoma associated with this infection. This association was established by sequencing the hypervariable regions of B cells present in the pre-neoplastic lesions and demonstrating that one of these sequences was identical to the hypervariable region seen in the B-cell lymhoma that eventually developed.[36]

Our laboratory used this same principle to demonstrate the progression of a multicentric B-cell lymphoma to multiple myeloma.[24] In this case, the dog originally presented with cytologically confirmed B-cell lymphoma and normal immunoglobulin levels. The dog was treated with a CHOP chemotherapy protocol and achieved clinical remission. Several months later the dog re-presented with a monoclonal gammopathy, lytic rib lesions, and plasma cells in multiple sites. The progression from multicentric B-cell lymphoma to multiple myeloma had not been reported in the literature, so we wanted to determine if these were 2 separate tumors. Sequencing of the hypervariable region of the immunoglobulin gene demonstrated that the B-cell lymphoma and the multiple myeloma were derived from the same clone. Although sequencing is not a routine part of PARR analysis, it is possible to tentatively conclude that 2 tumors in the same patient are related if the clonal PCR product is the same size. Therefore, the relatedness of 2 lymphoproliferative disorders appearing sequentially in the same patient is relatively simple to investigate.

PARR can be used to quantify tumor and monitor response to treatment

The PARR assay, in its current form, is not useful for clinical staging, in that cases of stage III lymphoma with PARR positive blood had similar outcomes to cases with PARR negative blood.[37] A modification of the PARR assay, however, has offered some useful insights into the response of dogs to treatment with chemotherapy.[26] The investigators in this study sequenced the hypervariable regions of the immunoglobulin gene involved in each case of B-cell lymphoma they followed. They then designed primers that would anneal specifically to the hypervariable region of each tumor; this is in contrast to the primers used for the standard PARR, which bind to the conserved regions in order to detect as many tumors as possible with as few primer combinations as possible. The advantage of making tumor specific primers is that the sensitivity for detecting tumor cells increases substantially, and the number of tumor cells can be quantified.

Only 1 dog was tested before treatment, so it is not possible to evaluate the magnitude of the initial response to chemotherapy. Blood from all dogs were tested during treatment, and at all times tumor was detectable in the peripheral blood, even if the patients achieved full clinical remission. In most cases, the number of tumor cells ranged between 1 and 10 cells/μL during remission, but those numbers increased drastically when coming out of clinical remission—achieving concentrations of 1000 cells/μL. An increase in the number of cells in the blood correlated very well with increasing lymph node size and loss of clinical remission.

While the production of tumor-specific primers may not be practical or affordable for a large number of owners, detecting minimal residual disease using this method can be useful in a research setting. For example, if it can be shown that the degree of tumor burden reduction in the earlier stages of treatment is correlated with eventual outcome, then quantifying tumor burden can be a useful way of testing the efficacy of novel chemotherapies without needing to follow a patient through the entire course of treatment. Quantifying the response to treatment may also be a first step toward understand why some tumor types have an overall poorer outcome.

PARR in the Diagnosis of Feline Intestinal Lymphoma

Feline intestinal lymphoma presents a pervasive diagnostic dilemma. Severe inflammatory bowel disease can have many of the histologic features of intestinal T-cell lymphoma, including significant increases in the T-cell population of the lamina propria and an increase in intraepithelial lymphocytes. Even with full-thickness biopsy samples, some cases can be difficult to diagnose. Establishing that the intestinal lymphocytic infiltrate is clonal may help distinguish between the 2 entities.

Several studies have now been reported in which clonality has been assessed in feline patients with histologically diagnosed lymphoma and histologically diagnosed inflammatory bowel disease. Moore and coworkers[38] examined 28 cases of intestinal

T-cell lymphoma and 9 cases of inflammatory bowel disease and found that 78% of the lymphoma cases had a clonal T-cell population (22 of 28), and none of the inflammatory bowel disease patients contained clonal T-cell populations. In a larger, more recent study, this same group looked at 120 cases that were chosen based on a histologic diagnosis of lymphoma[39] and found the same sensitivity for detecting clonal T-cell populations (78%). Sensitivity for detecting clonal B-cell populations in the less common B-cell lymphomas was 50%. Although clonality assessment proved helpful in making diagnostic decisions, this study also highlighted the importance of histopathology in predicting outcome in cases of feline lymphoma—patients whose lymphoma was classified as large cell had a median survival of 1.5 months, whereas the small cell lymphomas had a median survival of 28 months. Cases with mucosal involvement only also had a significantly better survival time than did cases with transmural involvement. Nonetheless, clonality assessment on mesenteric lymph node or intestinal aspirates may be a useful way to establish malignancy if owners are unwilling or unable to pursue more invasive diagnostics.

Refractory celiac sprue in human patients provides a potential parallel to feline inflammatory bowel disease. This is a subset of celiac disease that does not respond to gluten withdrawal. Refractory sprue does not have the histologic features of lymphoma. Nonetheless, in one early study, a majority of patients with this disease who have a clonally expanded T-cell population in their small intestine experienced a malignant course, eventually dying of malnutrition.[40] Thus, although they do not receive a histologic diagnosis of lymphoma, all the other features of the disease indicate malignancy. Subsequently, the presence of clonally expanded T-cell populations in patients with refractory sprue was shown to be 78% sensitive for the eventual development of histologically defined lymphoma.[41]

While the etiology of feline IBD and intestinal lymphoma is probably not the same as human refractory sprue, experience in the latter suggests that using a histologic diagnosis of lymphoma as the gold standard may warrant reconsideration. As yet there are no studies in which clonality has been assessed as an independent prognostic factor in a series of cases of severe inflammatory bowel disease, but such studies would be clinically very useful. Ultimately, a combination of histology, immunohistochemistry, and clonality determination may prove to be necessary to obtain accurate diagnostic and prognostic information in cases of feline intestinal disease.

Additional Comments About Clonality Testing

There are several applications that are not appropriate for any of the tests described here. These are not intended as a first-line diagnostic procedure and often are not necessary. For example, although PARR testing can provide lineage information (B vs T cell) when it is positive, if the diagnosis of lymphoma or leukemia is unambiguous, flow cytometry, immunocytochemistry, or immunohistochemistry is a better test to determine the phenotype because more information can be obtained. Therefore, PARR testing is less useful for confirmed cases of lymphoma. These assays are also not intended as screening tests for healthy animals, as they have not been evaluated in this capacity. These assays can, however, provide a wealth of clinically useful information (in resolving ambiguous cases) and be useful research tools for better understanding the biology of hematologic malignancy.

REFERENCES

1. London CA, Galli SJ, Yuuki T, et al. Spontaneous canine mast cell tumors express tandem duplications in the proto-oncogene c-kit. Exp Hematol 1999;27:689–97.

2. Ma Y, Longley BJ, Wang X, et al. Clustering of activating mutations in c-KIT's juxtamembrane coding region in canine mast cell neoplasms. J Inv Dermatol 1999; 112:165–70.

3. Letard S, Yang Y, Hanssens K, et al. Gain-of-function mutations in the extracellular domain of KIT are common in canine mast cell tumors. Mol Cancer Res 2008;6: 1137–45.

4. Jones CL, Grahn RA, Chien MB, et al. Detection of c-kit mutations in canine mast cell tumors using fluorescent polyacrylamide gel electrophoresis. J Vet Diagn Invest 2004;16:95–100.

5. Yamada O, Kobayashi M, Sugisaki O, et al. Imatinib elicited a favorable response in a dog with a mast cell tumor carrying a c-kit c.1523A>T mutation via suppression of constitutive KIT activation. Vet Immunol Immunopathol 2011;142:101–6.

6. Webster JD, Yuzbasiyan-Gurkan V, Kaneene JB, et al. The role of c-KIT in tumorigenesis: evaluation in canine cutaneous mast cell tumors. Neoplasia (New York) 2006;8: 104–11.

7. Webster JD, Yuzbasiyan-Gurkan V, Thamm DH, et al. Evaluation of prognostic markers for canine mast cell tumors treated with vinblastine and prednisone. BMC Vet Res 2008;4:32.

8. Downing S, Chien MB, Kass PH, et al. Prevalence and importance of internal tandem duplications in exons 11 and 12 of c-kit in mast cell tumors of dogs. Am J Vet Res 2002;63:1718–23.

9. Hahn KA, Ogilvie G, Rusk T, et al. Masitinib is safe and effective for the treatment of canine mast cell tumors. J Vet Intern Med 2008;22:1301–9.

10. London CA, Malpas PB, Wood-Follis SL, et al. Multi-center, placebo-controlled, double-blind, randomized study of oral toceranib phosphate (SU11654), a receptor tyrosine kinase inhibitor, for the treatment of dogs with recurrent (either local or distant) mast cell tumor following surgical excision. Clin Canc Res 2009;15:3856–65.

11. Romansik EM, Reilly CM, Kass PH, et al. Mitotic index is predictive for survival for canine cutaneous mast cell tumors. Vet Pathol 2007;44:335–41.

12. Scase TJ, Edwards D, Miller J, et al. Canine mast cell tumors: correlation of apoptosis and proliferation markers with prognosis. J Vet Intern Med 2006;20:151–8.

13. Zavodovskaya R, Chien MB, London CA. Use of kit internal tandem duplications to establish mast cell tumor clonality in 2 dogs. J Vet Intern Med 2004;18:915–7.

14. Isotani M, Yamada O, Lachowicz JL, et al. Mutations in the fifth immunoglobulin-like domain of kit are common and potentially sensitive to imatinib mesylate in feline mast cell tumours. Br J Haematol 2010;148:144–53.

15. Frost D, Lasota J, Miettinen M. Gastrointestinal stromal tumors and leiomyomas in the dog: a histopathologic, immunohistochemical, and molecular genetic study of 50 cases. Vet Pathol 2003;40:42–54.

16. Gregory-Bryson E, Bartlett E, Kiupel M, et al. Canine and human gastrointestinal stromal tumors display similar mutations in c-KIT exon 11. BMC Canc 2010;10: 559–68.

17. Delves PJ, Roitt IM. The immune system. First of two parts. N Engl J Med 2000;343: 37–49.

18. Blom B, Spits H. Development of human lymphoid cells. Annu Rev Immunol 2006; 24:287–320.

19. Swerdlow SH. Genetic and molecular genetic studies in the diagnosis of atypical lymphoid hyperplasias versus lymphoma. Hum Pathol 2003;34:346–51.

20. Vernau W, Moore PF. An immunophenotypic study of canine leukemias and preliminary assessment of clonality by polymerase chain reaction. Vet Immunol Immunopathol 1999;69:145–64.

21. Burnett RC, Vernau W, Modiano JF, et al. Diagnosis of canine lymphoid neoplasia using clonal rearrangements of antigen receptor genes. Vet Pathol 2003;40:32–41.
22. Tamura K, Yagihara H, Isotani M, et al. Development of the polymerase chain reaction assay based on the canine genome database for detection of monoclonality in B cell lymphoma. Vet Immunol Immunopath 2006;115:163–7.
23. Yagihara H, Tamura K, Isotania M, et al. Genomic organization of the T-cell receptor γ gene and PCR detection of its clonal rearrangement in canine T-cell lymphoma/leukemia. Vet Immunol Immunopathol 2007;115:375–82.
24. Burnett RC, Blake MK, Thompson LJ, et al. Evolution of a B-cell lymphoma to multiple myeloma after chemotherapy. J Vet Intern Med 2004;18:768–71.
25. Keller RL, Avery AC, Burnell RC, et al. Detection of neoplastic lymphocytes in peripheral blood of dogs with lymphoma by polymerase chain reaction for antigen receptor gene rearrangement. Vet Clin Pathol 2004;33:145–9.
26. Yamazaki J, Baba K, Goto-Koshino Y, et al. Quantitative assessment of minimal residual disease (MRD) in canine lymphoma by using real-time polymerase chain reaction. Vet Immunol Immunopathol 2008;126:321–31.
27. Chaubert P, Baur Chaubert AS, Sattler U, et al. Improved polymerase chain reaction-based method to detect early-stage epitheliotropic T-cell lymphoma (mycosis fungoides) in formalin-fixed, paraffin-embedded skin biopsy specimens of the dog. J Vet Diagn Invest 2010;22:20–9.
28. Valli VE, Vernau W, de Lorimier L-P, et al. Canine indolent nodular lymphoma. Vet Pathol 2006;43:241–56.
29. Weiss AT, Klopfleisch R, Gruber AD. T-cell receptor gamma chain variable and joining region genes of subgroup 1 are clonally rearranged in feline B- and T-cell lymphoma. J Comp Pathol 2011;144:123–34.
30. Ruslander DA, Gebhard DH, Tompkins MB, et al. Immunophenotypic characterization of canine lymphoproliferative disorders. In Vivo 1997;11:169–72.
31. Dobson JM, Blackwood LB, McInnes EF, et al. Prognostic variables in canine multicentric lymphosarcoma. J Sm Anin Pract 2001;42:377–84.
32. Ponce F, Magnol JP, Ledieu D, et al. Prognostic significance of morphological subtypes in canine malignant lymphomas during chemotherapy. Vet J 2004;167:158–66.
33. Rao S, Lana S, Eickhoff J, et al. Class II major histocompatibility complex expression and cell size independently predict survival in canine B-cell lymphoma. J Vet Intern Med 2011;25:1097–105.
34. Kyoda K, Nakamura S, Matano S, et al. Prognostic significance of immunoglobulin heavy chain gene rearrangement in patients with acute myelogenous leukemia. Leukemia 1997;11:803–6.
35. Affolter VK, Gross TL, Moore PF. Indolent cutaneous T-cell lymphoma presenting as cutaneous lymphocytosis in dogs. Vet Dermatol 2009;20:577–85.
36. Zucca E, Bertoni F, Roggero E, et al. Molecular analysis of the progression from Helicobacter pylori-associated chronic gastritis to mucosa-associated lymphoid-tissue lymphoma of the stomach. N Engl J Med 1998;338:804–10.
37. Lana SE, Jackson TL, Burnett RC, et al. Utility of polymerase chain reaction for analysis of antigen receptor rearrangement in staging and predicting prognosis in dogs with lymphoma. J Vet Intern Med 2006;20:329–34.
38. Moore PF, Woo JC, Vernau W, et al. Characterization of feline T cell receptor gamma (TCRG) variable region genes for the molecular diagnosis of feline intestinal T cell lymphoma. Vet Immunol Immunopathol 2005;106:167–78.

39. Moore PF, Rodriguez-Bertos A, Kass PH. Feline gastrointestinal lymphoma: mucosal architecture, immunophenotype, and molecular clonality. Vet Pathol 2011. [Epub ahead of print].

40. Cellier C, Delabesse E, Helmer C, et al. Refractory sprue, coeliac disease, and enteropathy-associated T-cell lymphoma. Lancet 2000;356:203–8.

41. Verbeek WH, Goerres MS, von Blomberg BM, et al. Flow cytometric determination of aberrant intra-epithelial lymphocytes predicts T-cell lymphoma development more accurately than T-cell clonality analysis in refractory celiac disease. Clin Immunol 2008;126:48–56.

42. Bao Y, Guo Y, Xiao S, et al. Molecular characterization of the VH repertoire in Canis familiaris. Vet Immunol Immunopathol 2010;137:64–75.

Neutropenia in Dogs and Cats: Causes and Consequences

Amy N. Schnelle, DVM*, Anne M. Barger, DVM, MS

KEYWORDS

• Neutropenia • Toxic neutrophils • Granulopoiesis

The neutrophil is a polymorphonuclear phagocytic granulocyte that plays a key role in the innate immune system and is the predominant leukocyte found in circulation. Cytologically, neutrophils are approximately 10 to 13 μm in diameter, with colorless or pale cytoplasm containing fine, neutral or pale pink granules, a multilobulated (2 to 5) nucleus, and dark purple, clumped chromatin. Neutrophils are produced in the bone marrow from the myeloid cell line, along with eosinophils and basophils, diverging from monocyte precursors. Granulopoiesis is mediated by granulocyte colony-stimulating factor (G-CSF), granulocyte-macrophage colony-stimulating factor (GM-CSF), interleukin (IL)-3, IL-2, IL-1, stem cell factor (SCF), IL-6, and IL-11,[1–3] which stimulate stem cell division and differentiation into myeloblasts, promyelocytes, myelocytes, metamyelocytes, band neutrophils, and, finally, segmented neutrophils. A portion of segmented neutrophils are retained in the bone marrow storage pool, while others are released into the peripheral blood. Release from the bone marrow is mediated by complement 5a (C5a), tumor necrosis factor (TNF)α, TNFβ, G-CSF, and GM-CSF, among others.[2,3] Here, the population divides into the circulating pool (CNP), which travels in the center column of flowing blood, and the marginated pool (MNP), which rolls along the endothelial surface, briefly and intermittently attaching to the surface of endothelial cells displaying appropriate markers. In dogs, the CNP:MNP is approximately 1:1, while in cats it is 1:3. Eventually, in health, circulating neutrophils will move out of the vasculature permanently into the tissues.

In infectious disease, neutrophils will marginate and extravasate, moving chemotactically by following C5a, IL-8, leukotriene B4 (LTB4), and platelet-activating factor (PAF) to the site of the stimulus.[2] This most often is bacteria, but fungal infections and sterile inflammatory conditions, such as bile peritonitis and panniculitis, will also attract neutrophils. Once there, the neutrophils phagocytose organisms and fuse the

---

The authors have nothing to disclose.
Department of Pathobiology, College of Veterinary Medicine, University of Illinois, 2001 South Lincoln Avenue, Urbana, IL 6102, USA
* Corresponding author.
E-mail address: aschnel2@illinois.edu

phagosome with a lysosome containing enzymes and microbicidal substances. These substances, along with the oxidative burst, are used to kill and to digest foreign pathogens.

Neutropenia is a decrease in the absolute number of neutrophils in circulation in the peripheral blood below 2900 cells/μL.[4] This change may be seen in situations of increased use, vascular sequestration (endotoxemia and anaphylaxis), immune-mediated destruction, and decreased or ineffective production. A false decrease in neutrophil numbers may be seen with in vitro changes, such as a clotted sample or potentially with EDTA-associated neutrophil aggregates.[5]

INCREASED USE

A marked increased demand for neutrophils can quickly annihilate the population available in circulation and storage without sufficient time for bone marrow compensation. Any severe suppurative inflammatory response has the potential to induce neutropenia. Acutely, endotoxin release by gram-negative bacteria into circulation induces increased margination of neutrophils in less than 1 hour via increased expression of adhesion molecules on the neutrophil surface,[6] resulting in neutropenia within the circulating pool.

A study by Brown and colleagues in 2001[7] evaluated causes of neutropenia in 232 dogs and 29 cats. Cases were classified as nonbacterial infectious disease (viral and fungal), increased demand, drug association, primary bone marrow disease, immune-mediated disease, and diseases of unclear etiology, which included cases of suspected but unconfirmed rickettsial disease. Among cats, 17% of cases of neutropenia were due to increased demand due to inflammation, bacterial sepsis, or endotoxemia from such causes as dog attack, endotoxemia, respiratory infection, and ulcerative dermatitis. They found that increased demand accounted for 10% of canine cases. Specific etiologies within the canine population included sepsis, pneumonias, peritonitis, and reproductive infections. Though a relatively small proportion was attributed to increased demand in this study, diseases with a viral or fungal origin made up more than 50% and parvoviral infections made up the bulk of this latter group. The increased consumption and loss secondary to gastrointestinal lesions and possible septicemia, along with endotoxic effects, were likely contributors to the pathogenesis of neutropenia in those cases, in addition to direct parvovirus-mediated destruction of myeloproliferative cells.[8]

DECREASED PRODUCTION

Decreased production of neutrophils or other cell lines may be seen with interference of cell replication, damage to precursors, or replacement of marrow populations. Damage or replacement of the hematopoietic population and supporting stroma of the bone marrow will induce variable cytopenias in the periphery; this includes primary or metastatic neoplasms, infectious organisms, dysplastic conditions, fibrosis, and necrosis. Bicytopenia or pancytopenia may also be present, with concurrent decreases in platelets, erythrocytes, and other leukocytes. Bone marrow insult from cytotoxic drugs or their metabolites is another potent way to induce cytopenias.

Chemotherapeutics target rapidly dividing cells via multiple mechanisms, including disruption of the mitotic spindle, inhibition of DNA, RNA, and protein synthesis, and by unknown mechanisms. Common offenders include doxorubicin and cyclophosphamide, but neutropenia has been reported as an adverse effect of many chemotherapeutic drugs. Of 29 drug-associated cases of neutropenia in one study, 19 were dogs being treated with one or more chemotherapeutic agents. The single feline drug-associated neutropenia case was receiving vincristine.[7] Azathioprine, a thiopurine antimetabolite used as an immunosuppressant, similarly can result in bone marrow suppression, particularly in cats, but dogs may be affected as well.[9–11]

Estrogen toxicity, via accidental ingestion, mismating or incontinence treatment, and estrogen-producing testicular (Sertoli) tumors in male dogs, results in myelosuppression with hypocellularity of all lines and pancytopenia.[12,13] In a case series of 8 dogs with estrogen toxicity secondary to Sertoli cell tumors, 2 dogs survived following castration and supportive care, while the remaining 5 died despite intervention. The surviving dogs showed hematologic improvement within 3 weeks and were normal at 5 months.[12] Aplastic anemia secondary to estradiol cyclopentylpropionate administration for urinary incontinence and prevention of pregnancy, as well as neutropenia secondary to concurrent administration of diethylstilbestrol, estradiol cypionate, and trimethoprime sulfate (TMS) in a dog have also been reported.[7,14]

A variety of adverse reactions to potentiated sulfonamides are well documented in the dog,[7,14–18] including a possible breed-associated Type III hypersensitivity response reported in 6 Doberman pinschers.[19] Neutrophils and other cell lines are notably affected in many cases, involving 27% of cases in one report.[16] The damage can range from mild neutropenia to agranulocytosis[17] or aplastic anemia.[14,15,18] It appears to be an idiosyncratic reaction, and patients can recover with discontinuation of treatment and supportive care, sometimes in as little as 24 hours.[17] One of these cases was treated concurrently with TMS and fenbendazole, while administration of the same drug combination in a normal dog did not have the same results.[15]

Other drugs with reported single or combination cytopenias involving neutropenias include phenylbutazone,[14,20] albenadazole in a dog and a cat,[21] chloramphenicol in cats,[22] captopril in a dog,[23] phenobarbital,[7,24] primidone,[24] cephalosporin in dogs,[25] methimazole in cats,[26] trimeprazine tartrate,[7] and quinidine.[14] Griseofulvin has been shown to induce neutropenia in cats infected with feline immunodeficiency virus (FIV), but normal cats in that study did not have the same response.[27] Nevertheless, hematologic and/or hepatic abnormalities may develop with the use of griseofulvin, but this appears to be an idiosyncratic reaction found only in a few cats.[28]

Another mechanism of decreased neutrophil production is myelophthisis, which is replacement of the normal bone marrow population with another cell type, such as neoplastic cells or fibrous tissue. Pancytopenia may be noted peripherally; a review of 51 cases of pancytopenia in dogs found 5 cases that were due to bone marrow infiltration of neoplastic cells, including malignant histiocytosis, lymphoblastic leukemia, and multiple myeloma.[13] In myelofibrosis, leukon and thrombon changes vary from case to case.[29] This same report mentions several cases of spontaneous myelofibrosis in intact female beagles in which severe nonregenerative anemia was the initial and most impressive clinical finding. Three dogs were discussed in detail, and all had a mild neutropenia. Antemortem bone marrow samples contained from 0% to 75% fibrosis in the sections examined. In all cases, erythroid precursors predominated with normal numbers of myeloid precursors despite neutropenia. Bone marrow necrosis was observed in the case without observed fibrosis.

Bone marrow necrosis may result in neutropenia. Causes include drug administration, sepsis, infectious organisms, and idiopathic causes. In an evaluation of 34 cases of bone marrow necrosis in dogs, 9 cases were considered idiopathic in origin, while the remaining cases were associated with disease conditions and drug exposures.[30] Neutropenia was more commonly present in dogs with a diagnosed etiology (56%), compared with idiopathic cases (33%) and cases without bone marrow necrosis (18%) that were neutropenic for other reasons. Drug exposures with bone marrow necrosis and neutropenia included phenobarbital, carprofen, metronidazole, cyclophosphamide, colchicine, and fenbendazole. A single case of heartworm disease with bone marrow necrosis also was neutropenic. Nonneutropenic cases of necrosis in this paper included blastomycosis, mast cell neoplasia, lupus erythematosus, lymphoma, mitotane treatment, and vincristine for megakaryoblastic leukemia.

Several congenital/hereditary defects affecting neutrophil production at the level of the bone marrow have been reported.

Grey collie syndrome or cyclic hematopoiesis is an autosomal recessive hereditary defect caused by a mutation in the *AP3B1* gene for the beta subunit of adaptor protein complex 3, which is responsible for shuttling of proteins, notably neutrophil elastase, from the Golgi apparatus to lysosomes.[31] The exact mechanism of feedback from this mutation to hematopoiesis is still unclear; functionally the mutation translates into waxing and waning neutrophil production, cycling every 11 to 14 days.[3] Left alone, this defect is fatal due to increased susceptibility to pathogens, and dogs frequently succumb to infections early in life, generally by 2 years of age.[32] Multiple treatments have been attempted, with administration of recombinant G-CSF (rG-CSF), human or canine, being one such treatment. Administration of human rG-CSF (rhG-CSF) is only a temporary stop-gap, however, since dogs develop antibodies against it in 14 to 21 days. These react not only with the administered medication but also with the dog's native G-CSF via cross-reactivity, leading to a drop in circulating neutrophil numbers.[33] This exacerbates the neutrophil production problem but appears to last only 4 months once rhG-CSF treatment is abandoned. Immune response against infused recombinant canine G-CSF does not appear to occur, as treatment at high doses induces a neutrophilia, without cyclical declines, that can be maintained for months with continued treatment.[34] Bone marrow transplantation has also reportedly had success in treating this defect,[35] although the availability, cost, and risks associated with this procedure are cause for consideration.

Trapped neutrophil syndrome of border collies is an autosomal recessive disorder caused by a mutation in Vesicle Protein Sorting 13B (*VPS13B*) and is analogous to Cohen syndrome in people. In dogs, this mutation results in myeloid hyperplasia, decreased release of mature neutrophils from the bone marrow, peripheral neutropenia, and increased susceptibility to pathogens.[36] The first 2 puppies described also had mild, nonregenerative anemia with circulating nucleated erythrocytes, as well as fractures and necrosis in multiple bones without expected concurrent inflammation.[36] Though the first cases were found in New Zealand and Australia and were linked by a common ancestor, testing of 5000 dogs from Europe, the United States, the United Kingdom, and Japan revealed 1100 carriers and 30 affected dogs.[37]

Additional abnormalities have been noted in other breeds. A study identified "physiologic" leukopenia in 65 of 180 healthy Belgian Tervurens in the United States, with neutrophil counts ranging from 1.15 to 12.20 $\times 10^3/\mu L$.[38] In contrast, a study of 94 dogs in Belgium reported leukopenia in only 1 dog.[39] This may represent a regional/genetic variant in the breed within the United States. Hereditary selective cobalamin malabsorption and deficiency have been associated with neutropenia in affected patients (a border collie and a family of giant schnauzers).[40,41]

Due to the presence of neutropenia in people affected with Chediak-Higashi (C-H) syndrome, a colony of 13 C-H cats was evaluated for neutropenia after discovery of an outside C-H cat that had recurring neutropenia at approximately 7-day intervals. The cats from the colony were found to have significantly ($P<.05$) lower (mean 8.609 $\pm$ 0.985 $\times 10^9/L$) absolute neutrophil counts compared with controls (mean 12.113 $\pm$ 1.363 $\times 10^9/L$). However, there was considerable overlap between groups, including 3 control cat data points that appeared to fall below the lowest C-H cat data point.[42]

Monocytic and granulocytic ehrlichiosis are diseases caused by invasion of peripheral leukocytes by gram-negative, obligate intracellular bacteria,[43] visualized by morulae within the cytoplasm of affected cells. Granulocytic ehrlichiosis is seen with infection by *Ehrlichia ewingii* and *Anaplasma phagocytophilum*, which was formerly known as separate organisms *Ehrlichia phagocytophila, E equi*, and the human granulocytic ehrlichiosis agent.[43] Primarily, *E ewingii* is transmitted by *Amblyomma americanum*, and *A phagocytophilum* is transmitted by *Ixodes* tick bites. Monocytic ehrlichiosis is caused by *Ehrlichia canis* that is transmitted by the brown dog tick (*Rhipicephalus sanguineus*).[44] Neutropenia has been reported in conjunction with both types of infection, though the incidence varies from study to study.[45–48]

There is variability in the reported incidence of neutropenia in cases of monocytic ehrlichiosis. Some authors report the majority of the cases as neutropenic,[45] while others observed only relative neutropenia.[46] Intuitively, one might suspect that granulocytic ehrlichiosis to have a higher incidence of neutropenia compared with monocytic ehrlichiosis; however, it is even more variable. Lilliehook and colleagues observed a transient decrease in neutrophil numbers with infection with *A phagocytophilum*, but absolute neutropenia did not occur and bone marrow evaluation revealed myeloid hyperplasia with left-shifting.[49] Kohn and colleagues report no cases of neutropenia among their 18 cases of *A phagocytophilum*, though in their discussion they mention other studies with an incidence of 13% among a combined 22 dogs.[43] Experimental infection of 7 dogs with *E ewingii* resulted in leukopenia in 4 dogs,[47] while a retrospective study of 15 naturally infected dogs found a single severely neutropenic case among the 13 dogs for which CBC results were available.[48]

Babesial infections have also been reported to be associated with neutropenia. These protozoal organisms infect erythrocytes and can be identified on peripheral blood smears and by polymerase chain reaction. Studies of dogs naturally infected with large *Babesia* spp showed a range of neutropenic patients from 36% to 73%.[50–52] A study of 5 dogs experimentally infected with small *Babesia gibsoni*–like organisms from Oklahoma identified mild neutropenia in 1 dog and severe neutropenia in 3 dogs at 1 week postinfection.[53] The cause of the neutropenia was unknown in these studies, but acute inflammatory response, systemic inflammatory response syndrome, pulmonary sequestration, and immune destruction were all speculated as possibilities.

The feline retroviruses, feline leukemia virus (FeLV) and FIV, have been noted causes of neutropenia in cats. However, not all infected cats are neutropenic and neutrophilia is seen in a substantial proportion of the retrovirus-positive population. In a retrospective study evaluating 3780 cats that were tested for FIV and FeLV, 90 were positive for FIV, 104 were positive for FeLV, and 5 were positive for both viruses. Neutropenia was observed in 26% of cats within each virus group, significantly higher rates compared with the 9% seen in the control group (cats that tested negative for both viruses); neutrophilia was noted in 31% of FIV-positive cats, 33% of FeLV-positive cats, and 30% of control cats.[54] Another recent study evaluated asymptomatic FIV-positive cats for hematologic changes and found that neutropenia was present in 13 of 50 cats, or 26%.[55] A slightly higher rate was found in another study, with neutropenia due to retrovirus infection accounting for 34% of the feline cases. Of that group, 70% were infected with FeLV and 30% were infected with FIV.[7]

Latent retroviral disease is sometimes blamed in cases of cytopenias in cats that test serologically retrovirus-negative. Stutzer and colleagues investigated the prevalence of latency by PCR testing of bone marrow samples from enrolled cats with nonregenerative cytopenias (anemia, leukopenia, thrombocytopenia) that were antigen negative with serologic FeLV ELISA testing.[56] Latent FeLV disease was found by

PCR in 2 of the 37 cats tested (both cats were anemic and neither was neutropenic nor thrombocytopenic); therefore, this appears to be rather uncommon. Severe erythropoietic hypoplasia was observed in both cases. Possible mechanisms include interference with regulatory pathways with incorporation of proviral DNA into the host cells, nascent expression of antigens on the cell surface recognized as foreign, leading to immune-mediated destruction, or an incidental finding of FeLV infection and cytopenia.[56]

The mechanism of neutropenia and other cytopenias in retroviral disease is likely multifactorial. Direct viral infection of bone marrow cells and stromal cells, neoplasia, infectious organisms secondary to suppressed immune function, and myelofibrosis are all possibilities. More specific mechanistic characterization is ongoing. In a 1989 case report, an FIV-infected cat is described with chronic leukopenia (>6 months), consisting of severe lymphopenia and mild neutropenia. A mild nonregenerative anemia was also present. Although bone marrow evaluation was normal, exposure of the cat's serum to cultured autologous bone marrow cells showed inhibition of colony-forming unit granulocyte-macrophage (CFU-GM) progenitors but not late colony-forming unit erythroid (CFU-E) or burst-forming unit erythroid (BFU-E) progenitors, suggesting a humoral inhibitory factor. However, this inhibition was not observed when bone marrow cultures from normal cats were exposed to serum from the infected cat, suggesting an alteration in the infected cat's cells, as well.[57] A 2010 study found that increased expression of FasL mRNA was correlated with onset of neutropenia, increases in proviral load, and large granular lymphocytosis in 5 cats experimentally infected with FIV.[58]

Canine parvovirus (CPV) and feline panleukopenia virus (FPV) are two well-known pathogens typically characterized by a depressed leukocyte count and, somewhat predictably, neutropenia in the clinical progression of disease. Viral infection of bone marrow precursors decimates this population,[59] leading to a paucity of cells in storage, as well as in the peripheral blood results, which is a particular concern in puppies with an inflamed gastrointestinal tract. However, it appears that pluripotent cells are spared.[60] In a recent study, the lack of cytopenias, specifically total leukocytes and lymphocyte counts, in puppies infected with CPV, were shown to have a positive predictive value of 100% for survival. The nonsurvivors had marked leukopenia at 24 and 48 hours postadmission, while survivors had median WBC counts that were within normal limits during hospitalization. In this study, total WBC, lymphocyte, monocyte, and eosinophil counts were more useful for prognosis than neutrophil number.[59] FPV, not surprisingly, also results in marked decreases in circulating WBCs, particularly neutrophils. The virus infects and replicates within early myeloid progenitor cells, resulting in cell death and decreased production.[61] As with CPV, severe diarrhea develops as the feline parvovirus replicates within the mitotically active intestinal crypt cells. Lymphoid tissue and bone marrow are also target organs of FPV, resulting in profound pancytopenia and sometimes thrombocytopenia.[62] Marked decreases in peripheral cells counts can be observed; leukocyte counts of 1000 to 2000 cells/μL and neutrophil counts of 200 cells/μL or even lower may be seen.[61] A study of 244 cats diagnosed with panleukopenia had a survival rate of 51.1%, and leukocyte and platelet counts were significantly lower in nonsurvivors. Of the total study population, 137 cats had neutrophil counts available in the record; 64 (46.7%) were neutropenic. Anorexia, diarrhea, and vomiting were the most common clinical signs recorded.[63]

DESTRUCTION

Immune-mediated neutropenia (IMN) is severe and unrelenting, and this condition may be primary, caused by an autoimmune response against mature, circulating neutrophils or precursors, or secondary, such as a Type II hypersensitivity response after drug administration. The key to diagnosis of IMN often depends on eliminating other differentials and observing a response to treatment with immunosuppressive therapies. Antineutrophil antibodies have been identified through indirect methods of agglutination and immunofluorescence, though these methods are not widely available.[64]

Few cases of suspected or confirmed IMN have been reported. Among these cases, the majority were diagnosed based on elimination of other etiologies and patient response to immunosuppressive therapies.[7,65–69] Others were diagnosed based on indirect methods (exposure of patient serum to washed neutrophils from the patient or healthy dogs) of immunofluorescence, detected by flow cytometry, or neutrophil agglutination, detected by manual evaluation.[65,70,71] None were diagnosed based on direct methods, evaluating patient neutrophils for bound antibody. A study of causes of pancytopenia in 51 dogs found 3 cases that were due to immune-mediated disease.[13] Based on the reports in the literature, IMN appears to be an infrequent disease that is challenging to diagnose, but unrecognized or unpublished cases may exist.

NEUTROPHIL MORPHOLOGY

With systemic inflammation, increased demand for neutrophils stimulates an increased mitotic rate of neutrophil precursors followed by a truncated maturation period and rapid release into circulation. The consequence of this response is the persistence of immature characteristics, such as cytoplasm with a basophilic appearance and the presence of Dohle bodies, small, blue-gray cytoplasmic structures made up of rough endoplasmic reticulum. Toxic granulation represents visible eosinophilic primary granules within the cytoplasm. Cytoplasmic vacuolation can also be seen, though this is less commonly noted than the aforementioned toxic changes and can occur with prolonged storage in EDTA. Giant neutrophils are also uncommon but are another recognized toxic change, indicative of cells that skipped a division cycle. The presence of toxic changes implies systemic inflammation, even in a patient with a normal neutrophil count and without bands. Prognostic information may also be derived from these changes. Studies separately evaluating neutrophil toxicity in cats and dogs revealed the prognostic value of these cytopathologic changes.[72,73] Among both dogs and cats, the duration of hospitalization and total cost of treatment were significantly higher in the 258 dogs and 150 cats assessed. The presence of neutrophil toxic changes and leukopenia were also each associated with a higher rate of fatality in dogs but not in cats.[72,73] The study in cats revealed that 43% of the cases had toxic changes in the neutrophils but normal leukocyte counts, neutrophil counts, and no bands. This evidence of inflammation would have been missed if only an automated CBC were performed in those cases.[73]

The presence of bands in a neutropenic patient is an indication that the bone marrow is reaching the last of its mature reserve cells and immature forms are being released early. Close monitoring of the CBC at this point may give clues to continued decline (increasing percentage of bands relative to segmented neutrophils) or indications of bone marrow recovery (resurgence of segmented neutrophils). The presence of bands and toxicity within the neutrophils is more suggestive of increased demand or an inflammatory response resulting in increased numbers of neutrophils in the tissue.

CONSEQUENCES

Consequences of neutropenia are somewhat dependent on the inciting cause. Situations of neutropenia due to increased use secondary to severe inflammation and infection, such as in a septic abdomen case, have many concurrent pathophysiologic changes that affect outcome. Disseminated intravascular coagulation, systemic inflammatory response syndrome, and multiple organ failure are all concerns in severely ill patients. In a study of 13 septic dogs, neutrophils showed an increased rate of phagocytic activity but a significantly downgraded phagolysosomal oxidative burst, possibly indicating a reduced ability to dispatch phagocytized bacteria.[74] Other sources contend that the decreased ability may be a protective measure to prevent serious vasculitis, as endotoxin-stimulated neutrophils also have a decreased ability to extravasate.[6] Neutropenia due to any cause exposes the patient to infection by loss of this important protective mechanism against infectious agents, particularly bacteria. Patients with immune-mediated conditions are generally on immunosuppressive therapy, which has similar risks in addition to medication side effects.

In approaching a neutropenic patient, several steps are recommended. It is critical to carefully record a thorough history, in order to assess whether there is recent toxin or drug exposures, travel history, traumatic events or injuries, as well as observed clinical signs. Palpation and imaging of the thorax and abdomen are important to determine if there is a souce of inflammation/infection. Ultrasound evaluation may be useful, especially for discovering fluid-filled pockets that could indicate an abscess. Tick titers may give an indication of exposure, and, though these do not prove a cause-and-effect relationship, they should be considered. Retroviral testing in cats is strongly recommended in neutropenic patients. Blood cultures may be helpful, especially if the patient is febrile. Sequential CBCs may be useful in tracking a decline, rebound, or lack of response. This may be especially useful when a nidus of infection or increased demand cannot be found and other mechanisms of neutropenia, such as a production problem, are rising up the differential list.

Bone marrow evaluation is a diagnostic to consider as a later step in the work up, especially once other etiologies have been ruled out and immune-mediated mechanisms are suspected. The examination of bone marrow may also be useful in drug reactions after withdrawal of the medication to assess evidence of recovery, if none is observed on the CBC. Bone marrow aspirates may be sufficient to diagnose myelophthisis due to some types of neoplasia and infectious agents, and results can lend support for a diagnosis of maturation arrest due to suspected immune-mediated conditions. Bone marrow core biopsies may be necessary in conditions in which aspirates are often insufficient, such as myelofibrosis, necrosis, hypoplasia, aplasia, and myelophthisis due to poorly exfoliating neoplasms.[75]

Diagnosing a drug-dependent neutropenia may be especially challenging. This requires obtaining a thorough history of drug/toxin exposures, comparing this with the onset of neutropenia, ruling out concurrent conditions, and monitoring the timing of recovery following withdrawal of the drug, if the damage is reversible.

Oncology patients undergoing chemotherapy are generally monitored closely during the expected nadir of their respective treatments, and prophylactic antibiotic therapy is recommended in asymptomatic animals with counts less than 1000 neutrophils/μL.[76] However, neutropenic oncology patients that are septic should be hospitalized for fluid therapy, intravenous antibiotics, and supportive care.[76] Thereafter, a decrease in dosage of the given chemotherapeutic at the next scheduled treatment is recommended.[76] The same type of broad-spectrum antibiotic therapy and supportive care also applies to animals that are septic for other reasons.

SUMMARY

Neutropenia is a serious hematopathologic change that should not be ignored. In almost all patients, it is an important primary or secondary indicator of significant underlying disease. While in some neutropenic patients the diagnostic work up will be simple, in others it is challenging. The value of examining a blood smear for toxic changes in neutrophils cannot be overemphasized; it may indicate the presence of systemic inflammation, as well as providing clues about prognosis and the extent of treatment the patient may require.

REFERENCES

1. Nelson RW, Couto CG. Leukopenia and leukocytosis. St Louis (MO): Mosby-Year Book; 1992. p. 912–7.
2. Stockham SL, Scott MA. Leukocytes. Ames (IA): Blackwell Publishing; 2008. p. 53–106.
3. Latimer KL, Prasse KW. Leukocytes. In: Latimer KL, Mahaffey EA, Prasse KW, editors. Duncan and Prasse's veterinary laboratory medicine: clinical pathology. 4th edition. Ames (IA): Blackwell Publishing Professional; 2003. p. 46–79.
4. Schultze AE. Interpretation of canine leukocyte responses. In: Weiss DJ, Wardrop KJ, editors. Schalm's veterinary hematology. 6th edition. Ames (IA): Blackwell Publishing Ltd.; 2010. p. 321–34.
5. Zandecki M, Genevieve F, Gerard J, et al. Spurious counts and spurious results on haematology analysers: a review. Part II: white blood cells, red blood cells, haemoglobin, red cell indices and reticulocytes. Int J Lab Hematol 2007;29:21–41.
6. Wagner J, Roth R. Neutrophil migration during endotoxemia. J Leuk Biol 1999;66(1): 10–24.
7. Brown MR, Rogers KS. Neutropenia in dogs and cats: a retrospective study of 261 cases. J Am Anim Hosp Assoc 2001;37:131–9.
8. Goddard A, Leisewitz AL, Christopher MM, et al. Prognostic usefulness of blood leukocyte changes in canine parvoviral enteritis. J Vet Intern Med 2008;22:309–16.
9. Beale KM, Altman D, Clemmons RR, et al. Systemic toxicosis associated with azathioprine administration in domestic cats. Am J Vet Res 1992;53:1236–40.
10. Paul AL, Shaw SP, Bandt C. Aplastic anemia in two kittens following a prescription error. J Am Anim Hosp Assoc 2008;44:25–31.
11. Rinkardt NE, Kruth SA. Azathioprine-induced bone marrow toxicity in four dogs. Can Vet J 1996;37:612–3.
12. Sherding RG, Wilson GP, Kociba GJ. Bone marrow hypoplasia in eight dogs with Sertoli cell tumor. J Am Vet Med Assoc 1981;178:497.
13. Weiss DJ, Evanson OA, Sykes J. A retrospective study of canine pancytopenia. Vet Clin Pathol 1999;28:83–8.
14. Weiss DJ, Klausner JS. Drug-associated aplastic anemia in dogs: eight cases (1984–1988). J Am Vet Med Assoc 1990;196:472.
15. Weiss DJ, Adams LG. Aplastic anemia associated with trimethoprim-sulfadiazine and fenbendazole administration in a dog. J Am Vet Med Assoc 1987;191:1119.
16. Trepanier L, Danhof R, Toll J, et al. Clinical findings in 40 dogs with hypersensitivity associated with administration of potentiated sulfonamides. J Vet Intern Med 2003; 17:647–52.
17. Trepanier LA. Idiosyncratic toxicity associated with potentiated sulfonamides in the dog. J Vet Pharmacol Ther 2004;27:129–38.

18. Fox LE, Ford S, Alleman AR, et al. Aplastic anemia associated with prolonged high-dose trimethoprim-sulfadiazine administration in two dogs. Vet Clin Pathol 1993;22:89–92.

19. Giger U, Werner LL, Millichamp NJ, et al. Sulfadiazine-induced allergy in six Doberman pinschers. J Am Vet Med Assoc 1985;186:479.

20. Watson AD, Wilson JT, Turner DM, et al. Phenylbutazone-induced blood dyscrasias suspected in three dogs. Vet Rec 1980;107:239.

21. Stokol T, Randolph JF, Nachbar S, et al. Development of bone marrow toxicosis after albendazole administration in a dog and cat. J Am Vet Med Assoc 1997;210):1753.

22. Watson AD. Further observations on chloramphenicol toxicosis in cats. Am J Vet Res 1980;41:293–4.

23. Holland M, Stobie D, Shapiro W. Pancytopenia associated with administration of captopril to a dog. J Am Vet Med Assoc 1996;208:1683.

24. Jacobs G, Calvert C, Kaufman A. Neutropenia and thrombocytopenia in three dogs treated with anticonvulsants. J Am Vet Med Assoc 1998;212:681–4.

25. Bloom JC, Thiem PA, Sellers TS, et al. Cephalosporin-induced immune cytopenia in the dog: demonstration of erythrocyte-, neutrophil-, and platelet-associated igg following treatment with cefazedone. Am J Hematol 1988;28:71–8.

26. Peterson ME, Kintzer PP, Hurvitz AI. Methimazole treatment of 262 cats with hyperthyroidism. J Vet Intern Med 1988;2:150–7.

27. Shelton GH, Grant CK, Linenberger ML, et al. Severe neutropenia associated with griseofulvin therapy in cats with feline immunodeficiency virus infection. J Vet Intern Med 1990;4:317–9.

28. Kunkle GA, Meyer DJ. Toxicity of high doses of griseofulvin in cats. J Am Vet Med Assoc 1987;191:322–3.

29. Reagan WJ. A review of myelofibrosis in dogs. Toxicol Pathol 1993;21:164–9.

30. Weiss D. Bone marrow necrosis in dogs: 34 cases (1996–2004). J Am Vet Med Assoc 2005;227:263–7.

31. Benson KF, Li F, Person RE, et al. Mutations associated with neutropenia in dogs and humans disrupt intracellular transport of neutrophil elastase. Nat Genet 2003;35:90.

32. Zinkl JG. The leukocytes. Vet Clin North Am Small Anim Pract 1981;11:237–61.

33. Hammond WP, Csiba E, Canin A, et al. Chronic neutropenia. A new canine model induced by human granulocyte colony-stimulating factor. J Clin Invest 1991;87:704–10.

34. Hammond W, Boone T, Donahue R, et al. A comparison of treatment of canine cyclic hematopoiesis with recombinant human granulocyte-macrophage colony-stimulating factor (GM-CSF), G-CSF interleukin-3, and canine G-CSF. Blood 1990;76:523–32.

35. Dale DC, Graw RG. Transplantation of allogenic bone marrow in canine cyclic neutropenia. Science 1974;183:83–4.

36. Allan FJ, Thompson KG, Jones BR, et al. Neutropenia with a probable hereditary basis in Border Collies. N Z Vet J 1996;44:67.

37. Shearman J, Wilton A. A canine model of cohen syndrome: trapped neutrophil syndrome. BMC Genom 2011;12:258.

38. Greenfield CL, Messick JB, Solter PF, et al. Results of hematologic analyses and prevalence of physiologic leukopenia in Belgian Tervuren. J Am Vet Med Assoc 2000;216:866–71.

39. Gommeren K, Duchateau L, Paepe D, et al. Investigation of physiologic leukopenia in Belgian Tervuren dogs. J Vet Intern Med 2006;20:1340–3.

40. Battersby IA, Giger U, Hall EJ. Hyperammonaemic encephalopathy secondary to selective cobalamin deficiency in a juvenile Border collie. J Small Anim Pract 2005;46:339–44.

41. Fyfe JC, Giger U, Hall CA, et al. Inherited selective intestinal cobalamin malabsorption and cobalamin deficiency in dogs. Pediatr Res 1991;29:24–31.
42. Prieur DJ, Collier LL. Neutropenia in cats with the Chediak-Higashi Syndrome. Can J Vet Res 1987;51:407–8.
43. Kohn B, Galke D, Beelitz P, et al. Clinical features of canine granulocytic anaplasmosis in 18 naturally infected dogs. J Vet Intern Med 2008;22:1289–95.
44. Groves MG, Dennis GL, Amyx HL, et al. Transmission of Ehrlichia canis to dogs by ticks (Rhipicephalus sanguineus). Am J Vet Res 1975;36:937.
45. Sacchini F, Cessford R, Robinson B. Outbreak of canine monocytic ehrlichiosis in Saudi Arabia. Vet Clin Pathol 2007;36:331–5.
46. Lorente C, Sainz A, Tesouro M. Immunophenotype of dogs with subclinical ehrlichiosis. Ann N Y Acad Sci 2008;1149:114–7.
47. Yabsley MJ, Adams DS, O'Connor TP, et al. Experimental primary and secondary infections of domestic dogs with Ehrlichia ewingii. Vet Microbiol 2011;150:315–21.
48. Goodman RA, Hawkins EC, Olby NJ, et al. Molecular identification of Ehrlichia ewingii infection in dogs: 15 cases (1997–2001). J Am Vet Med Assoc 2003;222:1102–7.
49. Lilliehook I. Diurnal variation of canine blood leukocyte counts. Vet Clin Pathol 1997;26:113–7.
50. Solano Gallego L, Trotta M, Carli E, et al. Babesia canis canis and Babesia canis vogeli clinicopathological findings and DNA detection by means of PCR-RFLP in blood from Italian dogs suspected of tick-borne disease. Vet Parasitol 2008;157:211–21.
51. Furlanello T, Fiorio F, Caldin M, et al. Clinicopathological findings in naturally occurring cases of babesiosis caused by large form Babesia from dogs of northeastern Italy. Vet Parasitol 2005;134:77–85.
52. Zygner W, Gjska O, Rapacka G, et al. Hematological changes during the course of canine babesiosis caused by large Babesia in domestic dogs in Warsaw (Poland). Vet Parasitol 2007;145:146–51.
53. Meinkoth J, Kocan AA, Loud S, et al. Clinical and hematologic effects of experimental infection of dogs with recently identified Babesia gibsoni-like isolates from Oklahoma. J Am Vet Med Assoc 2002;220:185–9.
54. Gleich S, Hartmann K. Hematology and serum biochemistry of feline immunodeficiency virus-infected and feline leukemia virus-infected cats. J Vet Intern Med 2009; 23:552–8.
55. Fujino Y, Horiuchi H, Mizukoshi F, et al. Prevalence of hematological abnormalities and detection of infected bone marrow cells in asymptomatic cats with feline immunodeficiency virus infection. Vet Microbiol 2009;136:217–25.
56. Stützer B, Müller F, Majzoub M, et al. Role of latent feline leukemia virus infection in nonregenerative cytopenias of cats. J Vet Intern Med 2010;24:192–7.
57. Shelton GH, Abkowitz JL, Linenberger ML, et al. Chronic leukopenia associated with feline immunodeficiency virus infection in a cat. J Am Vet Med Assoc 1989;194:253.
58. Sprague WS, TerWee JA, VandeWoude S. Temporal association of large granular lymphocytosis, neutropenia, proviral load, and FasL mRNA in cats with acute feline immunodeficiency virus infection. Vet Immunol Immunopathol 2010;134:115–21.
59. Goddard A, Leisewitz AL. Canine parvovirus. Vet Clin N Am Small Anim Pract 2010;40:1041–53.
60. Macartney L, McCandlish IA, Thompson H, et al. Canine parvovirus enteritis, 1: Clinical, haematological and pathological features of experimental infection. Vet Rec 1984;115:201–10.
61. Parrish CR. Pathogenesis of feline panleukopenia virus and canine parvovirus. Baillière's Clin Haematol 1995;8:57–71.

62. Truyen U, Addie D, Belák S, et al. Feline panleukopenia. ABCD guidelines on prevention and management. J Feline Med Surg 2009;11:538–46.

63. Kruse BD, Unterer S, Horlacher K, et al. Prognostic factors in cats with feline panleukopenia. J Vet Intern Med 2010;24:1271–6.

64. Wardrop KJ, Wilkerson MJ, Mastrorilli C. Testing for immune-mediated hematologic disease. In: Weiss DJ, Wardrop KJ, editors. Schalm's veterinary hematology. 6th edition. Ames (IA): Blackwell Publishing; 2010. p. 1106–13.

65. Vargo C, Taylor S, Haines D. Immune mediated neutropenia and thrombocytopenia in 3 giant schnauzers. Can Vet J 2007;48:1159–63.

66. Brown CD, Parnell NK, Schulman RL, et al. Evaluation of clinicopathologic features, response to treatment, and risk factors associated with idiopathic neutropenia in dogs: 11 cases (1990–2002). J Am Vet Med Assoc 2006;229:87–91.

67. Perkins MC, Canfield P, Churcher RK, et al. Immune-mediated neutropenia suspected in five dogs. Aust Vet J 2004;82:52–7.

68. McManus PM, Litwin C, Barber L. Immune-mediated neutropenia in 2 dogs. J Vet Intern Med 1999;13:372–4.

69. Maddison JE, Hoff B, Johnson RP. Steroid responsive neutropenia in a dog. J Am Anim Hosp Assoc 1983;19:881–6.

70. Weiss DJ. An indirect flow cytometric test for detection of anti-neutrophil antibodies in dogs. Am J Vet Res 2007;68:464–7.

71. Weiss DJ, Henson M. Pure white cell aplasia in a dog. Vet Clin Pathol 2007;36:373–5.

72. Aroch I, Klement E, Segev G. Clinical, biochemical, and hematological characteristics, disease prevalence, and prognosis of dogs presenting with neutrophil cytoplasmic toxicity. J Vet Intern Med 2005;19:64–73.

73. Segev G, Klement E, Aroch I. Toxic neutrophils in cats: clinical and clinicopathologic features, and disease prevalence and outcome: a retrospective case control study. J Vet Intern Med 2006;20:20–31.

74. Webb C, McCord K, Dow S. Neutrophil function in septic dogs. J Vet Intern Med 2007;21:982–9.

75. McSherry LJ. Techniques for bone marrow aspiration and biopsy. In: Ettinger SJ, Feldman EC, editors. Textbook of veterinary internal medicine: diseases of the dog and cat. 7th edition. St Louis (MO): Saunders Elsevier; 2010. p. 383–5.

76. Chun R, Garrett LD, Vail DM. Cancer chemotherapy. In: Withrow SJ, Vail DM, editors. Withrow & MacEwen's small animal clinical oncology. 4th edition. St Louis (MO): Saunders Elsevier; 2007. p. 163–92.

Hematologic Abnormalities in the Small Animal Cancer Patient

Michael O. Childress, DVM, MS

KEYWORDS

- Cancer • Hematology • Anemia • Thrombocytopenia
- Coagulopathy

Hematologic abnormalities are frequently encountered in small animal cancer patients, and may result from the direct effects of tumor growth or from paraneoplastic syndromes. Cancer-related hematologic disorders may be characterized by decreases or increases in the absolute numbers of circulating formed elements of the blood, alterations of hemostasis, or plasma protein dyscrasias. Hematologic abnormalities are more common in human cancer patients with hematopoietic malignancies or disseminated solid tumors than in patients with localized solid tumors.[1,2] The same situation is likely true in small animal cancer patients,[3,4] although epidemiologic data describing the prevalence of hematologic abnormalities in subpopulations of animals with specific tumor types are generally lacking. Small animal practitioners should be cognizant of the hematologic abnormalities that characterize neoplastic disorders for several reasons: (1) Hematologic abnormalities may be hallmarks of specific cancer types, and their identification may facilitate timely diagnosis. (2) Hematologic abnormalities may serve as biomarkers of response to cancer therapy or remission status. (3) Hematologic abnormalities may require therapy beyond that which is needed to address the underlying cancer. (4) Some hematologic abnormalities may be of prognostic relevance in patients with certain tumor types. This review will summarize the various hematologic abnormalities encountered in small animal cancer patients.

It should be noted from the outset that cancer therapy is one of the most common causes of hematologic alterations in dogs and cats with cancer. Cytotoxic chemotherapy, radiation therapy, and receptor tyrosine kinase inhibitors may all produce significant derangements of hematologic parameters. The hematologic side effects of cancer therapy have been described elsewhere[5–7] and will not be covered in this review.

The author has nothing to disclose.

Department of Veterinary Clinical Sciences, Purdue University School of Veterinary Medicine, 625 Harrison Street, West Lafayette, IN 47907-2026, USA

E-mail address: mochildr@purdue.edu

Vet Clin Small Anim 42 (2012) 123–155
doi:10.1016/j.cvsm.2011.09.009
0195-5616/12/$ – see front matter © 2012 Elsevier Inc. All rights reserved.

Table 1
Frequency of anemia at the time of diagnosis of various small animal tumors

Tumor Type	Frequency of Anemia (%)	References
Lymphoma (canine)	30–43	52,73,217–220
Lymphoma (feline)	43–58	139,221–224
Acute leukemia (canine)	87–98	91,225
Acute leukemia (feline)	100	50,51,164
Chronic lymphocytic leukemia (canine)	75–86	91,140
Multiple myeloma (canine)	68	191
Multiple myeloma (feline)	56–69	215,226
Histiocytic sarcoma (canine)		
Localized	0–46	227–229
Disseminated	53–94	38,230,231
Mast cell tumor (canine)		
Localized	5–9	147,232
Systemic	64–70	54,233
Hemangiosarcoma (canine)	28–72	234–237
Hemangiosarcoma (feline)	35–82	238–240

ABNORMAL DECREASES IN CIRCULATING BLOOD CELL CONCENTRATIONS
Anemia

Anemia is one of the most common hematologic abnormalities encountered in human cancer patients. Approximately 30% to 50% of patients with solid tumors and 40% to 70% of patients with hematopoietic tumors are anemic at the time of initiating cancer therapy.[8–10] The prevalence of anemia in these patient populations generally increases as cancer treatment progresses due to the myelosuppressive effects of cytotoxic chemotherapy and radiotherapy.[9–11] The true prevalence of anemia in small animal cancer patients is unknown; however, anemia is frequently identified in dogs and cats with a variety of cancers.[12] Anemia is especially common in patients with hematopoietic tumors and vascular tumors such as hemangiosarcoma. The reported frequencies of anemia associated with several small animal tumors at the time of diagnosis are listed in **Table 1**.

Cancer-related anemia may arise through several mechanisms and is often multifactorial in nature. The pathogenic mechanisms common to all anemias, including blood loss, increased red blood cell destruction (hemolysis), and decreased red blood cell production, may each play a role in cancer-related anemia. Tumoral hemorrhage may occur with a variety of cancers and may be acute or chronic in nature. Acute, severe tumoral hemorrhage is often seen with splenic hemangiosarcoma[13,14] but may also occur in patients with other malignant and benign splenic tumors,[12,14,15] hepatocellular carcinoma,[16] adrenal tumors,[17–19] and thyroid carcinoma.[20] Chronic, low-grade hemorrhage is seen with mucosal epithelial tumors, such as those of the gastrointestinal tract, nasal cavity, and urinary bladder.[21] These tumors are often quite friable and prone to bleed following even minimal trauma. Paraneoplastic syndromes may also contribute to hemorrhage in veterinary cancer patients—gastrointestinal ulceration and hemorrhage secondary to gastric hyperacidity are common in dogs and cats with mast cell tumor and gastrinoma. In such cases, excessive tumoral production of histamine and gastrin, respectively, are responsible for increased gastric acidity.[22–24]

Hemolytic anemias in cancer patients may be immune-mediated or non–immune-mediated. Immune-mediated hemolytic anemia (IMHA) is initiated by the binding of immunoglobulins, complement, or both to the erythrocyte membrane.[25,26] Erythrocytes coated with immunoglobulin or complement are subsequently recognized and destroyed by phagocytic cells in the spleen and liver (extravascular hemolysis). Binding of complement to the erythrocyte membrane also may also result in disrupted membrane permeability and intravascular hemolysis. Neoplasia is the most commonly identified underlying cause for IMHA in small animals.[25] Hematologic malignancies, such as lymphomas and leukemias, are the tumor types most frequently associated with IMHA in both small animals and humans.[2,12,25] Feline leukemia virus (FeLV) infection may cause IMHA in feline cancer patients.[27,28] The pathogenesis of IMHA in FeLV-infected cats is not entirely clear, but may result from cross-reactivity of antiviral antibodies with normal erythrocyte membrane antigens, or from an immune response directed against erythrocyte membrane antigens altered by viral infection of erythroid precursors in the bone marrow.[27,28] Concurrent infection with hemotropic *Mycoplasma* spp may also precipitate IMHA in FeLV-infected cats.[29,30]

Non–immune-mediated hemolytic anemias may arise in veterinary cancer patients due to microangiopathy, oxidative damage to erythrocytes, or tumor cell erythrophagocytosis. Microangiopathic hemolytic anemia (MAHA) is caused by pathologic changes, such as endothelial cell injury and fibrin deposition, in the systemic microvasculature.[12,31] These pathologic alterations cause shearing and destruction of erythrocytes as they attempt to traverse arterioles and capillaries. This type of hemolysis is characterized by increased numbers of fragmented erythrocytes (schistocytes) in the peripheral blood. The most common cause of MAHA in veterinary cancer patients is disseminated intravascular coagulation (DIC).[12] However, MAHA may also result from inherent abnormalities in tumor microvasculature, such as incomplete or absent endothelial coverage, tortuosity, variations in vascular caliber, and turbulent blood flow.[32,33] These vascular abnormalities are most notable in hemangiosarcoma,[33] but likely occur in many other tumor types.

Oxidative injury to red blood cells may also play a role in some cancer-related hemolytic anemias. Morphologic changes in erythrocytes that are characteristic of oxidative injury include eccentrocytosis and Heinz body formation. Eccentrocytes are erythrocytes in which the cell membrane has partially collapsed, causing hemoglobin to shift to one side of the cell, and a pale, eccentrically shaped clear zone to form on the opposite side. Heinz bodies are aggregates of denatured hemoglobin which accumulate along the internal surface of the erythrocyte cell membrane. Heinz bodies are the most common manifestation of oxidative damage to feline erythrocytes, while both Heinz bodies and eccentrocytes may be identified in canine blood following oxidative injury.[34] Eccentrocytes and erythrocytes bearing Heinz bodies may be destroyed by intravascular or extravascular hemolysis. Intravascular hemolysis results from a decrease in the deformability and increased fragility of the erythrocyte membrane, predisposing the cell to lysis within capillaries or vascular sinusoids. Extravascular hemolysis results from clustering of membrane band 3 proteins on the external surface of the cell membrane; these band 3 protein clusters are subsequently recognized and bound by autoantibodies and the cell is phagocytosed.[35] The overall importance of oxidative damage to cancer-related anemias in small animals is unknown, and other predisposing causes such as hyperthyroidism, diabetes mellitus, and exposure to oxidative toxins (eg, garlic, onions, acetaminophen) should be excluded in patients whose hemograms suggest oxidative erythrocyte injury. However, in a recent retrospective study of 60 dogs with eccentrocytosis, neoplasia was identified as an underlying cause in nine (15%); five of these nine dogs had T-cell

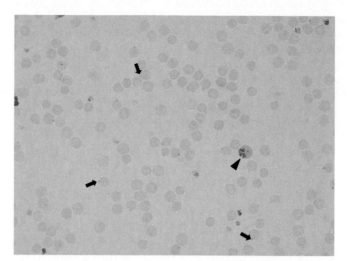

Fig. 1. Peripheral blood smear from a cat with high-grade gastric lymphoma (new methylene blue stain, original magnification ×100). Heinz bodies (*arrows*) are present on the surfaces of many erythrocytes. An aggregate reticulocyte (*arrowhead*) is also visible. The hematocrit was 26% (reference range 30% to 45%). Blood glucose concentration was 88 mg/dL (reference range 75 to 134) and total serum thyroxine concentration was 2.2 μg/dL (reference range 2.4 to 4.6). The cat had no history of exposure to oxidative toxins. Treatment with lomustine, L-asparaginase, and prednisone affected a complete remission of the lymphoma and the cat is alive 3 months later at the time of this report. The anemia resolved with remission of the cancer, although numerous Heinz bodies are persistently noted on blood smear evaluation.

lymphoma.[34] In another study of cats with Heinz body anemia, lymphoma was identified as a predisposing cause in 13 of 120 (10.8%) cats, and the association between lymphoma and Heinz body formation was statistically significant.[36] Lymphoma in these cats was identified as either gastrointestinal or multicentric in its anatomic distribution. The author has occasionally observed anemia in association with significant Heinz body formation in cats with gastrointestinal lymphoma (**Fig. 1**). An association between lymphoid malignancy and oxidative damage to erythrocytes has also been documented in humans.[37]

Tumor cell erythrophagocytosis is an uncommon cause of anemia in veterinary cancer patients. This type of anemia is most often identified in dogs with histiocytic sarcoma (**Fig. 2**), particularly of the hemophagocytic subtype.[38–40] Erythrophagocytosis is believed to be a primary cause for anemia in patients with this cancer, and the anemia is typically markedly regenerative. The mechanism for erythrophagocytosis by this tumor is uncertain, as dogs with hemophagocytic histiocytic sarcoma usually have negative direct antibody (Coomb's) test results.[38,40] Apart from histiocytic sarcoma, tumoral erythrophagocytosis is rarely observed in veterinary cancers. Erythrophagocytic behavior has been reported in association with canine and feline hepatosplenic lymphoma,[41,42] canine plasma cell tumors,[43,44] canine acute megakaryoblastic leukemia,[45] and feline mast cell tumors.[46–48] It is noteworthy that not all of the patients in these reports were anemic, and those that were sometimes had other explanations for their anemia, such as bone marrow infiltration by neoplastic cells. Therefore, the importance of erythrophagocytosis as a cause for anemia in patients with tumors other than histiocytic sarcoma is uncertain.

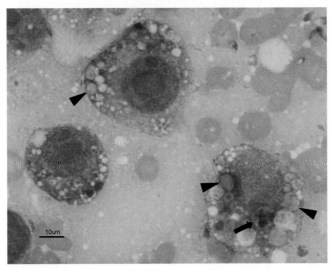

Fig. 2. Fine needle aspirate of a subcutaneous mass from a Golden retriever with dissemi-nated histiocytic sarcoma (Wright's stain, original magnification ×100). The neoplastic histiocytic cells contain numerous phagocytosed erythrocytes (*arrowheads*) in various stages degradation within phagolysosomes. A phagocytosed neutrophil (*arrow*) is also seen within the neoplastic cell at the bottom right of the image. Erythrophagocytosis is a common cause of anemia in dogs with disseminated histiocytic sarcoma.

Finally, nonregenerative anemias caused by decreased bone marrow production of erythrocytes must be considered. Indeed, hypoproliferative anemias are likely the most common anemias encountered in the veterinary cancer patient, and they may result from direct or indirect effects of cancer upon erythropoiesis. Cancers may directly inhibit bone marrow function by replacement of hematopoietic tissue with neoplastic tissue, a condition referred to as myelophthisis. Myelophthisis occurs with greatest frequency in patients with hematopoietic malignancies which originate in or readily metastasize to the bone marrow, such as acute leukemias,[49–51] lymphomas,[52] multiple myeloma,[53] mast cell tumor,[54] and disseminated histiocytic sarcoma.[38,55] Metastasis of solid tumors to bone marrow is well-documented in humans but is only rarely reported in small animal cancer patients.[56–58]

Indirect inhibition of bone marrow function may result from nutritional deficits of iron, folate, and vitamin B_{12} (cobalamin). Such deficiencies are frequently identified in anemic human cancer patients,[1,59,60] and their recognition is of great clinical importance as they may suggest a medical problem that requires attention (eg, chronic gastrointestinal hemorrhage causing iron deficiency anemia) or an anemia that may be correctable with nutritional supplementation. Nutritional deficiencies are infrequently reported to cause anemia in small animal cancer patients, although decreased serum levels of folate and cobalamin have been reported in cats with lymphomas, particularly lymphomas of the gastrointestinal tract.[61–63] To date, no studies have thoroughly evaluated whether supplementing these nutrients improves anemia or other clinical, hematologic, or biochemical parameters in these cats. Erythropoiesis may also be indirectly inhibited by myelosuppressive hormones elaborated by a tumor; estrogen produced by Sertoli cell tumors (and rarely interstitial cell tumors or seminomas) of the testis and granulosa cell tumors of the ovary may induce severe bone marrow hypoplasia and aplastic anemia.[64,65]

Perhaps the most important cause of nonregenerative anemia in cancer patients is the anemia of inflammatory disease (AID), also referred to as anemia of chronic disease. The prevalence of AID in human cancer patients is reportedly as high as 77%,[66] and some authors assert that it is a nearly universal feature of advanced cancer.[67] It is likely that AID is similarly prevalent in veterinary cancer patients.[12] AID is typically normocytic and normochromic and occurs in the face of normal bone marrow cellularity. It is characterized by inadequate production of erythropoietin (EPO), decreased response of erythroid progenitor cells in the marrow to EPO, shortened red blood cell survival time in circulation, and perturbations of iron storage and metabolism. The pathophysiology of AID is complex— in cancer patients, this disease is driven by inflammatory cytokines, including tumor necrosis factor (TNF)- α, interferon (IFN)-γ, interleukin (IL)-1β, IL-6, and IL-10, produced by leukocytes in response to the presence of a tumor.[8,66,68] A crucial downstream effector of these cytokines is hepcidin, a protein produced by the liver under the influence of IL-6. Hepcidin induces the internalization and lysosomal degradation of ferroportin, a membrane-bound protein whose function is to export iron from macrophages, hepatocytes, and duodenal enterocytes into the peripheral blood.[66,68] Hepcidin also reduces the expression of the divalent metal transporter-1 (DMT1) protein on the apical surface of duodenal enterocytes, reducing intestinal uptake of dietary iron.[68] These collaborative actions of hepcidin and inflammatory cytokines facilitate iron sequestration within reticuloendothelial cells and hepatocytes, resulting in hypoferremia and decreased availability of iron for erythropoiesis.

Anemia is a significant problem in clinical oncology. It contributes to fatigue, poor performance status, and diminished quality of life in human cancer patients. Moreover, anemia is frequently associated with poor treatment outcome and shortened survival times. A large meta-analysis showed that the relative risk of death was increased by 65% in anemic patients relative to nonanemic controls with a variety of cancer types.[69] The reasons for this phenomenon are unclear; one hypothesized mechanism is that anemia produces or exacerbates intratumoral hypoxia.[8,60] Cancer therapies that induce cytotoxicity through the generation of oxygen free radicals, such as radiation therapy, doxorubicin, and bleomycin, are less effective in the setting of hypoxia.[70] Hypoxia slows the progression of cancer cells through the cell cycle, further contributing to resistance to chemotherapy and radiotherapy, which are most active against rapidly dividing cells. Hypoxia also prevents the degradation of the HIF-1α transcription factor protein, allowing for the upregulation of several genes associated with cancer progression, angiogenesis, and metastasis.[8,60,70]

Although anemia is highly prevalent and of serious concern in human cancer patients, the optimal treatment of cancer-associated anemia has not been defined. Therapeutic options for anemia include iron supplementation, blood transfusion, and erythropoiesis stimulating agents (ESAs). The most commonly used ESAs are the recombinant human erythropoietins epoetin alfa (Epogen; Procrit) and darbepoetin alfa (Aranesp).[71] ESAs reduce transfusion requirements in anemic cancer patients,[1,2,8] and may also improve quality of life in patients with symptomatic anemia. Parenteral iron supplementation may enhance the bone marrow response to ESAs.[10] ESA use in cancer patients is controversial, and has been associated with thromboembolic events, development of antibodies to the ESA, increased risk of tumor progression, and shortened survival times.[8,71] ESAs are only labeled for the treatment of chemotherapy-related anemia, and their benefit in the treatment of AID and other cancer-associated anemias is unproven. The American Society of Clinical Oncology and American Society of Hematology recommend that ESAs be given at the lowest dose possible so as to achieve the lowest blood hemoglobin concentration (in many cases, approximately 10 g/dL) that allows avoidance of transfusion.[71] Further study is required to determine how best to manage anemia in human cancer patients.

The incidence, prevalence, clinical relevance, and optimal therapy of anemia in veterinary cancer patients are largely undefined. Although the frequency of anemia at the time of diagnosis is reported for several tumor types (see **Table 1**), large-scale studies describing the incidence, prevalence, and etiologies of anemia in dogs and cats with all cancer types have not been published. Furthermore, the effect of anemia on treatment outcome or prognosis for dogs and cats with cancer has not been examined across tumor types. Recent studies have identified anemia as an independent negative predictor of survival in dogs treated for lymphoma[72,73] and cats treated for nasal lymphoma[74] and soft tissue sarcoma.[75] Given the significance of anemia in human oncology, more thorough investigation of the epidemiology, pathogenesis, prognostic relevance, and treatment of anemia in canine and feline cancer patients is warranted.

Thrombocytopenia

Thrombocytopenia is frequently noted in veterinary cancer patients. Up to 36% of untreated canine cancer patients present with thrombocytopenia[76] and 39% of thrombocytopenic cats are diagnosed with underlying neoplasia.[77] Thrombocytopenia is especially common in dogs and cats with hematopoietic and vascular tumors.[32,76-78] The reported frequencies of thrombocytopenia associated with several small animal tumors at the time of diagnosis are listed in **Table 2**. The mechanisms underlying cancer-associated thrombocytopenia include decreased platelet production, increased platelet sequestration, increased platelet destruction, and increased platelet consumption or utilization.

Decreased production of platelets by the bone marrow is often associated with myelophthisis from hematologic malignancies such as lymphomas, acute leukemias, multiple myeloma, and disseminated histiocytic sarcoma. Acute megakaryoblastic

Table 2		
Frequency of thrombocytopenia at the time of diagnosis of various small animal tumors		
Tumor Type	**Frequency of Thrombocytopenia (%)**	**References**
Lymphoma (canine)	22–49	52,217,219,220
Lymphoma (feline)	10–18	222,223
Acute leukemia (canine)	46–90	91,225
Acute leukemia (feline)	92–100	51,164
Chronic lymphocytic leukemia (canine)	15–45	91,140
Multiple myeloma (canine)	33	191
Multiple myeloma (feline)	50	226
Histiocytic sarcoma (canine)		
Localized	0–22	227,229
Disseminated	56–88	38,230
Mast cell tumor (canine)		
Localized	9	147
Systemic	20–36	54,233
Hemangiosarcoma (canine)	25–75	33,234–237
Hemangiosarcoma (feline)	25–33	238,239

leukemia, a neoplastic proliferation of platelet precursors in the bone marrow, may be associated with thrombocytosis, but more commonly produces thrombocytopenia, which is often severe.[45,79,80] Thrombocytopenia resulting from decreased platelet production may also accompany estrogen-secreting testicular or ovarian tumors; the megakaryocytic lineage appears to be particularly susceptible to estrogen-induced aplasia.[64,65,79]

Thrombocytopenia secondary to increased platelet sequestration is a feature of splenic and hepatic malignancies, particularly those characterized by diffuse organomegaly. Approximately one third of the body's platelets are stored in the spleen, and any pathologic process resulting in splenomegaly will increase splenic blood pooling and enhance platelet sequestration.[79] Diffuse hepatosplenomegaly and consequent platelet sequestration may be seen in splenic or multicentric lymphomas and feline mast cell tumors.[79,81] Platelet sequestration may also occur in highly vascularized neoplasms, such as hemangioma and hemangiosarcoma, of the spleen, liver, and other anatomic sites.[79,81]

Increased platelet destruction may be immune-mediated or non–immune-mediated in nature. Cancer-associated immune-mediated thrombocytopenia (ITP), like IMHA, is most often associated with hematological malignancies in both humans and small animals. Chronic lymphocytic leukemia (CLL) and B-cell non-Hodgkin's lymphoma are cancers commonly associated with ITP in humans.[67] In dogs, ITP has been identified in association with lymphoma, multiple myeloma, and histiocytic sarcoma.[4,82,83] Although less frequent, ITP may also occur in patients with solid tumors.[84] Non–immune-mediated destruction of platelets most frequently occurs secondary to microangiopathy in cancer patients.[79,81]

Increased consumption or utilization of platelets is the final, and perhaps most significant, mechanism underlying cancer-related thrombocytopenia. Increased utilization of platelets occurs in patients with chronic low-grade hemorrhage, but should not result in thrombocytopenia until the regenerative capacity of the bone marrow has been exhausted.[79] Significant thrombocytopenia may also accompany acute, severe hemorrhage, such as that which occurs in patients with ruptured splenic tumors. However, thrombocytopenia associated with acute blood loss is self-limiting, and should resolve shortly after hemorrhage ceases.[85] In most cases, increased platelet consumption likely results from the hypercoagulable state that is extremely common in cancer patients.[86] Hypercoagulability may result in clinical thromboembolic disease in some patients, but in other cases it may manifest in more subtle ways. For instance, patients with chronic, compensated DIC may present with only mild thrombocytopenia, while lacking other clinical or clinicopathologic evidence of coagulopathy.[87] Experimental evidence supports the contention that chronic platelet consumption occurs in veterinary cancer patients. Platelet counts and kinetics in circulation were studied in a series of 52 tumor-bearing and 34 normal dogs.[88] Tumor-bearing dogs had significantly lower platelet counts than normal dogs, although moderate to severe thrombocytopenia was primarily seen in dogs with splenic or bone marrow disease. The mean survival time of circulating radiolabeled platelets in tumor-bearing dogs (3.5 days) was significantly shorter than that of normal control dogs (5.4 days).[88] Moreover, platelet survival time decreased in proportion to stage of disease—the mean platelet survival time for dogs with metastatic tumors (3.2 days) was significantly shorter than that for dogs with localized tumors (4.4 days).[88] Slichter and colleagues[89] report similar reductions in platelet survival in human cancer patients: platelet survival times in 77 patients with untreated malignancies averaged 2 to 4 days, depending upon type and stage of malignancy, while the mean platelet survival time in normal control patients was 9.5 days. Platelet survival was shortest (approximately 1 day) in patients with terminal cancer who died within two weeks of study enrollment. Interestingly, patients whose tumors showed a measurable response to therapy experienced corresponding increases in platelet survival.[89] These experimental observations suggest that a low-grade consumptive coagulopathy (ie, compensated DIC) is common, if not ubiquitous, in cancer patients, and the severity of this process is proportional to the stage of the cancer. Chronic, compensated DIC may therefore be the most common cause for thrombocytopenia in veterinary cancer patients.

It should be noted that thrombocytopenia occurs without an obvious underlying etiology in some cancer patients.[78,88] In a series of 214 thrombocytopenic dogs with cancer, 61% (130 of 214) had no identifiable explanation for their thrombocytopenia.[78] However, few dogs in this series were tested for antiplatelet antibodies, and thus ITP may have been underdiagnosed. Moreover, accelerated platelet consumption due to a hypercoagulable state was also likely underdiagnosed in this study, since platelet consumption has been historically challenging to diagnose without cumbersome tests such as radiolabeling studies, as described above. The increasing availability of global tests of coagulation, such as thromboelastography, may facilitate the diagnosis of hypercoagulability and help to identify the etiology of unexplained thrombocytopenia in canine and feline cancer patients. Further discussion of the hypercoagulable state and cancer follows later in this review.

Leukopenia

In the cancer patient, leukopenia is most often characterized by neutropenia.[4] Myelosuppressive cancer therapy (ie, chemotherapy and radiotherapy) is by far the most common cause of neutropenia in small animal oncology patients.[4] True cancer-associated neutropenia is less common, and usually is due to myelophthisis caused by hematopoietic malignancies.[49,51,53,90,91] Neutropenia is common in cats infected with FeLV or cats with late-stage feline immunodeficiency virus (FIV) infection, and in both cases neutropenia is often accompanied by other peripheral cytopenias.[27,28] Immune-mediated neutropenia may also occur in cancer patients. One report describes four dogs and three cats with untreated solid tumors and neutropenia of unknown origin.[4] No evidence of myelophthisis was apparent in any animal, and serologic testing for FeLV in all three cats was negative. Remission of the primary tumor resulted in resolution of the neutropenia in all seven animals. This clinical presentation suggests an immune-mediated origin of the neutropenia in these seven animals, although such cases are likely to be rare.

Bicytopenia and Pancytopenia

Bicytopenia is a reduction in the number of cells from two lineages in the blood while pancytopenia is a reduction the number of cells of all lineages. Multilineage cytopenias often result from decreased production of normal cells or increased production of abnormal cells in the bone marrow; thus, bone marrow evaluation is indicated in all cases of bi- or pancytopenia, especially if the cause of the cytopenias is not readily apparent.

Cytopenias in multiple cell lineages often indicate myelophthistic disease in the veterinary cancer patient. Bi- and pancytopenia occur frequently in patients with hematologic cancers, particularly acute leukemias.[49,51,90,91] Pancytopenia is also reported in dogs with lymphomas, myelodysplastic syndrome (MDS), multiple myeloma, and disseminated histiocytic sarcoma.[91,92] However, veterinarians treating cancer patients should be aware of etiologies other than myelophthisis for multilineage cytopenias. In a review of 51 pancytopenic dogs, by far the most common underlying etiology was chemotherapy administration (22 of 51; 43%).[92] Estrogen-induced bone marrow injury may cause pancytopenia in dogs with Sertoli cell tumors of the testis and granulosa cell tumors of the ovary.[64,65,92]

ABNORMAL INCREASES IN CIRCULATING BLOOD CELL CONCENTRATIONS
Erythrocytosis

Erythrocytosis is uncommon in veterinary cancer patients. When present, cancer-related erythrocytosis may be due to a primary myeloproliferative disease (ie, polycythemia vera) or may be a paraneoplastic syndrome. Paraneoplastic erythrocytosis is most often reported in dogs and cats with renal tumors.[93–101] Erythrocytosis associated with renal neoplasia is often attributed to increased serum EPO concentrations, and in some cases,[94,97] tumoral production of EPO has been documented. However, normal kidney tissue adjacent to a renal tumor may be induced to aberrantly produce EPO as it becomes compressed and hypoxic; this was recently demonstrated using immunohistochemistry in a dog with renal T-cell lymphoma.[97] Paraneoplastic erythrocytosis has also been reported in dogs with transmissible venereal tumor,[102] nasal fibrosarcoma,[103] and cecal leiomyosarcoma,[104] with ectopic tumoral production of EPO confirmed in the latter two cases.

Polycythemia vera (PV; also known as primary erythrocytosis) is a rare myeloproliferative disease (MPD) that causes erythrocytosis in dogs and cats.[105–107] It is characterized by a clonal proliferation of erythroid progenitor cells in the bone marrow, independent of serum EPO concentrations. PV is a diagnosis of exclusion, and distinguishing it from other causes of erythrocytosis is challenging. Patients with PV typically have marked increases in hematocrit (usually >65%), erythrocyte count, and hemoglobin concentration, in the face of normal arterial oxygen saturation.[105] Splenomegaly may also be present, although this is not as common in dogs and cats as it is in humans with PV.[105] Bone marrow is often hypercellular in patients with PV; however, the cellularity may also be normal, and bone marrow evaluation does not reliably differentiate PV from other causes of erythrocytosis. Measurement of serum EPO concentrations is the most reliable method for diagnosing PV in patients with erythrocytosis.[105,108] EPO concentrations should be low to undetectable in patients with PV, whereas they will be increased in patients with erythrocytosis of nearly all other etiologies.

Because erythrocytosis is uncommonly associated with canine and feline cancers, its identification should prompt a search for other underlying causes. Erythrocytosis may be either relative or absolute. Relative erythrocytosis is caused by a decrease in plasma volume and subsequent hemoconcentration, such as would occur in a dehydrated patient.[108] Transient relative erythrocytosis can also be produced by splenic contraction. Absolute erythrocytosis refers to an increase in a patient's total red blood cell mass. Absolute erythrocytosis may be further characterized as primary or secondary. Primary erythrocytosis is synonymous with polycythemia vera, and has already been discussed. Secondary erythrocytosis is associated with increased production of EPO, which in turn may be appropriate or inappropriate.[108] An appropriate increase in EPO production occurs in response to hypoxemia and is seen in patients that have adapted to high-altitude environments or patients with chronic pulmonary disease, cyanotic heart disease, or hemoglobinopathies. Inappropriate EPO production occurs irrespective of tissue hypoxia, and is associated primarily with renal (and rarely extrarenal) neoplasia, as well as non-neoplastic renal disease.[108,109]

Thrombocytosis

Although thrombocytosis occurs in up to 60% of human cancer patients,[110] it is infrequently documented in association with cancer in the veterinary literature.[101,111–113] However it is possible that the true incidence of thrombocytosis in veterinary cancer patients is underrecognized or underreported. In one retrospective study of dogs and cats with thrombocytosis, neoplasia was the most commonly diagnosed concurrent disease.[111]

The etiology of thrombocytosis in dogs and cats may be classified as physiologic, reactive, or neoplastic.[112,114] Physiologic thrombocytosis results from splenic contraction under the influence of epinephrine. Thrombocytosis secondary to splenic contraction is typically transient, lasting only 15 to 30 minutes.[112] Physiologic thrombocytosis also occurs in splenectomized patients, since the lack of a spleen eliminates a normal site for sequestration of circulating platelets. Thrombocytosis following splenectomy may be transient or persistent.

Reactive thrombocytosis occurs in response to inflammatory cytokines or hematopoietic growth factors. Cytokines known to stimulate thrombopoiesis include IL-1α IL-3, IL-6, and IL-9.[114] Thrombopoietin (TPO), produced by the liver and kidney, is the primary thrombopoietic growth factor, although stromal cell-derived factor-1 (SDF-1), stem cell factor, granulocyte-macrophage colony-stimulating factor (GM-CSF), and EPO often act in concert with TPO to stimulate thrombopoiesis.[114] Reactive thrombocytosis also occurs in response to iron deficiency and hyperadrenocorticism, although the mechanisms underlying the association between these diseases and thrombocytosis are unclear.[114]

Both physiologic and reactive thrombocytosis may occur in patients with cancer. Anemic cancer patients with thrombocytosis should be screened for microcytosis and hypochromasia, which may suggest iron deficiency.[21,115] Thrombocytosis is commonly seen in patients with chronic MPDs, and may result from alterations in the cytokine milieu in the bone marrow microenvironment. Apparent paraneoplastic thrombocytosis has been documented in dogs and cats with a variety of tumors, including lymphomas, malignant melanoma, nasal adenocarcinoma, primary central nervous system tumors, mast cell tumor, mesothelioma, spinal osteosarcoma, primary lung carcinoma, thymoma, intestinal plasma cell tumor, and renal adenocarcinoma.[101,111–113,115] Thrombocytosis was noted in 18 (46%) of 39 dogs with massive hepatocellular carcinoma in one study.[116] It is likely that many of these cases of "paraneoplastic" thrombocytosis are simply examples of reactive thrombocytosis in response to the underlying inflammation induced by a neoplasm, although thrombocytosis due to possible EPO-producing renal tumors was reported in two cats.[101]

True neoplastic thrombocytosis occurs in essential thrombocythemia (ET), a chronic MPD characterized by persistent thrombocytosis (by definition $\geq$600,000/μL, and often >1,000,000/μL) and clonal proliferation of megakaryocytes in the bone marrow.[114] Humans with ET often present with spontaneous hemorrhage or thrombosis, but these clinical signs are uncommon in dogs and cats with the disease.[117] Diagnosis of ET is made by excluding other causes of reactive or physiologic thrombocytosis, and by careful assessment of peripheral blood smears and bone marrow cytology and histopathology samples. In particular, acute megakaryoblastic leukemia[80] and other chronic MPDs,[118–121] which all may present with thrombocytosis, must be excluded by bone marrow examination. Only a few dogs and cats with ET are reported in the veterinary literature[122–126]; therefore, more common causes of thrombocytosis should be given higher consideration in animals presenting with this hematologic abnormality.

Leukocytosis

Leukocytosis attributable to absolute increases in the numbers of any of the leukocyte subsets (granulocytes, lymphocytes, monocytes) in the blood may occur in cancer patients. However, in most cases, leukocytosis in canine and feline cancer patients can be attributed to the etiologies for leukocytosis in any patient[4]; neutrophilic leukocytosis may be attributable to acute or chronic inflammation or tissue necrosis associated with cancer, or may be attributable to stress; lymphocytosis may occur with chronic inflammation or from excitement and epinephrine release; monocytosis may occur with chronic inflammation, tumoral or tissue necrosis, or stress; and eosinophilia or basophilia may be secondary to allergic or parasitic diseases. In general, these pathophysiologic processes should be given primary consideration in any cancer patient with leukocytosis. However, certain types of leukocytosis, which are often paraneoplastic in nature, may be a hallmark of specific malignancies, thereby assisting in timely diagnosis or in assessment of cancer remission status. In other cases, leukocytosis may be of prognostic relevance. These specific examples of cancer-related leukocytosis will be discussed in further detail.

Paraneoplastic neutrophilic leukocytosis is reported in association with adenomatous rectal polyps, renal tumors, pulmonary carcinoma, intestinal T-cell lymphoma, and metastatic fibrosarcoma in dogs,[115,127–132] and in pulmonary squamous cell carcinoma and dermal tubular adenocarcinoma in cats.[131,133] Circulating neutrophil counts in these animals were extremely high (range 74,347 to 202,522 cells/μL), and the neutrophilia was often accompanied by a left shift, monocytosis, and eosinophilia. Neutrophilic leukocytosis of this magnitude is often referred to as a leukemoid response because it may be challenging to distinguish from chronic myelogenous leukemia (CML). CML is sometimes characterized by a disorderly left shift and the presence of granulocytes having abnormal morphology in the bone marrow. While cytochemical staining may assist in the differentiation of CML from a leukemoid response, in human patients, a distinction between neoplastic versus reactive neutrophilic leukocytosis has not been shown using this procedure.[134] Leukemoid responses are defined by extreme neutrophilic leukocytosis (neutrophils $\geq$50,000 to 100,000 cells/μL), usually with a pronounced, but orderly, left shift. They may occur in patients with chronic localized infections (eg, pyometra), *Hepatozoon canis* infection, IMHA, and CD11/CD18 neutrophil protein adhesion deficiency, as well as cancer patients.[135] Paraneoplastic leukemoid responses are usually attributed to ectopic production of GM-CSF or granulocyte colony-stimulating factor (G-CSF) by a tumor, and tumoral production of these cytokines has been documented in small animal cancer patients.[131,132] GM-CSF stimulates the proliferation of hematopoietic precursors for the neutrophil, monocyte, and eosinophil lineages,[136] and this may explain the monocytosis and eosinophilia that can accompany neutrophilic leukocytosis in a leukemoid response. The clinical significance of paraneoplastic leukemoid responses is debatable; some sources claim that they are of little importance, and in many cases a leukemoid response will resolve with appropriate therapy for the underlying cancer. However, two reports[137,138] show extreme neutrophilic leukocytosis of any etiology to be associated with a high mortality rate. In these two reports, patients with neoplasia were at increased risk of death compared to patients with other diseases.

In addition to neutrophils, increased numbers of lymphocytes, monocytes, eosinophils, and basophils may characterize the leukocytosis seen in cancer patients.

Lymphocytosis occurs primarily in patients with lymphoid malignancies such as lymphomas, acute lymphoblastic leukemia (ALL), and CLL.[49,50,52,139–142] Indeed, neoplasia is the most common cause of persistent lymphocytosis in dogs and cats.[143] High-grade lymphomas with circulating lymphocytosis (ie, stage V lymphoma) and ALL are both characterized by large or intermediate size, immature lymphoblasts in circulation, whereas the lymphocytosis in low-grade lymphomas or CLL is characterized by small, mature lymphocytes.[143] The degree of lymphocytosis in patients with CLL may be considerable (**Fig. 3**), although this disease is often identified incidentally in patients with minimal to no clinical signs. Benign, paraneoplastic lymphocytosis may be observed in dogs and cats with thymomas.[142,143]

Monocytosis is uncommonly documented in small animal cancer patients, but may occur in patients with MPDs, particularly those of a monocytic lineage.[144–146] Monocytosis may also be observed in patients with leukemoid responses, as previously noted.

Eosinophilia is also uncommon in veterinary cancer patients and is most often noted in dogs and cats with mast cell tumors[147–150] and lymphomas,[116,151–154] particularly T-cell lymphomas. Mast cells produce the eosinophilopoietic cytokine IL-5 as well as eosinophil chemotactic factors,[155] and these likely are responsible for the eosinophilia seen in patients with mast cell tumors. In humans, the production of IL-5 by T-cell lymphomas has been documented,[116,151,152] and it is hypothesized that this occurs in small animal T-cell lymphomas as well. Paraneoplastic eosinophilia is rare in patients with solid tumors, but has been documented in dogs with oral fibrosarcoma,[156] and mammary carcinoma,[157] and in cats with oral squamous cell carcinoma[4] and transitional cell carcinoma.[158] Eosinophilic leukemia is a rare chronic MPD characterized by marked peripheral eosinophilia and eosinophil infiltrates in bone marrow and visceral organs.[159–161] The presence of immature eosinophil precursors in circulation and in tissues helps to distinguish this cancer from benign idiopathic hypereosinophilic syndrome. Eosinophilia, like monocytosis, may be seen in patients with leukemoid responses.

Basophilia is very rarely encountered in veterinary oncology patients. When noted, it usually occurs in dogs and cats with mast cell tumors.[147,148,150] Basophilia is also occasionally reported in association with chronic MPDs.[123,124] Rare cases of basophilic leukemia, a chronic MPD characterized by marked basophilia, are reported in dogs and cats.[120,121,162–164]

Abnormal Cells in Circulation

In addition to perturbations in the circulating numbers of normal blood cells, the hemogram of the veterinary cancer patient may occasionally be characterized by the presence of cells that do not circulate under normal physiologic conditions. This is most apparent, and often striking, in dogs and cats with acute leukemias, MPDs, and MDS.[49–51,90,119] These diseases are characterized by abnormal proliferation of immature hematopoietic precursor cells in the bone marrow, with subsequent release of these cells into circulation. Other hematopoietic neoplasms affecting the bone marrow, such as lymphoma[52,141] and, rarely, multiple myeloma[53] and histiocytic sarcoma[165] may also present with a leukemic blood profile.

Mast cells may occasionally be seen in the circulation of dogs and cats with mast cell tumors,[46,48,148] particularly those with visceral or bone marrow metastasis. In health, mast cells are only found in solid organs, and are most numerous in the mucosae of the respiratory and gastrointestinal tracts, where they function as mediators of the innate immune response.[156] The appearance of mast cells in the peripheral blood is always pathologic.[166] However, circulating mastocythemia is not

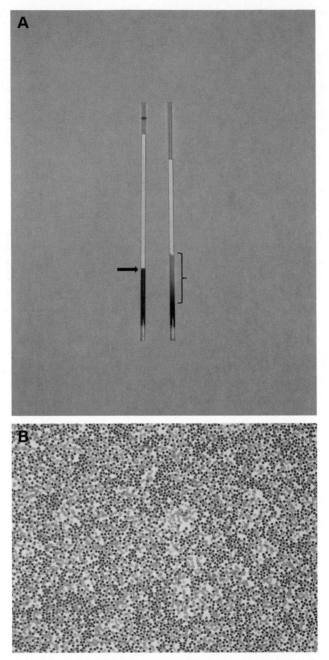

Fig. 3. (*A*) Spun microhematocrit tubes from a dog with chronic lymphocytic leukemia (*right*) and from a normal dog (*left*). Note the marked discrepancy in the size of the buffy coat of the affected dog (*bracket*) compared to that of the normal dog (*arrow*). (*B*) Peripheral blood smear from the same dog (Wright's stain, original magnification ×20). The peripheral lymphocyte count was 930,000/μL. Remarkably, the dog had relatively few clinical signs apart from mild lethargy and inappetance at the time of diagnosis. A partial remission was achieved with chlorambucil and prednisone chemotherapy, but the dog died of acute renal failure 2 months after diagnosis.

specific for mast cell neoplasia, and may occur in patients with acute inflammatory diseases, trauma, regenerative anemia, inflammatory skin disease, and non–mast cell neoplasia.[167–169] These conditions should be ruled out in a patient with circulating mastocythemia without an apparent mast cell tumor. Moreover, patients with mast cell tumor and circulating mastocythemia should be carefully staged for the presence of visceral or marrow metastasis.

Metarubricytosis, or the presence of nucleated red blood cells (nRBCs) in circulation, is occasionally noted in veterinary cancer patients. Under normal conditions, nRBCs are prevented from entering circulation by the sinusoidal and vascular endothelium of the bone marrow. In highly regenerative anemias, early release of nRBCs may occur in response to accelerated hematopoiesis (appropriate metarubricytosis).[170] Such cases are characterized by marked polychromasia and reticulocytosis. Metarubricytosis in the absence of anemia, or that is disproportionate to the degree of polychromasia/reticulocytosis present, is pathologic (inappropriate metarubricytosis) and is believed to be an indicator of injury to the sinusoidal or vascular endothelium of the bone marrow, allowing premature entrance of nRBCs into the peripheral blood.[170,171] Inappropriate metarubricytosis may therefore be noted in patients with primary or metastatic bone marrow malignancies, such as leukemias, lymphomas, and other hematopoietic neoplasms.[51,52,119] If the presence of nRBCs in blood extends to less mature erythroid precursors, including erythroblasts, the possibility of an acute erythroid leukemia should be considered. Metarubricytosis also occurs frequently in patients with hemangiosarcoma,[14,171,172] although the mechanism behind this is less clear. A regenerative response to tumor-associated hemorrhage is a plausible explanation, although metarubricytosis associated with hemangiosarcoma is often marked (>100 nRBCs/100 white blood cells), and may occur in patients with only mild anemia. Splenic disease may also cause metarubricytosis, as the spleen is responsible for clearing nRBCs inappropriately released into circulation[14]; however, metarubricytosis is documented in patients with hemangiosarcoma at extrasplenic locations.[171,173] Recent findings on the ontogeny of hemangiosarcoma may serve to elucidate the mechanism for metarubricytosis associated with this cancer. Hemangiosarcoma has long been known to express antigens consistent with endothelial cell differentiation (eg, CD31, factor VIII-related antigen).[174] Lamerato-Kozicki and colleagues[175] recently demonstrated that hemangiosarcoma also expresses antigens consistent with early hematopoietic differentiation (eg, CD34, CD45). This suggests the possibility of a bone marrow stem cell niche for this neoplasm, and the proliferation of neoplastic hemangiosarcoma cells in the bone marrow may explain the inappropriate metarubricytosis noted in some patients with this cancer. Gross and microscopic lesions of hemangiosarcoma in the bone marrow are identified at necropsy in some,[173] but not all,[171] affected dogs; however, it is doubtful that complete postmortem examination of the bone marrow occurred in all reported cases. The hematopoietic origin of this cancer is an intriguing hypothesis that merits further investigation.

COAGULOPATHIES IN CANCER PATIENTS

Disorders of coagulation are common in both veterinary and human cancer patients, and both hypocoagulable and hypercoagulable states may occur. In humans, thromboembolic disease associated with hypercoagulability is much more common than bleeding tendencies associated with hypocoagulability.[110,176] Limited data suggest a similar pattern in dogs and cats with cancer. In a group of 36 dogs with various tumors, 18 (50%) were found to be hypercoagulable (relative to normal control dogs) using tissue factor–activated thromboelastography (TEG).[177] In the same study, only 6 dogs (17%) were hypocoagulable. However, relatively few large-scale studies detailing the prevalence and types of hemostatic abnormalities in veterinary cancer patients are available. In both small animal and human patients, laboratory evidence of coagulopathy is extremely common, while frank hemorrhage or thromboembolic disease are seen much less frequently. In humans, laboratory evidence of altered hemostasis is present in up to 98% of patients with cancer,[178] although clinically apparent coagulopathies only occur in 15% to 30%.[110,176,178-180] In a report[76] describing 100 dogs with untreated tumors, 83% had one or more laboratory abnormalities consistent with altered hemostasis. Dogs with clinical evidence of bleeding were excluded from this report and, in general, dogs and cats with clinically apparent cancer-related coagulopathies are described only in case reports or small case series.[33,181-187] The pathogenesis and clinical syndromes associated with hypocoagulability and hypercoagulability are described in further detail later. DIC, which may be associated with either hypercoagulability or hypocoagulability, depending on its stage of evolution, shall be considered separately.

Hypocoagulability

Hypocoagulability and associated hemorrhagic diatheses may occur due to decreases in platelet numbers, alterations in platelet function, decreased concentrations or functional alterations of plasma clotting proteins, tumoral production of anticoagulant substances, alterations in plasma viscosity, or combinations of these.[181] The etiology and prevalence of cancer-associated thrombocytopenia have already been discussed. Thrombocytopathy associated with decreased platelet function is most commonly seen in association with paraproteinemia in small animal cancer patients. Paraproteinemia occurs in patients with multiple myeloma, Waldenstrom's macroglobulinemia, and lymphomas and leukemias of the B-cell lineage.[53,181] In these diseases, immunoglobulins or immunoglobulin fragments elaborated by tumor cells coat platelets and decrease their adhesiveness to vascular walls. Immunoglobulin (Ig) A and IgM paraproteinemias are particularly associated with this type of thrombocytopathy.[181] Platelet dysfunction may occur in patients with MPDs such as polycythemia vera and essential thrombocythemia.[110,122] Acquired von Willebrand's disease is an important cause of thrombocytopathy in human cancer patients, particularly those with lymphoid malignancy[110,181]; however, this disorder has not been documented in veterinary cancer patients.

Numerous qualitative and quantitative alterations in plasma clotting proteins are described in human cancer patients. These include acquired hemophilia A (associated with autoantibodies to factor VIII), isolated clotting factor deficiencies, and production of abnormal or dysfunctional clotting factors.[110] Vitamin K deficiency also occurs with some frequency in humans cancer patients due to malnutrition, diarrhea, hepatic metastasis or dysfunction, hepatobiliary obstruction, prolonged antibiotic use (which depopulates vitamin K–producing enteric bacteria), and oral anticoagulant therapy.[110,181] The most common cause of clotting factor dysfunction in veterinary oncology is likely the production of heparin by mast cell tumors.[181,188] Heparin functions as a cofactor for antithrombin, and the combined activity of these molecules inactivates factor X, preventing the conversion of prothrombin to thrombin.[189] Prolonged bleeding may be encountered following fine needle aspirate, biopsy, or surgical excision of mast cell tumors. Spontaneous hemorrhage may also be observed in some patients (**Fig. 4**). Only sporadic reports of other clotting factor deficiencies or dysfunction in veterinary cancer patients exist. Prekallikrein deficiency was documented in a dog with renal transitional cell carcinoma[183] and factor V

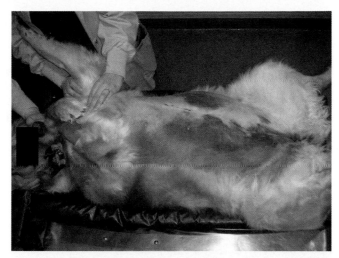

Fig. 4. Massive subcutaneous hemorrhage in a golden retriever with a large, recurrent, subcutaneous, high-grade mast cell tumor of the right thoracic wall (not readily apparent in the photograph). The surgical scar corresponding to the site of the original tumor is apparent on the ventral midline. Spontaneous hemorrhage may have resulted from heparin release by the neoplastic mast cells.

deficiency was reported in a dog with nasal adenocarcinoma,[184] although this dog was suspected to have underlying acute DIC.

Hemorrhagic diathesis may also be a consequence of increased blood viscosity. Significant increases in viscosity alter the rheologic properties of blood, leading to sludging in the microvasculature. This in turn causes overdistention and rupture of capillaries, resulting in hemorrhage.[181,190] Hyperviscosity may also result in hemorrhage by preventing the conversion of fibrinogen to fibrin.[181] Hyperviscosity is most commonly seen in patients with extreme increases in plasma protein concentrations secondary to immunoglobulin-producing tumors.[53,190] Although dysproteinemias are the most often cited cause of hyperviscosity in veterinary cancer patients, it should be recognized that pathologic increases in the absolute numbers of any of the formed elements of the blood may also produce hyperviscosity and subsequent hemorrhage.[190] The hematocrit makes the greatest contribution to blood viscosity, and viscosity rises logarithmically with increases in hematocrit.[190] It is therefore understandable that extreme increases in hematocrit, as may be seen in paraneoplastic erythrocytosis and polycythemia vera,[106] are associated with microvascular hemorrhage. Due to the relative infrequency of leukocytes in the blood relative to erythrocytes, leukocytosis rarely results in hyperviscosity. However, extreme leukocytosis (>100,000 cells/μL), which may occur in patients with leukemias and leukemoid reactions, is associated with hyperviscosity in humans.[190]

Hypercoagulability

The association between malignancy and thrombosis has been recognized for nearly 150 years, since Armand Trousseau described a syndrome of migratory venous thromboembolism in patients with gastric carcinoma.[179] Thromboembolic disease is the second-leading cause of death in human cancer patients.[179] The incidence of clinically apparent venous thromboembolism in humans with cancer is 15%,[180,192]

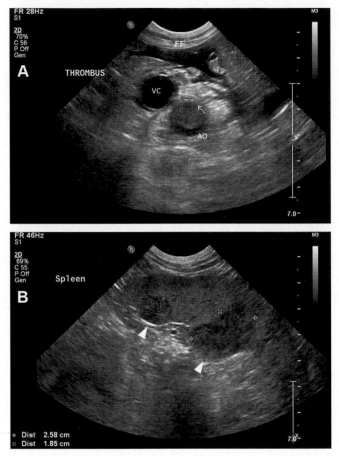

Fig. 5. Ultrasonographic images from a Labrador retriever presented for acute collapse and paraplegia. (*A*) Transverse images of the caudal abdomen show a large thrombus (*white arrow*) nearly completely occluding the lumen of the aorta (AO). The caudal vena cava (VC) is seen to the left of the aorta. A small amount of free fluid (FF) is seen at the top of the image. Fluid analysis was consistent with a modified transudate, which likely developed as a result of increased arterial hydrostatic pressure. (*B*) Multiple heteroechoic splenic masses (*arrowheads*) were also identified ultrasonographically. At necropsy a 4-cm thrombus was identified in the caudal abdominal aorta and extending into the external iliac arteries. The splenic masses were confirmed as hemangiosarcoma, and metastases were identified in the lungs, right atrium, and left kidney. Coagulopathies are extremely common in dogs with hemangiosarcoma, and up to 50% present with evidence of DIC.

and thrombosis is detectable in approximately one-half of cancer patients at autopsy.[176] The clinical manifestations of thromboembolic disease in human cancer patients include deep venous thrombosis (DVT), pulmonary thromboembolism (PE), migratory superficial thrombophlebitis (Trousseau's syndrome), nonbacterial thrombotic endocarditis, and DIC. Arterial thromboembolism also occurs in cancer patients (**Fig. 5**) but is less common than venous thrombosis. The incidence of thromboembolic disease in veterinary cancer patients is unknown; however, underlying neoplasia was identified in 3 (27%) of 11 dogs with portal vein thrombosis,[193] 43 (54%) of 80 dogs with splenic vein thrombosis,[194] and 14 (30%) of 47 dogs with PE[195] in three separate reports. Cancer therefore appears to be a major cause of thromboembolic disease in small animals, and it is reasonable to believe that thromboembolic disease may contribute significantly to morbidity and mortality in small animal cancer patients.

The pathogenesis of thromboembolism in cancer is complex and multifactorial, but may be generally conceptualized in the context of Virchow's classic triad of patho-logic conditions necessary for thrombus formation: (1) hemodynamic stasis or perturbations in blood flow, (2) vascular injury or dysfunction, and (3) hypercoagula-bility of the blood.[192,196] A major cause for hemodynamic derangement in cancer patients is the morphologic abnormality of tumor vasculature previously de-scribed.[32,33] Blood flow may be further perturbed by hyperviscosity or by tumoral invasion or compression of normal blood vessels. Vascular injury is most obviously manifested by direct tumoral invasion into vessels, but tumors may also mediate functional rather than structural vascular alterations. Inflammatory cytokines, such as IL-1 and TNF-α, elaborated by a tumor or by the host immune response to a tumor, cause endothelial cells to lose their natural antithrombotic properties, and become prothrombotic.[192] These cytokines upregulate endothelial cell production of von Willebrand's factor, platelet-activating factors, and tissue factor, while downregulat-ing the expression of thrombomodulin and the activation of protein C, thus favoring platelet adherence and fibrin deposition. Hypercoagulability in cancer patients occurs through structural and functional alterations in the cellular and soluble protein constituents of the blood. As previously discussed, platelet turnover is accelerated in cancer patients,[88] and this likely results in part from increased rates of platelet activation and aggregation.[86,192] Cancer cells and cancer cell extracts have been shown to cause direct platelet activation in vitro, and plasma concentrations of platelet activation biomarkers, such as P-selectin and β-thromboglobulin, are in-creased in cancer patients.[192] Cancer cells may also activate the coagulation cascade through the production of tissue factor or cancer procoagulant, a unique cancer-associated protein that directly activates factor X.[176]

Evidence of hypercoagulability in veterinary cancer patients is sparse. Shortening of the prothrombin time (PT) or activated partial thromboplastin time (aPTT), which may imply a hypercoagulable state, were documented in 43% of dogs with mammary carcinoma[197] and 14% of dogs with a variety of malignancies.[76] In vitro platelet aggregometry was used to assess platelet function in dogs with lymphoma[198] as well as dogs with various cancers.[199] In both studies, platelet aggregation in response to agonists (collagen, adenosine diphosphate, or platelet-activating factor) was signifi-cantly greater in dogs with neoplasia than in healthy control dogs. TEG, which provides a global functional assessment of the cellular and plasma protein compo-nents of hemostasis, may be a more sensitive method for detection of hypercoagu-lability than other currently available tests. Fifty percent (18 of 36) of dogs with untreated neoplasia were shown to be hypercoagulable using TEG.[177] TEG also documented hypercoagulability in a similar proportion (9 of 16; 56%) of dogs with untreated lymphoma.[200] The latter two studies suggest that hypercoagulability may be quite common in small animal cancer patients, although the clinical implications of this are unknown.

For many years, thrombosis was considered primarily an epiphenomenon associ-ated with cancer but not causally associated with oncogenesis. Recent experimental data suggest that this paradigm requires revision, and that activation of coagulation may be an intrinsic and necessary step in cancer progression. Fibrin deposition around emerging neoplastic foci forms a provisional extracellular matrix, and is hypothesized to be a critical early event in tumor progression.[176,201] This fibrin matrix provides a scaffold upon which angiogenesis may proceed, and also serves to recruit and trap macrophages and other leukocytes. Inflammatory cytokines produced by these immune effector cells amplify the activation of coagulation in the tumor microenvironment, driving continued tumor progression in a vicious cycle. Boccaccio and colleagues[201] provided evidence linking coagulation and early events in oncogenesis using a mouse model in which an activated MET oncogene was targeted to the liver. The development of grossly apparent liver tumors in these mice was preceded by a profound thrombohemorrhagic syndrome, suggesting that widespread activation of coagulation is an early event in MET-induced oncogenesis. Gene microarray analysis showed that MET activation was associated with upregulation of plasminogen activator inhibitor type-1 (PAI-1) and cyclooxygenase 2 (COX-2), two genes associated with inflammation and thrombogenesis. Compellingly, treatment of these mice with inhibitors of PAI-1 (XR5118) or COX-2 (rofecoxib) prolonged survival, prevented the emergence of a coagulopathy, and in some cases elicited tumor regression.[201] Activation of the coagulation cascade may also facilitate the metastatic process. The formation of fibrin–platelet–tumor cell complexes increases the adherence of circulating cancer cells to the endothelium, thereby enhancing metastatic efficiency.[176] Platelet coating may also serve to protect tumor cells from immunosurveillance. Amirkhosravi and colleagues[202] demonstrated the significance of coagulation in the trapping of circulating tumor cells by injecting MC28 fibrosarcoma cells into the tail vein of Lister rats. Subsequent electron microscopy demonstrated that tumor cells were deposited in complexes incorporating platelets and fibrin within the pulmonary capillaries. Anticoagulant therapy significantly abrogated this process.[201] Thus, a hypercoagulable state may promote cancer at many stages in its evolution. This would suggest a therapeutic role for anticoagulation, not solely for the prevention of cancer-associated thrombosis but also as a means of halting tumor progression. This is an active area of investigation in both animal models and human cancer patients.

Disseminated Intravascular Coagulation

DIC is a syndrome associated with excessive activation of the coagulation cascade, leading to widespread microthrombosis and multiorgan failure.[87] Although DIC is initially characterized by hypercoagulability and thrombosis (peracute DIC), eventual consumption of platelets and clotting factors leads to uncontrollable hemorrhage in the terminal stages of the disorder (acute DIC). Peracute and acute DIC may be preceded by a smoldering, asymptomatic form of the disorder (chronic DIC). Chronic DIC is common, if not ubiquitous, in patients with advanced or metastatic tumors,[87,176,192] and is a manifestation of the hypercoagulable state that commonly accompanies cancer.

The diagnosis of DIC is challenging, particularly so for the chronic form. Typically a constellation of clinical and clinicopathologic abnormalities must be present in order to make a confident diagnosis of DIC. Assessment of platelet count, red blood cell morphology (presence of schistocytes), PT, aPTT, plasma concentrations of fibrinogen, fibrin degradation products (FDPs) and D-dimers, as well as antithrombin (AT) activity is necessary to diagnose DIC.[87] Alterations in these clinicopathologic parameters, combined with characteristic clinical signs, often facilitates the diagnosis of acute or peracute DIC. On the contrary, patients with chronic DIC often have no clinical signs and may show only subtle alterations in laboratory tests of hemostasis, making the accurate diagnosis of this syndrome particularly vexing.[87,176] Global tests of hemostatic function, such as TEG,[203] may serve to better identify cancer patients with chronic DIC, but still require validation in a clinical setting. The reader is directed to Chapter 15 of this VCNA edition for a more detailed discussion of the laboratory diagnosis of DIC in dogs and cats.

DIC is diagnosed relatively frequently in small animal cancer patients, and indeed neoplasia is the most common cause of DIC in dogs.[204] One report estimated the incidence of DIC in dogs with neoplasia to be approximately 10%.[205] DIC is especially common in dogs with hemangiosarcoma, of which up to 50% may present with DIC on initial evaluation.[33,205] DIC is also associated with mammary gland carcinoma (particularly inflammatory mammary carcinoma)[205–207] and pulmonary adenocarcinoma[205] in dogs. It should be noted that the cited studies were designed primarily to detect the acute form of DIC, and thus the true incidence of DIC in these patients was likely underestimated.

DYSPROTEINEMIAS

Although perturbations in plasma protein concentrations are common in small animal cancer patients, the most diagnostically relevant of these is hyperglobulinemia. The identification hyperglobulinemia, particularly if marked or persistent, should prompt further characterization of the serum protein profile using electrophoresis. Serum protein electrophoresis separates the serum proteins into distinct groups based upon electrical charge and size. In dogs and cats, six protein groups, corresponding to albumin, and globulins of the α_1, α_2, β_1, β_2, and γ classes are separated using agarose gel electrophoresis.[208] The concentrations of serum proteins corresponding to these groups are plotted on an electrophoretogram. Hyperglobulinemia characterized by a broad-based peak in the α, β, or γ regions of the electrophoretogram is indicative of an increased concentration of globulins of multiple classes, and this is typically seen in patients with acute or chronic inflammatory diseases of numerous etiologies. On the contrary, hyperglobulinemia characterized by a tall, narrow peak is consistent with a monoclonal gammopathy, for which the list of possible etiologies is much shorter.[209]

Monoclonal gammopathies are pathologic increases in the concentrations of serum globulins produced by a single clone of B-lymphocytes or plasma cells. Monoclonal gammopathies may be characterized by increased concentrations of IgG, IgA, or IgM. Although monoclonal gammopathies are often characterized by spikes in the γ region of the electrophoretogram, clinicians should be aware that IgA and IgM may segregate in the β_2 region, and monoclonal gammopathies of these immunoglobulin classes would produce spikes in the β rather than the γ region.[208] In both dogs and cats, monoclonal gammopathies most often indicate the presence of a neoplasm the B-lymphocyte lineage. These include multiple myeloma, solitary plasmacytoma, Waldenstrom's macroglobulinemia, B-cell lymphomas, and chronic B-cell lymphocytic leukemia.[53] Nonlymphoid neoplasms are also rarely associated with monoclonal gammopathy.[53] Reported non-neoplastic causes of monoclonal gammopathy in dogs include ehrlichiosis, leishmaniasis, heartworm disease, chronic pyoderma, and plasmacytic gastroenterocolitis.[53,209,210] Idiopathic monoclonal gammopathy is also reported in the dog.[211] The most common non-neoplastic etiology of monoclonal gammopathy in cats is feline infectious peritonitis, although monoclonal gammopathy has also been reported in cats with ehrlichiosis and anaplasmosis.[212]

Multiple myeloma is the most common cause of monoclonal gammopathy in the dog,[209] and the same is likely true in cats.[212,213] This disease is classically defined as a systemic neoplastic proliferation of plasma cells in the bone marrow. However, recent evidence suggests that feline multiple myeloma primarily evolves at extramedullary sites such as the skin, oral cavity, and abdominal viscera.[214] The paraprotein (also referred to as the M-component) produced by the neoplastic cell population may be a whole immunoglobulin molecule or an immunoglobulin fragment. Fragments consisting of immunoglobulin light chains may pass through the glomerular filtration barrier and be detected in the urine as Bence-Jones proteins.[53]

Monoclonal gammopathies evoke a spectrum of clinical and clinicopathologic abnormalities. Precipitation of immunoglobulin light chains within nephrons may lead to tubular obstruction and eventual renal failure and azotemia.[53] Bleeding diatheses are common in patients with monoclonal gammopathy; hemorrhage may result from immunoglobulin coating of platelets, which interferes with release of platelet factor 3 and platelet aggregation.[53] Hemorrhage may also result from distension and rupture of microvessels secondary to plasma hyperviscosity.[53,191] The microvasculature of the eye and central nervous system appear to be especially prone to this complication. Hyperviscosity also increases cardiac workload, resulting in compensatory myocardial hypertrophy and possible heart failure.[53,213] Fortunately, in many cases the deleterious physiological consequences of monoclonal gammopathy can be reversed with appropriate treatment of the underlying neoplasm and correction of the associated paraproteinemia. Approximately 90% of dogs[191] and 60% of cats[215] with multiple myeloma will experience remission of their cancer following chemotherapy. B-cell lymphomas and chronic lymphocytic leukemias are also typically chemoresponsive.

SUMMARY

Veterinarians will encounter hematologic abnormalities routinely while treating small animal cancer patients. Some of these abnormalities, such as monoclonal gammopathy, are relatively rare and highly associated with specific neoplasms. Thus, their detection should compel a search for underlying cancer. Other hematologic abnormalities, such as anemia or thrombocytopenia, are very common in cancer patients, and their identification should prompt clinicians to consider the different mechanisms by which they may have arisen and whether further diagnostic tests are needed to fully characterize their etiology. Although cancer-related hematologic abnormalities are frequently described in the veterinary literature, the incidence, prevalence, and clinical significance of these abnormalities are less well-defined. Anemia and coagulopathies are major causes of morbidity and mortality in human cancer patients, and may have a tremendous impact on disease progression and tumor response to antineoplastic therapy. It is plausible that the same is true for veterinary cancer patients, given the pathological and biological similarity between human and small animal tumors.[216] Future studies should address the epidemiology and clinical significance of these, and perhaps other, hematologic abnormalities in order to determine whether therapeutic intervention to correct them may improve patient outcomes.

ACKNOWLEDGMENTS

The author would like to gratefully acknowledge Drs Craig Thompson and Katie Boes for their technical assistance in preparation of the photomicrographs featured in this review.

REFERENCES

1. Glaspy J. Disorders of blood cell production in clinical oncology. In: Abeloff MD, Armitage JE, Niederhuber JE, et al, editors. Abeloff's clinical oncology. 4th edition. Philadelphia: Churchill Livingstone; 2008. p. 677–92.

2. Kaufman RM, Anderson KC. Hematologic complications and blood bank support. In: Hong WK, Bast RC, Hait WN, et al, editors. Cancer medicine. 8th edition. Shelton (CT): PMPH-USA; 2010. p. 1797–812.

3. Couto CG. Hematologic abnormalities in small animal cancer patients. Part I. Red blood cell abnormalities. Compend Contin Educ Vet 1984;6:1059–68.

4. Couto CG. Hematologic abnormalities in small animal cancer patients. Part II. White blood cell, platelet, and combined abnormalities. Compend Contin Educ Vet 1985; 7:21–30.

5. Rosenthal R. Chemotherapy-induced myelosuppression. In: Kirk RW, editor. Kirk's current veterinary therapy X. Philadelphia: WB Saunders; 1989. p. 494–7.

6. Barger AM, Grindem CB. Hematologic abnormalities associated with cancer therapy. In: Feldman BF, Zinkl JG, Jain MC, editors. Schalm's veterinary hematology. 5th edition. Baltimore: Lippincott Williams & Wilkins; 2000. p. 676–81.

7. Axiak SM, Carreras JK, Hahn KA, et al. Hematologic changes associated with half-body irradiation in dogs with lymphoma. J Vet Intern Med 2006;20:1398–401.

8. Spivak JL, Gascón P, Ludwig H. Anemia management in oncology and hematology. Oncologist 2009;14(suppl 1):43–56.

9. Ludwig H, Van Belle S, Barrett-Lee P, et al. The European cancer anaemia survey (ECAS): a large, multinational, prospective survey defining the prevalence, incidence, and treatment of anaemia in cancer patients. Eur J Cancer 2004;40:2293–306.

10. Birgegård G, Gascón P, Ludwig H. Evaluation of anemia in patients with multiple myeloma and lymphoma: findings of the European Cancer Anemia Survey. Eur J Haematol 2006;77:378–86.

11. Tchekmedyian NS. Anemia in cancer patients: Significance, epidemiology, and current therapy. Oncology (Williston Park) 2002;16(Suppl 10):17–24.

12. Madewell BR, Feldman BF. Characterization of anemias associated with neoplasia in small animals. J Am Vet Med Assoc 1980;176:419–25.

13. Prymak C, McKee LJ, Goldschmidt MH, et al. Epidemiologic, clinical, pathologic, and prognostic characteristics of splenic hemangiosarcoma and splenic hematoma in dogs: 217 cases (1985). J Am Vet Med Assoc 1988;193:706–12.

14. Smith AN. Hemangiosarcoma in dogs and cats. Vet Clin North Am Small Anim Pract 2003;33:533–52.

15. Weinstein MJ, Carpenter JL, Schunk CJM. Nonangiogenic and nonlymphomatous sarcomas of the canine spleen: 57 cases (1975–1987). J Am Vet Med Assoc 1989;195:784–8.

16. Aronsohn MG, Dubiel B, Roberts B, et al. Prognosis for acute nontraumatic hemoperitoneum in the dog: A retrospective analysis of 60 cases (2003–2006). J Am Anim Hosp Assoc 2009;45:72–7.

17. Pintar J, Breitschwerdt EB, Hardie EM, et al. Acute nontraumatic hemoabdomen in the dog: A retrospective analysis of 39 cases (1987–2001). J Am Anim Hosp Assoc 2003;39:518–22.

18. Whittemore JC, Preston CA, Kyles AE, et al. Nontraumatic rupture of an adrenal gland tumor causing intra-abdominal hemorrhage or retroperitoneal hemorrhage in four dogs. J Am Vet Med Assoc 2001;219:329–33.

19. Gilson SD, Withrow SJ, Wheeler SJ, et al. Pheochromocytoma in 50 dogs. J Vet Intern Med 1994;8:228–32.

20. Slensky KA, Volk SW, Schwarz T, et al. Acute severe hemorrhage secondary to arterial invasion in a dog with thyroid carcinoma. J Am Vet Med Assoc 2003;223:649–53.

21. Harvey JW, French TW, Meyer DJ. Chronic iron deficiency anemia in dogs. J Am Anim Hosp Assoc 1982;18:946–60.

22. Ishiguro T, Kadosawa T, Takagi S, et al. Relationship of disease progression and plasma histamine concentrations in 11 dogs with mast cell tumors. J Vet Intern Med 2003;17:194–8.

23. Fox LE, Rosenthal RC, Twedt DC, et al. Plasma histamine and gastrin concentrations in 17 dogs with mast cell tumors. J Vet Intern Med 1990;4:242–6.

24. Simpson KW, Dykes NL. Diagnosis and treatment of gastrinoma. Semin Vet Med Surg (Small Anim) 1997;12:274–81.

25. McCullough S. Immune-mediated hemolytic anemia: Understanding the nemesis. Vet Clin North Am Small Anim Pract 2003;33:1295–315.

26. Balch A, Mackin A. Canine immune-mediated hemolytic anemia: Pathophysiology, clinical signs, and diagnosis. Compend Contin Educ Vet 2007;29:217–25.

27. Shelton GH, Linenberger ML. Hematological abnormalities associated with retroviral infections in the cat. Semin Vet Med Surg (Small Anim) 1995;10:220–33.

28. Linenberger ML, Abkowitz JL. Haematological disorders associated with feline retroviral infections. Baillière's Clin Haematol 1995;8:73–112.

29. Harrus S, Klement E, Aroch I, et al. Retrospective study of 46 cases of feline haemobartonellosis in Israel and their relationship with FeLV and FIV infections. Vet Rec 2002;151:82–5.

30. Sykes JE. Feline hemotropic mycoplasmas. Vet Clin North Am Small Anim Pract 2010;40:1157–70.

31. Martinez J. Microangiopathic hemolytic anemia. In: Beutler E, Lichtman MA, Coller BS, et al, editors. Williams hematology. 6th edition. New York: McGraw-Hill; 2001. p. 623–6.

32. Fukumura D, Jain R. Tumor microvasculature and microenvironment: Targets for anti-angiogenesis and normalization. Microvasc Res 2007;74:72–84.

33. Hammer AS, Couto CG, Swardson C, et al. Hemostatic abnormalities in dogs with hemangiosarcoma. J Vet Intern Med 1991;5:11–4.

34. Caldin M, Carli E, Furlanello T, et al. A retrospective study of 60 cases of eccentrocytosis in the dog. Vet Clin Pathol 2005;34:224–31.

35. Thrall MA. Regenerative anemia. In: Thrall MA, Baker DC, Campbell TW, et al, editors. Veterinary hematology and clinical chemistry. Philadelphia: Lippincott Williams & Wilkins; 2004. p. 95–119.

36. Christopher MM. Relationship of endogenous Heinz bodies to disease and anemia in cats: 120 cases (1978–1987). J Am Vet Med Assoc 1989;194:1089–95.

37. Pavri RS, Gupta AD, Baxi AJ, et al. Further evidence for oxidative damage to hemoglobin and red cell membrane in leukemia. Leuk Res 1983;7:729–33.

38. Moore PF, Affolter VK, Vernau W. Canine hemophagocytic histiocytic sarcoma: A proliferative disorder of CD11d+ macrophages. Vet Pathol 2006;43:632–45.

39. Moore PF, Rosin A. Malignant histiocytosis of Bernese mountain dogs. Vet Pathol 1986;23:1–10.

40. Dobson J, Villiers E, Roulois A, et al. Histiocytic sarcoma of the spleen in flat-coated retrievers with regenerative anaemia and hypoproteinaemia. Vet Rec 2006;158:825–9.

41. Fry MM, Vernau W, Pesavento PA, et al. Hepatosplenic lymphoma in a dog. Vet Pathol 2003;40:556–62.

42. Carter JE, Tarigo JL, Vernau W, et al. Erythrophagocytic low-grade extranodal T-cell lymphoma in a cat. Vet Clin Pathol 2008;37:416–21.

43. Marks SL, Moore PF, Taylor DW, et al. Nonsecretory multiple myeloma in a dog: Immunohistologic and ultrastructural observations. J Vet Intern Med 1995;9:50–4.

44. Yearley JH, Stanton C, Olivry T, et al. Phagocytic plasmacytoma in a dog. Vet Clin Pathol 2007;36:293–6.

45. Ledieu D, Palazzi X, Marchal T, et al. Acute megakaryoblastic leukemia with erythrophagocytosis and thrombosis in a dog. Vet Clin Pathol 2005;34:52–6.
46. Madewell BR, Gunn C, Gribble DH. Mast cell phagocytosis of red blood cells in a cat. Vet Pathol 1983;20:638–40.
47. Madewell BR, Munn RJ, Phillips LP. Endocytosis of erythrocytes in vivo and particulate substances in vitro by feline neoplastic mast cells. Can J Vet Res 1987;51:517–20.
48. Allan R, Halsey TR, Thompson KG. Splenic mast cell tumor and mastocytaemia in a cat: case study and literature review. N Z Vet J 2000;48:117–21.
49. Leifer CE, Matus RE. Lymphoid leukemia in the dog. Vet Clin North Am Small Anim Pract 1985;15:723–30.
50. Cotter SM, Essex M. Animal model: Feline acute lymphoblastic leukemia and aplastic anemia. Am J Pathol 1977;87:265–8.
51. Blue JT, French TW, Kranz JS. Non-lymphoid hematopoietic neoplasia in cats: A retrospective study of 60 cases. Cornell Vet 1988;78:21–42.
52. Madewell BR. Hematological and bone marrow cytological abnormalities in 75 dogs with malignant lymphoma. J Am Anim Hosp Assoc 1986;22:235–40.
53. MacEwen EG, Hurvitz AI. Diagnosis and management of monoclonal gammopathies. Vet Clin North Am Small Anim Pract 1977;7:119–33.
54. Marconato L, Bettini G, Giacoboni C, et al. Clinicopathological features and outcome for dogs with mast cell tumors and bone marrow involvement. J Vet Intern Med 2008;22:1001–7.
55. Affolter VK, Moore PF. Localized and disseminated histiocytic sarcoma of dendritic cell origin in dogs. Vet Pathol 2002;39:74–83.
56. Pickens EH, Kim DY, Gaunt S, et al. Unique radiographic appearance of bone marrow metastasis of an insulin-secreting beta-cell carcinoma in a dog. J Vet Intern Med 2005;19:350–4.
57. Smith DA, Hill FWG. Metastatic malignant mesothelioma in a dog. J Comp Path 1989;100:97–101.
58. Kelly WR, Wilkinson GT, Allen PW. Canine angiosarcomas (lymphangiosarcoma): A case report. Vet Pathol 1981;18:224–7.
59. Birgegård G, Aapro MS, Bokemeyer C, et al. Cancer-related anemia: Pathogenesis, prevalence, and treatment. Oncology 2005;68(Suppl 1):3–11.
60. Grotto HZW. Anaemia of cancer: an overview of mechanisms involved in its pathogenesis. Med Oncol 2008;25:12–21.
61. Kiselow MA, Rassnick KM, McDonough SP, et al. Outcome of cats with low-grade lymphocytic lymphoma: 41 cases (1995–2005). J Am Vet Med Assoc 2008;232: 405–10.
62. Simpson KW, Fyfe J, Cornetta A, et al. Subnormal concentrations of serum cobalamin (Vitamin B_{12}) in cats with gastrointestinal disease. J Vet Intern Med 2001;15: 26–32.
63. Ruaux CG, Steiner JM, Williams DA. Early biochemical and clinical responses to cobalamin supplementation in cats with signs of gastrointestinal disease and severe hypocobalaminemia. J Vet Intern Med 2005;19:155–60.
64. Morgan RV. Blood dyscrasias associated with testicular tumors in the dog. J Am Anim Hosp Assoc 1982;18:970–5.
65. McCandlish IAP, Munro CD, Breeze RG, et al. Hormone producing ovarian tumours in the dog. Vet Rec 1979;105:9–11.
66. Weiss G, Goodnough LT. Anemia of chronic disease. N Engl J Med 2005;352: 1011–23.

67. Staszewski H. Hematological paraneoplastic syndromes. Semin Oncol 1997;24: 329–33.
68. McCown JL, Specht AJ. Iron homeostasis and disorders in dogs and cats: A review. J Am Anim Hosp Assoc 2011;47:151–60.
69. Caro JJ, Salas M, Ward A, et al. Anemia as an independent prognostic factor for survival in patients with cancer: A systematic quantitative review. Cancer 2001;91: 2214–21.
70. Snyder SA, Dewhirst MW, Hauck ML. The role of hypoxia in canine cancer. Vet Comp Oncol 2008;6:213–23.
71. Rizzo JD, Brouwers M, Hurley P, et al. American Society of Clinical Oncology/ American Society of Hematology clinical practice guideline update on the use of epoetin and darbepoetin in adult patients with cancer. J Clin Oncol 2010;33:4996– 5010.
72. Abbo AH, Lucroy MD. Assessment of anemia as an independent predictor of response to chemotherapy and survival in dogs with lymphoma: 96 cases (1993– 2006). J Am Vet Med Assoc 2007;231:1836–42.
73. Miller AG, Morley PS, Rao S, et al. Anemia is associated with decreased survival time in dogs with lymphoma. J Vet Intern Med 2009;23:116–22.
74. Haney SM, Beaver L, Turrel J, et al. Survival analysis of 97 cats with nasal lymphoma: A multi-institutional retrospective study (1986–2006). J Vet Intern Med 2009;23:287–94.
75. Mayer MM, Treur PL, LaRue SM. Radiotherapy and surgery for feline soft tissue sarcoma. Vet Radiol Ultrasound 2009;50:669–72.
76. Madewell BR, Feldman BF, O'Neill S. Coagulation abnormalities in dogs with neoplastic disease. Thromb Haemost 1980;44:35–8.
77. Jordan HL, Grindem CB, Breitschwerdt EB. Thrombocytopenia in cats: A retrospective study of 41 cases. J Vet Intern Med 1993;7:261–5.
78. Grindem CB, Breitschwerdt EB, Corbett WT, et al. Thrombocytopenia associated with neoplasia in dogs. J Vet Inter Med 1994;8:400–5.
79. Chisholm-Chait A. Mechanisms of thrombocytopenia in dogs with cancer. Compend Contin Educ Vet 2000;22:1006–18.
80. Comazzi S, Gelain ME, Bonfanti U, et al. Acute megakaryoblastic leukemia in dogs: A report of three cases and review of the literature. J Am Anim Hosp Assoc 2010;46:327–35.
81. Helfand SC. Platelets and neoplasia. Vet Clin North Am Small Anim Pract 1988;18: 131–56.
82. Jain NC, Switzer JW. Autoimmune thrombocytopenia in dogs and cats. Vet Clin North Am Small Anim Pract 1981;11:421–34.
83. Dircks BH, Schuberth H, Mischke R. Underlying diseases and clinicopathologic variables of thrombocytopenic dogs with and without platelet-bound antibodies detected by use of a flow cytometric assay: 83 cases (2004–2006). J Am Vet Med Assoc 2009;235:960–6.
84. Helfand SC, Couto CG, Madewell BR. Immune-mediated thrombocytopenia associated with solid tumors in dogs. J Am Anim Hosp Assoc 1985;21:787–94.
85. Thomas JS. Non-immune-mediated thrombocytopenia. In: Weiss DJ, Wardrop KJ, editors. Schalm's veterinary hematology. 6th edition. Philadelphia: Blackwell Publishing; 2010. p. 596–604.
86. Caine GJ, Stonelake PS, Lip GYH, et al. The hypercoagulable state of malignancy: Pathogenesis and current debate. Neoplasia 2002;4:465–73.
87. Thomason JD, Calvert CA, Greene CE. DIC: Diagnosing and treating a complex disorder. Vet Med 2005;100:670–8.

88. O'Donnell MR, Slichter SJ, Weiden PL, et al. Platelet and fibrinogen kinetics in canine tumors. Cancer Res 1981;41:1379–83.
89. Slichter SJ, Harker LJ. Hemostasis in malignancy. Ann NY Acad Sci 1974;230: 252–61.
90. Adam F, Villiers E, Watson S, et al. Clinical pathological and epidemiological assessment of morphologically and immunologically confirmed canine leukemia. Vet Comp Oncol 2009;7:181–95.
91. Tasca S, Carli E, Caldin M, et al. Hematologic abnormalities and flow cytometric immunophenotyping results in dogs with hematopoietic neoplasia: 210 cases (2002–2006). Vet Clin Pathol 2009;38:2–12.
92. Weiss DJ, Evanson OA, Sykes J. A retrospective of canine pancytopenia. Vet Clin Pathol 1999;28:38–88.
93. Bryan JN, Henry CJ, Turnquist SE, et al. Primary renal neoplasia of dogs. J Vet Intern Med 2006;20:1155–60.
94. Durno AS, Webb JA, Gauthier MJ, et al. Polycythemia and inappropriate erythropoietin concentrations in two dogs with renal T-cell lymphoma. J Am Anim Hosp Assoc 2011;47:122–8.
95. Snead EC. A case of bilateral renal lymphosarcoma with secondary polycythaemia and paraneoplastic syndromes of hypoglycaemia and uveitis in an English Springer Spaniel. Vet Comp Oncol 2005;3:139–44.
96. Crow SE, Allen DP, Murphy CJ, et al. Concurrent renal adenocarcinoma and polycythemia in a dog. J Am Anim Hosp Assoc 1995;31:29–33.
97. Peterson ME, Zanjani ED. Inappropriate erythropoietin production from a renal carcinoma in a dog with polycythemia. J Am Vet Med Assoc 1981;179:995–6.
98. Nelson RW, Hager D, Zanjani ED. Renal lymphosarcoma with inappropriate erythropoietin production in a dog. J Am Vet Med Assoc 1983;182:1396–7.
99. Gorse MJ. Polycythemia associated with renal fibrosarcoma in a dog. J Am Vet Med Assoc 1988;192:793–4.
100. Henry CJ, Turnquist SE, Smith A, et al. Primary renal tumors in cats: 19 cases (1992-1998). J Feline Med Surg 1999;1:165–70.
101. Klainbart S, Segev G, Loeb E, et al. Resolution of renal adenocarcinoma-induced secondary inappropriate polycythaemia after nephrectomy in two cats. J Feline Med Surg 2008;10:264–8.
102. Cohen D. The canine transmissible venereal tumor: A unique result of tumor progression. Adv Cancer Res 1985;43:75–112.
103. Couto CG, Boudrieau RJ, Zanjani ED. Tumor-associated erythrocytosis in a dog with nasal fibrosarcoma. J Vet Intern Med 1989;3:183–5.
104. Sato K, Hikasa Y, Morita T, et al. Secondary erythrocytosis associated with high plasma erythropoietin concentrations in a dog with cecal leiomyosarcoma. J Am Vet Med Assoc 2002;220:486–90.
105. McGrath CJ. Polycythemia vera in dogs. J Am Vet Med Assoc 1974;164:1117–22.
106. Peterson ME, Randolph JF. Diagnosis of canine primary polycythemia and management with hydroxyurea. J Am Vet Med Assoc 1982;180:415–8.
107. Evans LM, Caylor KB. Polycythemia vera in a cat and management with hydroxyurea. J Am Anim Hosp Assoc 1995;31:434–8.
108. Nitsche EK. Erythrocytosis in dogs and cats: Diagnosis and management. Compend Contin Educ Vet 2004;26:104–19.
109. Waters DJ, Prueter JC. Secondary polycythemia associated with renal disease in the dog: Two case reports and review of literature. J Am Anim Hosp Assoc 1988;24: 109–14.

110. DeSancho MT, Rand JH. Coagulopathic complications of cancer patients. In: Hong WK, Bast RC, Hait WN, et al, editors. Cancer medicine. 8th edition. Shelton (CT): PMPH-USA; 2010. p. 1813–22.

111. Hammer AS. Thrombocytosis in dogs and cats: A retrospective study. Comp Haematol Intl 1991;1:181–6.

112. Rizzo F, Tappin SW, Tasker S. Thrombocytosis in cats: a retrospective study of 51 cases (2000-2005). J Feline Med Surg 2007;9:319–25.

113. Hogan DF, Dhaliwal RS, Sisson DD, et al. Paraneoplastic thrombocytosis-induced systemic thromboembolism in a cat. J Am Anim Hosp Assoc 1999;35:483–6.

114. Stokol S. Essential thrombocythemia and reactive thrombocytosis. In: Weiss DJ, Wardrop KJ, editors. Schalm's veterinary hematology. 6th edition. Philadelphia: Blackwell Publishing; 2010. p. 605–11.

115. Marchetti V, Benetti C, Citi S, et al. Paraneoplastic hypereosinophilia in a dog with intestinal T-cell lymphoma. Vet Clin Pathol 2005;34:259–63.

116. Liptak JM, Dernell WS, Monnet E, et al. Massive hepatocellular carcinoma in dogs: 48 cases (1992–2002). J Am Vet Med Assoc 2004;225:1225–30.

117. Bass MC, Schultze AE. Essential thrombocythemia in a dog: Case report and literature review. J Am Anim Hosp Assoc 1998;34:197–203.

118. Degen MA, Feldman BF, Turrel JM, et al. Thrombocytosis associated with a myeloproliferative disorder in a dog. J Am Vet Med Assoc 1989;194:1457–9.

119. Harvey JW. Myeloproliferative disorders in dogs and cats. Vet Clin North Am Small Anim Pract 1981;11:349–81.

120. Mears EA, Raskin RE, Legendre AM. Basophilic leukemia in a dog. J Vet Intern Med 1997;11:92–4.

121. MacEwen EG, Drazner FH, McClelland AJ, et al. Treatment of basophilic leukemia in a dog. J Am Vet Med Assoc 1975;166:376–80.

122. Dunn JK, Heath MF, Jefferies AR, et al. Diagnostic and hematologic features of probable essential thrombocythemia in two dogs. Vet Clin Pathol 1999;28:131–8.

123. Hopper PE, Mandell CP, Turrel JM, et al. Probable essential thrombocythemia in a dog. J Vet Intern Med 1989;3:79–85.

124. Mizukoshi T, Fujino Y, Yasukawa K, et al. Essential thrombocythemia in a dog. J Vet Med Sci 2006;68:1203–6.

125. Simpson JW, Else RW, Honeyman P. Successful treatment of suspected essential thrombocythaemia in the dog. J Small Anim Pract 1990;31:345–8.

126. Hammer AS, Couto CG, Getzy D, et al. Essential thrombocythemia in a cat. J Vet Intern Med 1990;4:87–91.

127. Thompson JP, Christopher MM, Ellison GW, et al. Paraneoplastic leukocytosis associated with a rectal adenomatous polyp in a dog. J Am Vet Med Assoc 1992;201:737–8.

128. Knottenbelt CM, Simpson JW, Chandler ML. Neutrophilic leukocytosis in a dog with a rectal tumor. J Small Anim Pract 2000;41:457–60.

129. Lappin MR, Latimer KS. Hematuria and extreme neutrophilic leukocytosis in a dog with renal tubular carcinoma. J Am Vet Med Assoc 1988;192:1289–92.

130. Peeters D, Clercx C, Thiry A, et al. Resolution of paraneoplastic leukocytosis and hypertrophic osteopathy after resection of a renal transitional cell carcinoma producing granulocyte-macrophage colony-stimulating factor in a young bull terrier. J Vet Intern Med 2001;15:407–11.

131. Sharkey LC, Rosol TJ, Gröne A, et al. Production of granulocyte colony-stimulating factor and granulocyte-macrophage colony-stimulating factor by carcinomas in a dog and a cat with paraneoplastic leukocytosis. J Vet Intern Med 1996;10:405–8.

132. Chinn DR, Myers RK, Matthews JA. Neutrophilic leukocytosis associated with metastatic fibrosarcoma in a dog. J Am Vet Med Assoc 1985;186:806–9.
133. Dole RS, MacPhail CM, Lappin MR. Paraneoplastic leukocytosis with mature neutrophilia in a cat with pulmonary squamous cell carcinoma. J Feline Med Surg 2004;6:391–5.
134. Dotti G, Garattini E, Borleri G, et al. Leucocyte alkaline phosphatase identifies terminally differentiated normal neutrophils and its lack in chronic myelogenous leukemia is not dependent on p210 tyrosine kinase activity. Br J Haematol 1999; 105:163–72.
135. Schultze AE. Interpretation of canine leukocyte responses. In: Weiss DJ, Wardrop KJ, editors. Schalm's veterinary hematology. 6th edition. Philadelphia: Blackwell Publishing; 2010. p. 321–34.
136. Kaushansky K, O'Hara PJ, Berkner K, et al. Genomic cloning, characterization, and multilineage growth-promoting activity of human granulocyte-macrophage colony-stimulating factor. Proc Natl Acad Sci USA 1986;83:3101–5.
137. Lucroy MD, Madewell BR. Clinical outcome and associated diseases in dogs with leukocytosis and neutrophilia: 118 cases (1996–1998). J Am Vet Med Assoc 1999;214:805–7.
138. Lucroy MD, Madewell BR. Clinical outcome and diseases associated with extreme neutrophilic leukocytosis in cats: 104 cases (1991–1999). J Am Vet Med Assoc 2001;218:736–9.
139. Gabor LJ, Canfield PJ, Malik R. Haematological and biochemical findings in cats in Australia with lymphosarcoma. Aust Vet J 2000;78:456–61.
140. Leifer CE, Matus RE. Chronic lymphocytic leukemia in the dog: 22 cases (1974–1984). J Am Vet Med Assoc 1986;189:214–7.
141. Raskin RE, Krehbiel JD. Prevalence of leukemic blood and bone marrow in dogs with multicentric lymphoma. J Am Vet Med Assoc 1989;194:1427–9.
142. Avery AC, Avery PR. Determining the significance of persistent lymphocytosis. Vet Clin North Am Small Anim Pract 2007;37:267–82.
143. Batlivala TP, Bacon NJ, Avery AC, et al. Paraneoplastic T cell lymphocytosis associated with thymoma in a dog. J Small Anim Pract 2010;51:491–4.
144. Raskin RE, Krehbiel JD. Myelodysplastic changes in a cat with myclomonocytic leukemia. J Am Vet Med Assoc 1985;187:171–4.
145. Shimoda T, Shiranaga N, Mashita T, et al. Chronic myelomonocytic leukemia in a cat. J Vet Med Sci 2000;62:195–7.
146. Rossi G, Gelain ME, Foroni S, et al. Extreme monocytosis in a dog with chronic monocytic leukemia. Vet Rec 2009;165:54–6.
147. Endicott MM, Charney SC, McKnight JA, et al. Clinicopathological findings and results of bone marrow aspiration in dogs with cutaneous mast cell tumors: 157 cases (1999–2002). Vet Comp Oncol 2007;5:31–7.
148. O'Keefe DA, Couto CG, Burke-Schwartz C, et al. Systemic mastocytosis in 16 dogs. J Vet Intern Med 1987;1:75–80.
149. Peaston AE, Griffey SM. Visceral mast cell tumor with eosinophilia and eosinophilic peritoneal and pleural effusions in a cat. Aust Vet J 1994;71:215–7.
150. Bortnokski HB, Rosenthal RC. Gastrointestinal mast cell tumors and eosinophilia in two cats. J Am Anim Hosp Assoc 1992;28:271–5.
151. Lapointe J-M, Higgins RJ, Kortz GD, et al. Intravascular malignant T-cell lymphoma (malignant angioendotheliomatosis) in a cat. Vet Pathol 1997;34:247–50.
152. Barrs VR, Beatty JA, McCandlish IA, et al. Hypereosinophilic paraneoplastic syndrome in a cat with intestinal T-cell lymphosarcoma. J Small Anim Pract 2002;43: 401–5.

153. Cave TA, Gault EA, Argyle DJ. Feline epitheliotrophic T-cell lymphoma with para-neoplastic eosinophilia—immunochemotherapy with vinblastine and recombinant interferon a2b. Vet Comp Oncol 2004;2:91–7.

154. Tomiyasu H, Fujino Y, Ugai J, et al. Eosinophilic infiltration into splenic B-cell high-grade lymphoma in a dog. J Vet Med Sci 2010;72:1367–70.

155. London CA. Mast cell tumors in the dog. Vet Clin North Am Small Anim Pract 2003;33:473–89.

156. Couto CG. Tumor-associated eosinophilia in a dog. J Am Vet Med Assoc 1984;184:837.

157. Losco PE. Local and peripheral eosinophilia in a dog with anaplastic mammary carcinoma. Vet Pathol 1986;23:536–8.

158. Sellon RK, Rottman JB, Jordan HL. Hypereosinophilia associated with transitional cell carcinoma in a cat. J Am Vet Med Assoc 1992;201:591–3.

159. Gelain ME, Antoniazzi E, Bertazzolo W, et al. Chronic eosinophilic leukemia in a cat: cytochemical and immunophenotypical features. Vet Clin Pathol 2006;35:454–9.

160. Huibregtse BA, Turner JL. Hypereosinophilic syndrome and eosinophilic leukemia: A comparison of 22 hypereosinophilic cats. J Am Anim Hosp Assoc 1994;30:591–9.

161. Ndikuwera J, Smith DA, Obwolo MJ, et al. Chronic granulocytic leukaemia/eosino-philic leukaemia in a dog? J Small Anim Pract 1992;33:553–7.

162. Mahaffey EA, Brown TP, Duncan JR, et al. Basophilic leukemia in a dog. J Comp Path 1987;97:393–9.

163. Alroy J. Basophilic leukemia in a dog. Vet Pathol 1972;9:90–5.

164. Henness AM, Crow SE. Treatment of feline myelogenous leukemia: four case reports. J Am Vet Med Assoc 1977;171:263–6.

165. Rossi S, Gelain ME, Comazzi S. Disseminated histiocytic sarcoma with peripheral blood involvement in a Bernese Mountain dog. Vet Clin Pathol 2009;38:126–30.

166. Bookbinder PF, Butt MT, Harvey HJ. Determination of the number of mast cells in lymph node, bone marrow, and buffy coat cytologic specimens from dogs. J Am Vet Med Assoc 1992;200:1648–50.

167. McManus PM. Frequency and severity of mastocytaemia in dogs with and without mast cell tumors: 120 cases (1995–1997). J Am Vet Med Assoc 1999;215:355–7.

168. Stockham SL, Basel DL, Schmidt DA. Mastocytemia in dogs with acute inflamma-tory diseases. Vet Clin Pathol 1986;15:16–21.

169. Cayatte SM, McManus PM, Miller WH, et al. Identification of mast cells in buffy coat preparations from dogs with inflammatory skin diseases. J Am Vet Med Assoc 1995;206:325–6.

170. Stockham SL, Scott MA. Erythrocytes. In: Stockham SL, Scott MA, editors. Funda-mentals of veterinary clinical pathology. Ames (IA): Iowa State Press; 2002. p. 85–154.

171. Shull RM. Inappropriate marrow release of hematopoietic precursors in three dogs. Vet Pathol 1981;18:569–76.

172. Johnson KA, Powers BE, Withrow SJ, et al. Splenomegaly in dogs: Predictors of neoplasia and survival after splenectomy. J Vet Intern Med 1989;3:160–6.

173. Kleine LJ, Zook BC, Munson TO. Primary cardiac hemangiosarcomas in dogs. J Am Vet Med Assoc 1970;157:326–37.

174. Sharkey LC, Modiano JF. Bone marrow-derived sarcomas. In: Weiss DJ, Wardrop KJ, editors. Schalm's veterinary hematology. 6th edition. Philadelphia: Blackwell Publishing; 2010. p. 447–50.

175. Lamerato-Kozicki AR, Helm KM, Jubala CM, et al. Canine hemangiosarcoma originates from hematopoietic precursors with potential for endothelial differentia-tion. Exp Hematol 2006;34:870–8.

176. Francis JL, Biggerstaff J, Amirkhosravi A. Hemostasis and malignancy. Semin Thromb Hemost 1998;24:93–109.
177. Kristensen AT, Wiinberg B, Jessen LR, et al. Evaluation of human recombinant tissue factor-activated thromboelastography in 49 dogs with neoplasia. J Vet Intern Med 2008;22:140–7.
178. Sun NCJ, McAfee WM, Hum GJ, et al. Hemostatic abnormalities in malignancy, a prospective study of one hundred eight patients. Part I. Coagulation studies. Am J Clin Pathol 1979;71:10–6.
179. Rickles FR, Edwards RL. Activation of blood coagulation in cancer: Trousseau's syndrome revisited. Blood 1983;62:14–31.
180. Doitcher SR. Diagnosis, treatment, and prevention of cancer-related venous thrombosis. In: Abeloff MD, Armitage JE, Niederhuber JE, et al, editors. Abeloff's clinical oncology. 4th edition. Philadelphia: Churchill Livingstone; 2008. p. 693–715.
181. O'Keefe DA, Couto CG. Coagulation abnormalities associated with neoplasia. Vet Clin N Am Small Anim Pract 1988;18:157–68.
182. Slappendel RJ, de Maat CEM, Rijnberk A, et al. Spontaneous consumption coagulopathy in a dog with thyroid cancer. Thromb Diath Haemorrh 1970;24:129–35.
183. Chinn DR, Dodds WJ, Selcer BA. Prekallikrein deficiency in a dog. J Am Vet Med Assoc 1986;188:69–71.
184. Prasse KW, Hoskins JD, Glock RD, et al. Factor V deficiency and thrombocytopenia in a dog with adenocarcinoma. J Am Vet Med Assoc 1972;160:204–7.
185. Jones DRE, Gruffydd-Jones TJ, McCullagh KG. Disseminated intravascular coagulation in a dog with thoracic neoplasia. J Small Anim Pract 1980;21:303–9.
186. Hargis AM, Feldman BF. Evaluation of hemostatic defects secondary to vascular tumors in dogs: 11 cases (1983–1988). J Am Vet Med Assoc 1991;198:891–4.
187. Ihle SL, Baldwin CJ, Pifer SM. Probable recurrent femoral artery thrombosis in a dog with intestinal lymphosarcoma. J Am Vet Med Assoc 1996;280:240–2.
188. Hottendorf GH, Nielsen SW, Kenyon AJ. Canine mastocytoma: I. Blood coagulation time in dogs with mastocytoma. Pathol Vet 1965;2:129–41.
189. Fox PR, Petrie J-P, Hohenhaus AE. Peripheral vascular disease. In: Ettinger SJ, Feldman EC, editors. Textbook of veterinary internal medicine. 6th edition. St Louis: Elsevier Saunders; 2005. p. 1145–65.
190. Somer T, Meiselman HJ. Disorders of blood viscosity. Ann Med 1993;24:31–9.
191. Matus RE, Leifer CE, MacEwen EG, et al. Prognostic factors for multiple myeloma in the dog. J Am Vet Med Assoc 1986;188:1288–92.
192. Yip GYH, Chin BSP, Blann AD. Cancer and the prothrombotic state. Lancet Oncol 2002;3:27–34.
193. Van Winkle TJ, Bruce E. Thrombosis of the portal vein in eleven dogs. Vet Pathol 1993;30:28–35.
194. Laurenson MP, Hopper K, Herrera MA, et al. Concurrent diseases and conditions in dogs with splenic vein thrombosis. J Vet Intern Med 2010;24:1298–304.
195. LaRue MJ, Murtaugh RJ. Pulmonary thromboembolism in dogs: 47 cases (1986–1987). J Am Vet Med Assoc 1990;197:1368–72.
196. Rickles FR. Mechanisms of cancer-induced thrombosis. Pathophysiol Haemost Thromb 2006;35:103–10.
197. Stockhaus C, Kohn B, Rudolph R, et al. Correlation of haemostatic abnormalities with tumor stage and characteristics in dogs with mammary carcinoma. J Small Anim Pract 1999;40:326–31.
198. Thomas JS, Rogers KS. Platelet aggregation and adenosine triphosphate secretion in dogs with untreated multicentric lymphoma. J Vet Intern Med 1999;13:319–22.

199. McNiel EA, Ogilvie GK, Fettman MJ, et al. Platelet hyperfunction in dogs with malignancies. J Vet Intern Med 1997;11:178–82.

200. Kol A, Marks SL, Skorupski KA, et al. Serial thromboelastographic monitoring of dogs with multicentric lymphoma [abstract 36]. In: Research Abstract Program of the 2010 ACVIM Forum. Anaheim (CA), 2010. p. 22.

201. Boccaccio C, Sabatino G, Medico E, et al. The MET oncogene drives a genetic programme linking cancer to haemostasis. Nature 2005;434:396–400.

202. Amirkhosravi M, Francis JL. Procoagulant effects of the MC28 fibrosarcoma cell line in vitro and in vivo. Br J Haematol 1993;85:736–44.

203. Wiinberg B, Jensen AL, Johansson PI, et al. Thromboelastographic evaluation of hemostatic function in dogs with disseminated intravascular coagulation. J Vet Intern Med 2008;22:357–65.

204. Feldman BF, Madewell BR, O'Neill S. Disseminated intravascular coagulation: Antithrombin, plasminogen, and coagulation abnormalities in 41 dogs. J Am Vet Med Assoc 1981;179:151–4.

205. Maruyama H, Miura T, Sakai M, et al. The incidence of disseminated intravascular coagulation in dogs with malignant neoplasia. J Vet Med Sci 2004;66:573–5.

206. Susaneck SJ, Allen TA, Hoopes J, et al. Inflammatory mammary carcinoma in the dog. J Am Anim Hosp Assoc 1983;19:971–6.

207. Marconato L, Romanelli G, Stefanello D, et al. Prognostic factors for dogs with mammary inflammatory carcinoma: 43 cases (2003-2008). J Am Vet Med Assoc 2009;235:967–72.

208. Stockham SL, Scott MA. Proteins. In: Stockham SL, Scott MA, editors. Fundamentals of veterinary clinical pathology. Ames (IA): Iowa State Press; 2002. p. 251–76.

209. Giraudel JM, Pagès J-P, Guelfi J-F. Monoclonal gammopathies in the dog: A retrospective study of 18 cases (1986–1999) and literature review. J Am Anim Hosp Assoc 2002;38:135–47.

210. De Caprariis D, Sasanelli M, Paradies P, et al. Monoclonal gammopathy associated with heartworm disease in a dog. J Am Anim Hosp Assoc 2009;45:296–300.

211. Hoenig M, O'Brien JA. A benign hypergammaglobulinemia mimicking plasma cell myeloma. J Am Anim Hosp Assoc 1988;24:688–90.

212. Taylor SS, Tappin SW, Dodkin SJ, et al. Serum protein electrophoresis in 155 cats. J Feline Med Surg 2010;12:643–53.

213. Boyle TE, Holowaychuk MK, Adams AK, et al. Treatment of three cats with hyperviscosity syndrome and congestive heart failure using plasmapheresis. J Am Anim Hosp Assoc 2011;47:50–5.

214. Mellor PJ, Haugland S, Smith KC, et al. Histopathologic, immunohistochemical, and cytologic analysis of feline myeloma-related disorders: further evidence for primary extramedullary development in the cat. Vet Pathol 2008;45:159–73.

215. Hanna F. Multiple myeloma in cats. J Feline Med Surg 2005;7:275–87.

216. Paoloni M, Khanna C. Translation of new cancer treatments from pet dogs to humans. Nat Rev Cancer 2008;8:147–56.

217. Simon D, Nolte I, Eberle N, et al. Treatment of dogs with lymphoma using a 12-week, maintenance-free combination chemotherapy protocol. J Vet Intern Med 2006;20: 948–54.

218. Lucroy MD, Christopher MM, Kraegel SA, et al. Anemia associated with canine lymphoma. Comp Hematol Int 1998;8:1–6.

219. Zemann BI, Moore AS, Rand WM, et al. A combination chemotherapy protocol (VELCAP-L) for dogs with lymphoma. J Vet Intern Med 1998;12:465–70.

220. Moore AS, Cotter SM, Rand WM, et al. Evaluation of a discontinuous treatment protocol (VELCAP-S) for canine lymphoma. J Vet Intern Med 2001;15:348–54.

221. Mooney SC, Hayes AA, Matus RE, et al. Renal lymphoma in cats: 28 cases (1977–1984). J Am Vet Med Assoc 1987;191:1473–7.
222. Krick EL, Little L, Patel R, et al. Description of clinical and pathological findings, treatment and outcome of feline large granular lymphocyte lymphoma (1996–2004). Vet Comp Oncol 2008;6:102–10.
223. Spodnick GJ, Berg J, Moore FM, et al. Spinal lymphoma in cats: 21 cases (1976–1989). J Am Vet Med Assoc 1992;200:373–6.
224. Mahoney OM, Moore AS, Cotter SM, et al. Alimentary lymphoma in cats: 28 cases (1988–1993). J Am Vet Med Assoc 1995;207:1593–8.
225. Matus RE, Leifer CE, MacEwen EG. Acute lymphoblastic leukemia in the dog: A review of 30 cases. J Am Vet Med Assoc 1983;183:859–62.
226. Patel RT, Caceres A, French AF, et al. Multiple myeloma in cats: a retrospective study. Vet Clin Pathol 2005;34:341–52.
227. Skorupski KA, Clifford CA, Paoloni MC, et al. CCNU for the treatment of dogs with histiocytic sarcoma. J Vet Intern Med 2007;21:121–6.
228. Fidel J, Schiller I, Hauser B, et al. Histiocytic sarcomas in flat-coated retrievers: a summary of 37 cases (November 1998–March 2005). Vet Comp Oncol 2006;4: 63–74.
229. Skorupski KA, Rodriguez CO, Krick EL, et al. Long-term survival in dogs with localized histiocytic sarcoma treated with CCNU as adjuvant to local therapy. Vet Comp Oncol 2009;7:139–44.
230. Abadie J, Hedan B, Cadieu E, et al. Epidemiology, pathology, and genetics of histiocytic sarcoma in the Bernese Mountain dog breed. J Hered 2009;100(suppl 1): S19–27.
231. Schultz RM, Puchalski SM, Kent M, et al. Skeletal lesions of histiocytic sarcoma in nineteen dogs. Vet Radiol Ultrasound 2007;48:539–43.
232. Gieger TL, Théon AP, Werner JA, et al. Biologic behavior and prognostic factors for mast cell tumors of the canine muzzle: 24 cases (1990–2001). J Vet Intern Med 2003;17:687–92.
233. Takahashi T, Kadosawa T, Nagase M, et al. Visceral mast cell tumors in dogs: 10 cases (1982–1997). J Am Vet Med Assoc 2000;216:222–6.
234. Kim SE, Liptak JM, Gall TT, et al. Epirubicin in the adjuvant treatment of splenic hemangiosarcoma in dogs: 59 cases (1997–2004). J Am Vet Med Assoc 2007;231: 1550–7.
235. Wood CA, Moore AS, Gliatto JM, et al. Prognosis for dogs with stage I or II splenic hemangiosarcoma treated by splenectomy alone: 32 cases (1991–1993). J Am Anim Hosp Assoc 1998;34:417–21.
236. Locke JE, Barber LG. Comparative aspects and clinical outcomes of canine renal hemangiosarcoma. J Vet Intern Med 2006;20:962–7.
237. Shiu K-B, Flory AB, Anderson CL, et al. Predictors of outcome in dogs with subcutaneous or intramuscular hemangiosarcoma. J Am Vet Med Assoc 2011;238: 472–9.
238. Culp WTN, Drobatz KJ, Glassman MM, et al. Feline visceral hemangiosarcoma. J Vet Intern Med 2008;22:148–52.
239. Kraje AC, Mears EA, Hahn KA, et al. Unusual metastatic behavior and clinicopathologic findings in eight cats with cutaneous or visceral hemangiosarcoma. J Am Vet Med Assoc 1999;214:670–2.
240. Scavelli TD, Patnaik AK, Mehlhaff CJ, et al. Hemangiosarcoma in the cat: Retrospective evaluation of 31 surgical cases. J Am Vet Med Assoc 1985;187:817–9.

Neutrophil Function in Small Animals

Shannon Jones Hostetter, DVM, PhD

KEYWORDS

• Neutrophil • Function • Granule • NETs
• Inherited neutrophil disorders

Neutrophils, one of the primary effector cells of mammalian innate immunity, serve as the initial defense against bacterial and fungal pathogens. They are highly mobile phagocytes that are rapidly recruited to sites of injury, inflammation, or infection via a variety of chemokines, cytokines, and other mediators.[1] Once there, they serve to control and contain infection through both antimicrobial and proinflammatory functions. The importance of the neutrophil in immunity is illustrated by diseases and conditions that result in decreased neutrophil function, resulting in increased susceptibility to infection and disease. Recent research has also highlighted neutrophils as a link between innate and adaptive immunity, and an effector cell in the resolution of inflammation.[2,3] Despite their critical role in host defense against infectious disease, neutrophils can be deleterious to host health in certain circumstances. The same powerful neutrophil-derived proteases and mediators that are so effective at killing pathogens can also cause substantial native tissue damage. Neutrophils have evolved several strategies to mitigate damage to host tissue, including the packaging of proteases and other potent substances in granules that are under controlled release. In this review, the role of neutrophils in innate immunity will be discussed, including how neutrophils are recruited to sites of inflammation and how they kill microbes. Additionally, a brief discussion of the evolving role of neutrophils in other aspects of immunity and host health is included. Finally, the major inherited disorders of neutrophil function relevant to veterinary medicine are conferred.

NEUTROPHIL GRANULES AND THEIR CONTENTS

Neutrophils package and store the proteins utilized to migrate into tissues and fight invading pathogens in cytoplasmic granules. This strategy allows more controlled release of potentially toxic mediators into the external environment and restricts the interactions of certain substances with one another in the cytoplasm. Classically,

---

The author has nothing to disclose.
Department of Veterinary Pathology, Iowa State University, College of Veterinary Medicine, Christiansen Drive, Ames, IA 50011, USA
E-mail address: smjones@iastate.edu

Vet Clin Small Anim 42 (2012) 157–171
doi:10.1016/j.cvsm.2011.09.010
0195-5616/12/$ – see front matter © 2012 Elsevier Inc. All rights reserved.

neutrophil production of three distinct granules is described, each containing a specific subset of proteins. The first granule to be produced during neutrophil development beginning at the promyelocyte stage is the primary granule, also known as the azurophilic granule, and this is the only granule that contains myeloperoxidase (MPO). Secondary granules, also referred to as specific granules, and tertiary granules, also known as gelatinase granules, are formed sequentially during neutrophil maturation and lack MPO. Secondary granules are formed during the myelocyte stage, and tertiary granules during the metamyelocyte and band stages.[1,4] Recently, new studies have shown that both primary and secondary granules can be further divided into subsets based on variation in granule contents.[2,5] For example, some primary granules have high levels of defensins ("defensin-rich"), while others have low levels ("defensin-poor").[5] Defensins are a class of potent antimicrobial peptide found in primary granules. These subsets arise due to timing of granule formation during neutrophil development, since granule protein synthesis is under tight chronological control. The theory that granule content heterogeneity is a result of when proteins are formed has been termed the "targeting by timing of biosynthesis" hypothesis.[6,7]

Following granule development, secretory vesicles are produced via endocytosis. Secretory vesicles contain plasma proteins, adhesion molecules, and others substances that are rapidly assimilated into the plasma membrane to allow for attachment to the vascular endothelium and subsequent tissue migration.[2] The rapid integration of receptors from secretory vesicles into the plasma membrane allows neutrophils to more readily respond to cues from the environment as well, such as chemoattractants.[1] Secretory vesicles and tertiary granules are the most readily released following neutrophil stimulation, followed by secondary granules. Primary granules, which contain MPO and other potentially damaging substances, are last to be released, thereby minimizing native tissue damage during neutrophil activation. Although some overlap exists in the function of these granule proteins, their overall function can be summarized as follows: secretory vesicles contain proteins and receptors that contribute to neutrophil adhesion to vascular endothelium; tertiary (gelatinase) granules contain matrix metalloproteases and receptors necessary for diapedesis and migration; secondary (specific) granules contain antimicrobial substances (proteases, antimicrobial peptides, etc), and matrix metalloproteases that are secreted both into the phagocytic vacuole and the extracellular space to thwart pathogens and aid migration, respectively; primary (azurophilic) granules contain proteolytic enzymes and antimicrobial peptides that are secreted into the phagocytic vacuole to kill microorganisms[1,2,4] A partial list of neutrophil granule and secretory vesicle contents is listed in **Table 1**.

NEUTROPHIL RECRUITMENT

For neutrophils to fulfill their role as effector cells in innate immunity, they must first reach the site of pathogen invasion. The site of neutrophil extravasation is determined by endothelial cell activation predominantly in postcapillary venules. Exposure of endothelial cells to proinflammatory mediators, such as cytokines (tumor necrosis factor [TNF]α, interleukin [IL]-β, etc), upregulates expression of several adhesion molecules including integrins (intercellular adhesion molecule [ICAM] and vascular cell adhesion molecule [VCAM]) and selectins (E and P selectin) on the endothelial cell surface.[8,9] The ligands and adhesion molecules in neutrophils that mediate initial contact with endothelial cells are located in clusters associated with microvilli along the cell membrane to facilitate interaction with the endothelial cell receptors.[10] Specifically, L-selectin, E-selectin ligand-1 (ESL-1), and P-selectin glycoprotein

Table 1
A partial list of contents for the different neutrophil granules as well as secretory vesicles

Primary Granules	Secondary Granules	Tertiary Granules	Secretory Vesicles
Antimicrobial	*Adhesion Molecules*	*Adhesion Molecules*	*Adhesion Molecules*
Myeloperoxidase	β_2-Integrins	β_2-Integrins	β_2-ntegrins
Lysozyme	*NADPH Oxidase*	*NADPH Oxidase*	*NADPH Oxidase*
Defensins	gp91^{phox}/p22^{phox}	gp91^{phox}/p22^{phox}	gp91^{phox}/p22^{phox}
Bactericidal permeability- inducing protein (BPI)	*Antimicrobial*	*Antimicrobial*	*Enzymes*
Enzymes	Lysozyme	Lysozyme	Prcteinase 3
Elastase	Lactoferrin	*Enzymes*	Alkaline phosphatase
Cathepsin G	Vitamin B$_{12}$ binding protein	Gelatinase	*Receptors*
Proteinase 3	*Enzymes*	Acetyltransferase	Complement, TNF, IFN, IL-1, IL-10,
Sialidase	Alkaline phosphatase	Acid phosphatase	⁻GFβ, fMLP, others
α-Mannosidase	Gelatinase	*Receptors*	*Misc. Factors*
β-Glucoronidase	Collagenase (type IV)	u-PA, TNF, complement, others	De:ay accelerating factor
Collagenase (nonspecific)	Sialidase	*Misc. Factors*	Azurocidin
Phospholipase A$_2$	Phospholipase A$_2$	β_2-Microglobulin	Plasma proteins
Misc. Factors	*Receptors*		
Azurocidin	u-PA, TNF, complement, fibronectin, thrombospondin, others		
α$_1$-Antitrypsin	*Misc. Factors*		
	β_2-Microglobulin		
	Pentraxin-3		
	Plasminogen activator		

Factors are subdivided based on their function and/or structure.[4,89,90]

ligand-1 (PSGL-1) on neutrophils interact with P and E selectin and integrins to mediate the processes of initial tethering and rolling.[1,8] These initial interactions between ligands and receptors initiate a signaling cascade in neutrophils that ultimately leads to integrin expression and cytoskeletal rearrangements to facilitate firm adhesion and diapedesis.[11]

Classically, three steps have been described for neutrophil diapedesis: rolling, activation, and firm adhesion.[9,12] In recent years, however, several additional steps involved in neutrophil extravasation have been described. These new steps are as follows, with inclusion of the classic steps for sequential reference: capture, rolling, slow rolling, activation, spreading, arrest, intravascular crawling, and transcellular and paracellular migration.[9,13] The initial capture (tethering) of neutrophils by activated endothelium, as mentioned above, precedes rolling and involves interactions of selectins and PSGL-1. Likewise, slow rolling is also mediated by the catch and release interactions of selectins and their ligands, as neutrophils attach and detach during the rolling process.[12] This process is an intermediate step between initial tethering and firm adhesion that serves to reduce the velocity of the neutrophil as it rolls along the endothelium, thereby facilitating firm adhesion.

Recent evidence has shown that firm adhesion to the vessel wall, slow-rolling along the endothelial surface, and transmigration through the vessel are mediated, at least in part, by β_2-integrins.[14,15] The β_2-integrins are a family of transmembrane cell surface proteins present on neutrophils as well as other white blood cells such as monocytes and lymphocytes. The process of integrin expression on the cell surface is triggered by chemokine exposure during the activation phase. The β_2-integrins exist as heterodimers, consisting of an α and a β subunit, which are noncovalently associated. There is only one β subunit common to all the β_2-integrins, CD18. It is the α subunit (CD11) that distinguishes the three particular proteins in the β_2-integrin family, namely leukocyte functional antigen-1 (LFA-1), Mac-1 (also known as complement receptor 3 or CR3), and p150,95 (also known as CR4). Each of these molecules contains a different α subunit that imparts a different function to the heterodimer. LFA-1 and Mac-1 both bind the intercellular adhesion molecules 1 and 2 (ICAM-1 and -2). The interaction of LFA-1 and Mac-1 on the leukocyte with ICAM on the endothelial cells is imperative for both slow rolling and firm adhesion of the cell to the endothelial surface and the subsequent migration through the endothelium.[15–17] Finally, the β_2-integrins mediate intravascular crawling, the novel step preceding endothelial transmigration in which neutrophils hone in on a specific site for extravasation. Expression levels of these adhesion molecules may also help determine the mode of extravasation, as blocking expression led to enhanced transcellular over paracellular migration.[14]

Neutrophils respond to a plethora of signals from the environment in the process of chemotaxis, choreographing their migration from the bloodstream to their final destination in tissues. Chemotaxis is coordinated via chemoattractants, diffusible molecules that direct responsive cells to the site of production. These chemoattractants are detected by membrane-associated G protein–coupled receptors. The vast array of chemoattractants directing neutrophil recruitment is derived from a variety of sources, including other cells (platelets, macrophages, neutrophils, endothelial cells, etc), complement components, invading pathogens, and damaged tissue. Examples of potent chemoattractants for neutrophils include IL-8, activated complement components C5a and C3a, platelet activating factor, bacterial derived N-formyl peptides such as fMLP, and leukotrienes, particularly LTB$_4$.[18,19] It is molecules such as these that are sensed by neutrophils, thereby guiding them to the site where they will ultimately fulfill their effector functions.

MICROBIOCIDAL MECHANISMS

Once they have reached their destination, activated neutrophils release antimicrobial products, produce reactive oxygen species, and generate proinflammatory cytokines to kill microbes and control infection. The first step in this process involves priming and activation of these phagocytes, which occurs via detection of both pathogen and host derived signals recognized by the neutrophil as a call to arms.

Priming and Activation

Neutrophil priming and activation are required for full cell functionality, including maximized generation of the oxidative burst, and enhanced phagocytosis and degranulation. Priming precedes activation and sensitizes the cell to secondary signals, which promote activation. The requirement for priming is beneficial for limiting native tissue damage, since neutrophils are only triggered to release their cytotoxic granule contents when properly signaled to do so. Many of the chemoattractants discussed earlier also serve as priming agents; therefore, priming of neutrophils often occurs well before the cell reaches its destination.[20]

Activation of primed neutrophils occurs via exposure to numerous substances, including cytokines (interferon [IFN], TNF), chemokines, and pathogen-derived products such as lipopolysaccharides (LPS). Neutrophils are equipped with several membrane-associated pattern recognition receptors (PRRs) that detect pathogen-associated molecular patterns (PAMPs) released from infectious agents. Examples of neutrophil PRRs include Toll-like receptors (TLRs) and lectins, and signaling through these receptors is critical for cellular activation and execution of effector functions.[21,22] Neutrophils can also respond to damage-associated molecular patterns (DAMPs), also referred to as alarmins, which are released from cells and tissues secondary to necrosis or other forms of tissue damage. Several classes of receptors recognize DAMPs, including TLRs and the intracellular NOD-like receptors. Detection of DAMPs via these receptors, similar to PAMPs, results in neutrophil recruitment and activation.[18]

Phagocytosis and Intracellular Killing

Phagocytosis is an active, receptor-mediated process by which pathogens are engulfed by the neutrophil and entrapped within a membrane bound vacuole called the phagosome. Opsinization of organisms with substances such as specific antibody or complement facilitates this process. For example, in addition to their function in leukocyte adhesion, the β_2-integrins Mac-1 and p150.95 also serve as complement receptors (CR3 and CR4) that bind the inactivated complement component C3b (iC3b). iC3b binds to the surface of pathogens and serves as an opsonin. When iC3b bound to the pathogen is subsequently bound to CR3 on the neutrophil, this interaction can stimulate phagocytosis of the pathogen by the neutrophil.[23,24] Subsequently, a chain of events transpires within the neutrophil ultimately leading to microbe killing within the phagolysosome. Neutrophils also possess a variety of receptors allowing them to recognize pathogens directly, such as the TLRs, thereby bypassing the opsonization as a requirement for phagocytosis.[24]

Several events rapidly occur both during and following phagocytosis that quickly and efficiently destroy the microbe. First, primary/azurophilic and secondary/specific granules fuse with the membrane of the phagosome during development to ensure the arrival of granule contents within the phagosome.[24,25] There is rapid assembly of the NADPH oxidase, whose activity is necessary for the respiratory burst and generation of reactive oxygen species (ROS) and whose formation coincides with degranulation. The NADPH oxidase is composed of several membrane-associated and cytosolic parts, which are not associated in a resting or primed neutrophil. During neutrophil activation, however, the components of this enzyme come together to form a functional enzyme. The membrane-associated cytochrome b_{558} complex is composed of two components: $gp91^{phox}$ and $p22^{phox}$. During assembly, the cytosolic components $p40^{phox}$, $p47^{phox}$, and $p67^{phox}$ group with the membrane-bound b_{558} complex to create a functional NADPH oxidase.[8,26] The NADPH oxidase primary function is to generate superoxide ion and release it into the phagocytic vacuole. Superoxide then combines with other molecules, such as hydrogen peroxide, to create additional ROS. Myeloperoxidase released into the phagosome from primary/azurophilic granules works in concert with ROS to cause oxidation of halides. The bactericidal properties of neutrophils have long been linked to their generation of ROS during the oxidative burst and in vitro experiments have demonstrated the direct bactericidal properties of these ROS; however, more recent evidence suggests that a main function of the ROS may be to activate and augment the functions of proteases and other granule-derived bactericidal proteins.[27] Of the more potent antimicrobial molecules released into the phagolysosome are the neutral proteinases elastase, proteinase-3 and cathepsin G. Their importance in microbial killing has been demonstrated in studies with knockout mice.[27] Other important antimicrobial molecules from granules include antimicrobial peptides, whose mechanism of action typically involves disrupting the cell membrane and azurocidin.[28]

Neutrophil Extracellular Traps (NETs)

Within the past decade, a novel and unexpected weapon has been added to the neutrophil arsenal against microbial invaders. In 2004, Brinkmann and colleagues[29] discovered that activated neutrophils create extracellular structures composed of granule proteins and histones on a scaffold of DNA that ensnare and subsequently kill surrounding bacteria. These structures, termed "neutrophil extracellular traps" or "NETs" by the investigators, were characterized via electron microscopy and immunofluorescence. Scanning electron microscopy revealed that NETs are composed of both smooth and globular domains that intertwine to create larger bundles with diameters up to 50 nm. Ensnarement of both gram-positive and gram-negative pathogens in NETs led to degradation of bacterial virulence factors at the hands of extracellular neutrophil elastase and potentially other neutrophil-derived proteases. It was also determined that the formation of NETs was necessary for extracellular bacterial killing, presumably through concentration of granule-derived proteases within the NET scaffold. Extracellular bacteria that become ensnared within the NET are therefore exposed to high concentrations of bactericidal molecules, including proteases and histones, which mediate bacterial killing. The formation of NETs in vivo was confirmed via histopathologic analysis of tissues from both a rabbit model of shigellosis and human appendicitis. The authors proposed that NETs contribute to control of infection not only via direct microbial killing but also by entrapment and localization of bacteria. NETs may also serve as an important means of limiting the migration of proteases and histones into native tissues to mitigate neutrophil-induced tissue damage.[29]

Since their initial discovery, NET formation by neutrophils has been described in numerous diverse species along the phylogenetic scale, including zebrafish, chickens, mice, rabbits, cattle, and humans.[29–32] NETs are formed rapidly proceeding neutrophil activation via several pathways. Neutrophil activation via LPS, phorbol myristate acetate (PMA), or IL-8 led to morphologic changes in neutrophils consistent with activation and subsequent NET formation.[29] The complement protein C5a can also induce NET formation but only in mature neutrophils previously exposed to interferon.[34] Toll-like receptors (TLRs) and Fcγ receptors also may trigger NET formation.[35] Formation of NETs can occur as early as 10 minutes following neutrophil activation, a time point that has lead researchers to postulate that NET formation is an active process in viable cells rather than a passive component of apoptosis.[29,33] More recent studies, however, have observed NET formation via microscopy occurring as part of an active cell-death program secondary to activation with PMA.[36] This process, which is unrelated to either apoptosis or necrosis and is dependent on ROS, has been coined "netosis." It is possible that both mechanisms for NET formation play a role in the innate immune response, depending on the specific pathogen and/or host environment. A variety of pathogens are susceptible to entrapment and subsequent killing by NETs, including both gram-positive and gram-negative bacteria such as *Staphylococcus aureus* and *Shigella flexneri*, as well as both the yeast and hyphae forms of *Candida albicans*.[29,37] In contrast, other pathogens resist killing in NETs through a variety of mechanisms.[38,39]

ROLE IN IMMUNE RESPONSE, INFLAMMATION, AND COAGULATION

Although neutrophils are traditionally recognized as key players in the innate immune response through their roles in phagocytosis and pathogen destruction, in recent years their additional diverse and complex functions in host health and defense have come to light. Numerous neutrophil-derived products further promote inflammation through the recruitment of other immune cells to sites inflammation. For example, azurocidin, a serine protease found in both secretory vesicles and primary granules that has previously been discussed for its antimicrobial properties, recruits monocytes to areas of inflammation. Additionally, azurocidin activates macrophages to induce proinflammatory cytokine release and augment phagocytosis.[40] Some granule products, such as pentraxin 3 (PTX3), serve to both augment and dampen the innate immune response. PTX3, which is stored in specific granules, binds the surface of pathogens and serves as an opsonin, and can also activate complement, emphasizing its role in innate immunity; however, PTX3 can also limit neutrophil recruitment to sites of inflammation by binding P-selectin on endothelial cells, thereby reducing neutrophil rolling. PTX3 may have an additional role in tissue repair and remodeling, as recent evidence suggests it plays a role in angiogensis.[41–43] In addition to the role their preformed products play in the modulation of the immune response, stimulated neutrophils also actively produce and secrete a variety of cytokines, chemokines, and other mediators that contribute to both the immune response and tissue repair. For example, neutrophil production of proinflammatory cytokines/chemokines (TNFα, IL-1β, and IL-8), anti-inflammatory/immunomodulatory cytokines (IL-10, transforming growth factor [TGF]β), and growth factors (VEGF, HGF) is recognized.[44]

Recently, it was shown that the neutrophil serine proteases, elastase and cathepsin-G, are critically linked to coagulation and thrombus formation in vivo.[45] In this study, elastase and cathepsin G knockout mice were used to demonstrate that these neutrophil-derived proteases were critically important in intravascular fibrin deposition and clot formation. Additionally, elastase and cathepsin G derived specifically from both murine and human neutrophils interact with platelets to enhance factor X activation. These proteases also work to promote coagulation via proteolytic inactivation of tissue factor pathway inhibitor (TFPI). Taken together, these findings clearly identify a role of neutrophils in coagulation and thrombus formation. It was theorized by the authors that this could aid in limiting pathogen dissemination and infection, by entrapment of bacteria that gain access to the bloodstream within a thrombus.

INHERITED DISORDERS OF NEUTROPHIL FUNCTION IN VETERINARY MEDICINE
Bovine Leukocyte Adhesion Deficiency

Bovine leukocyte adhesion deficiency (BLAD) is an immunodeficiency described in Holsteins and is inherited as an autosomal recessive trait. The molecular basis for BLAD has been determined to be a result of deficient expression of CD11/CD18 on leukocytes, as in the human disease counterpart.[46] The reduced surface expression of CD11/CD18 is due to a heritable defect in the CD18 allele. This defect is a point mutation in a single base that results in an amino acid substitution in the CD18 protein and directly results in decreased surface expression of CD11/CD18.[46,47] Neutrophils isolated from calves homozygous for BLAD have decreased ability to phagocytose and destroy pathogens such as the yeast C albicans.[48] BLAD neutrophils also are unable to successfully transmigrate across the endothelium of blood vessels, thereby confining them to the bloodstream. This contributes to the characteristic clinical signs in cattle with BLAD, which are similar to those that are observed in other species with LAD: chronic bacterial and fungal infections with a lack of noticeable pus formation. Laboratory and histopathologic findings include persistent, marked neutrophilia with normal neutrophil morphology and an absence of neutrophilic inflammation in most tissues, respectively.[46,49]

The clinical disease in cattle is first observed in young calves and is characterized by marked gingivitis with gingival recession, oral ulcers, and stunted growth. As the animals age, the severity of the clinical signs usually progresses as they develop more serious infections, such as pneumonia. Cattle with BLAD will typically suffer from chronic diarrhea due to inflammation and bacterial overgrowth in the intestinal tract.[50] Patients with BLAD typically die from severe infections by 1 year of age. Based on the clinical course of BLAD and the negligible degree of CD11/CD18 expression on BLAD leukocytes, it has been correlated to the severe phenotype of its human disease counterpart. Calves suspected of having BLAD can be rapidly diagnosed using flow cytometry. Although clinical therapies are not practical or cost-effective in this species, definitive diagnosis of clinically affected animals and heterozygous carriers is useful for identifying affected bloodlines in the Holstein breed.[46,49,50]

Canine Leukocyte Adhesion Deficiency

Canine leukocyte adhesion deficiency (CLAD) is an autosomal recessive inherited defect in CD11/CD18 expression described in Irish setters and Irish setter crosses. Affected dogs typically have less than 2% of CD11b/CD18 on their neutrophils as identified using flow cytometry. Their neutrophil function was found to be substantially decreased as these neutrophils exhibited decreased adhesion and failed to ingest particles opsonized with either C3b or IgG.[51,52] The cause of the disease is a single missense mutation in the β_2-integrin gene (CD18 specifically) resulting in an amino acid substitution on the CD18 protein.[53]

The clinical features of the immunodeficiency in dogs are similar to those in cattle and include recurrent bacterial infections that respond poorly to antibiotic therapy, gingivitis, fever, omphalophlebitis, enlarged peripheral lymph nodes, and persistent marked neutrophilia. Additionally, affected dogs have an increased occurrence of bone lesions (eg, osteomyelitis, periostitis, and cranial mandibular osteopathy) and mild persistent pneumonia. Notably, the lesions lack a significant neutrophilic component since affected neutrophils are unable to migrate into the tissues in response to infection. Puppies afflicted with CLAD exhibit signs of illness from birth, including umbilical cord infections, inappetance, poor weight gain, weakness, and

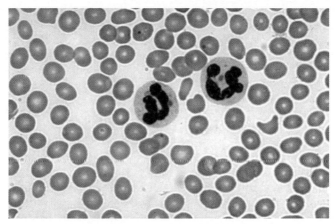

Fig. 1. Peripheral blood from a cat with Chediak-Higashi syndrome, depicting the characteristic large cytoplasmic inclusions within neutrophils (Wright's stain, ×100 oil magnification). (*Courtesy* Dr Claire Andreasen.)

skin wounds. The prognosis for CLAD is grave, and affected dogs either succumb to bacterial infections or are euthanized prior to maturity.[52,54,55]

Chediak-Higashi Syndrome

Chediak-Higashi syndrome (CHS) is a rare genetic disorder with autosomal recessive inheritance that affects the skin, eyes, hair, platelets, granulocytes, and nervous system. Characteristics of the disease in human beings include albinism, nervous system abnormalities, bleeding tendency, persistent neutropenia, immunodeficiency, photophobia, and development of lymphoma during childhood. Affected individuals have characteristic large inclusions in peripheral blood granulocytes, and abnormal melanin granules (**Fig. 1**).[56] A similar syndrome has been identified in several other species, including mink, cattle, mice, rats, and a killer whale.[57]

CHS was first described in Persian cats during the 1970s. Affected cats were from a single family and were yellow eyed with blue smoke coloring. These cats had the characteristic peroxidase-positive cytoplasmic inclusions within neutrophils and other granulocytes shown to be lysosomes.[57,58] CHS cats are photophobic and have prolonged bleeding times compared with healthy controls due to both impaired platelet aggregation and a storage pool deficiency.[59] Neutrophil function also is impaired in CHS cats, as evidenced by decreased in vitro chemotaxis, migration and phagocytosis.[60] Affected cats also tend to be neutropenic.[56]

Partial albino Hereford cattle, Japanese black cattle, and Aleutian mink with CHS have an increased susceptibility to infections and characteristic granulocytic inclusions.[61] CHS has also been described in Brangus cattle.[62] Neutrophil function studies in CHS cattle found a markedly reduced capacity for bacterial killing, despite normal phagocytic activity, that was attributed to failure or delay of primary granule fusion with the phagolysosome.[63] Cattle with CHS also have bleeding tendencies secondary to platelet dysfunction.[64]

Birman Cat Neutrophil Granulation Anomaly

This hereditary anomaly of neutrophil granulation in Birman cats was first described by Hirsh and Cunningham[65] in 1984. Affected cats had fine granules within the cytoplasm that stained eosinophilic with Romanowsky stains. Granulation of other leukocytes was not observed, and no other noticeable defects were identified. The authors compared neutrophil ultrastructure and function in affected cats to those of healthy controls and found no significant differences in phagocytosis, oxidative burst, and bactericidal activity. These cats did not exhibit evidence of immunodeficiency, and it was concluded that the cytoplasmic granules were enlarged lysosomes.[65]

Canine Cyclic Hematopoiesis (Cyclic Hematopoiesis of Gray Collie Dogs; Gray Collie Syndrome)

Canine cyclic hematopoiesis (CH) is an autosomal recessive disorder resulting in cyclic fluctuations in neutrophil, eosinophil, platelet, and reticulocyte counts and was first described in the late 1960s.[66] Clinically, the disease is associated with hypopigmentation (gray coat color) and is characterized by 11- to 14-day cycles in the neutrophil count that result in severe infection and death during the nadir period.[67–69] Platelet, reticulocyte, eosinophil, and monocyte counts also fluctuate cyclically in peripheral blood. Hematopoietic activity cycles in the bone marrow to correlate with the deficiencies observed in peripheral blood, leading investigators to conclude that the cytopenias were secondary to decreased production.[70–72] Canine CH has been used as an animal model for both cyclic neutropenia and severe congenital neutropenia in human beings, despite the fact that canine CH more closely resembles Hermansky-Pudlak syndrome type 2, another hereditary cause of neutropenia in human beings. Cyclic neutropenia and most cases of severe congenital neutropenia are both caused by mutations in the gene encoding for neutrophil elastase, *ELA2*.[73–75] In contrast, the genetic basis for both canine CH and Hermansky-Pudlak syndrome type 2 is a mutation in the β subunit of the adapter protein complex-3. This complex is responsible for trafficking of proteins following their formation in the Golgi to lysosomes and other storage complexes, including neutrophil elastase trafficking to primary granules.[76,77] Indeed, dogs with CH had decreased amounts of enzymatically active mature neutrophil elastase and increased amounts of elastase precursor proteins.[76,78]

Pelger-Huet

Pelger-Huet is a congenital neutrophil disorder characterized by hyposegmentation of granulocytes in peripheral blood. It exhibits autosomal dominant inheritance, and has been described in dogs, rabbits, horses, cats, and human beings.[79–83] In most species, Pelger-Huet manifests solely as decreased nuclear lobulation in granulocytes in heterozygotes, despite a mature condensed chromatin pattern (**Fig. 2**). Nuclear morphology ranges from round to bean shaped to dumbbell shaped, and therefore may be mistaken for a degenerative left shift. Affected homozygotes, described in rabbits, cats, and human beings, exhibit more profound hyposegmentation of granulocytes, as well as other abnormalities including chondrodyplasia and developmental abnormalities.[84,85] The cause for the anomaly has been identified as multiple mutations in the gene encoding for the lamin B receptor, a nuclear envelope protein.[84] Recent studies indicate that the lamin B receptor is necessary for morphologic maturation of granulocytes, but not functional maturation.[86]

Although decreased neutrophil function has previously been described in neutrophils from Pelger-Huet patients, most studies in the more current veterinary literature suggest affected neutrophils are fully functional. Neutrophils isolated from dogs with Pelger-Huet anomaly showed normal adherence and responsiveness to chemotaxins, were able to migrate into tissues, and retained full microbiocidal and phagocytic functions. Additionally, affected dogs have no known predisposition to infection.[87]

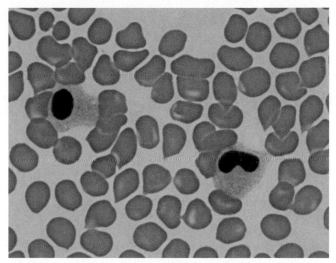

Fig. 2. Peripheral blood from an Australian shepherd with Pelger-Huet. Note the hyposegmentation (bean-shaped and round nuclei) in neutrophils despite the mature chromatin pattern (Wright's stain, ×100 oil magnification).

Similarly, neutrophils from an Arabian mare with Pelger-Huet anomaly exhibited similar adhesion molecule expression and neutrophil function based on phagocytosis and oxidative burst assays compared to controls.[81] Pelger-Huet has been identified in the following breeds: Australian shepherds, English springer spaniels, Doberman pinschers, blue heelers, fox hounds, Samoyeds, German shepherds, coonhounds, and Arabian horses.[4,79,81,88]

SUMMARY

Neutrophils are highly mobile phagocytes that serve as the initial effectors against pathogens and are actively recruited to sites of inflammation. Chemoattractants guide them toward the inflammation, and their interaction with endothelial cells directs them through postcapillary venules and into the tissues. Once they have reached their destination, they can efficiently kill many microbes via phagocytosis, extracellular release of granule contents, and the formation of NETs. They also actively produce cytokines and other mediators to promote or suppress inflammation, repair tissues, and modulate the immune response. The importance of neutrophil function in host health is emphasized through discussion of inherited disorders of neutrophil function such as leukocyte adhesion deficiency and cyclic hematopoiesis.

REFERENCES

1. Borregaard N, Sorensen OE, Theilgaard-Monch K. Neutrophil granules: a library of innate immunity proteins. Trends Immunol 2007;28:340.
2. Hager M, Cowland JB, Borregaard N. Neutrophil granules in health and disease. J Intern Med 2010;268:25.
3. Nathan C. Neutrophils and immunity: challenges and opportunities. Nat Rev Immunol 2006;6:173.
4. Weiss DJ, Wardrop KJ, Schalm OW. Schalm's veterinary hematology. 6th edition. Ames (IA): Wiley-Blackwell; 2010.

5. Faurschou M, Sorensen OE, Johnsen AH, et al. Defensin-rich granules of human neutrophils: characterization of secretory properties. Biochim Biophys Acta 2002; 1591:29.

6. Borregaard N, Theilgaard-Monch K, Sorensen OE, et al. Regulation of human neutrophil granule protein expression. Curr Opin Hematol 2001;8:23.

7. Le Cabec V, Cowland JB, Calafat J, et al. Targeting of proteins to granule subsets is determined by timing and not by sorting: The specific granule protein NGAL is localized to azurophil granules when expressed in HL-60 cells. Proc Natl Acad Sci U S A 1996;93:6454.

8. Borregaard N. Neutrophils, from marrow to microbes. Immunity 2010;33:657.

9. Ley K, Laudanna C, Cybulsky MI, et al. Getting to the site of inflammation: the leukocyte adhesion cascade updated. Nat Rev Immunol 2007;7:678.

10. Steegmaier M, Borges E, Berger J, et al. The E-selectin-ligand ESL-1 is located in the Golgi as well as on microvilli on the cell surface. J Cell Sci 1997;110(Pt 6):687.

11. Barreiro O, Sanchez-Madrid F. Molecular basis of leukocyte-endothelium interactions during the inflammatory response. Rev Esp Cardiol 2009;62:552.

12. Smith GS. Neutrophils. In: Feldman BV, Zinkl JG, Jain NC, editors. Schalm's veterinary hematology. 5th edition. Philadelphia: Lippincott Williams & Wilkins; 2000.

13. Woodfin A, Voisin MB, Nourshargh S. Recent developments and complexities in neutrophil transmigration. Curr Opin Hematol 2010;17:9.

14. Phillipson M, Heit B, Colarusso P, et al. Intraluminal crawling of neutrophils to emigration sites: a molecularly distinct process from adhesion in the recruitment cascade. J Exp Med 2006;203:2569.

15. Zarbock A, Ley K. Mechanisms and consequences of neutrophil interaction with the endothelium. Am J Pathol 2008;172:1.

16. Dunne JL, Ballantyne CM, Beaudet AL, et al. Control of leukocyte rolling velocity in TNF-alpha-induced inflammation by LFA-1 and Mac-1. Blood 2002;99:336.

17. Shaw JM, Al-Shamkhani A, Boxer LA, et al. Characterization of four CD18 mutants in leucocyte adhesion deficient (LAD) patients with differential capacities to support expression and function of the CD11/CD18 integrins LFA-1, Mac-1 and p150,95. Clin Exp Immunol 2001;126:311.

18. McDonald B, Kubes P. Cellular and molecular choreography of neutrophil recruitment to sites of sterile inflammation. J Mol Med (Berl) 2011;89(11):1079–88.

19. Springer TA. Traffic signals for lymphocyte recirculation and leukocyte emigration: the multistep paradigm. Cell 1994;76:301.

20. Swain SD, Rohn TT, Quinn MT. Neutrophil priming in host defense: role of oxidants as priming agents. Antioxid Redox Signal 2002;4:69.

21. Bourgeois C, Majer O, Frohner IE, et al. Fungal attacks on mammalian hosts: pathogen elimination requires sensing and tasting. Curr Opin Microbiol 2010;13:401.

22. Parker LC, Whyte MK, Dower SK, et al. The expression and roles of Toll-like receptors in the biology of the human neutrophil. J Leukoc Biol 2005;77:886.

23. Mayadas TN, Cullere X. Neutrophil β2 integrins: moderators of life or death decisions. Trends Immunol 2005;26:388.

24. Nordenfelt P, Tapper H. Phagosome dynamics during phagocytosis by neutrophils. J Leukoc Biol 2011;90(2):271–84.

25. Naucler C, Grinstein S, Sundler R, et al. Signaling to localized degranulation in neutrophils adherent to immune complexes. J Leukoc Biol 2002;71:701.

26. Sheppard FR, Kelher MR, Moore EE, et al. Structural organization of the neutrophil NADPH oxidase: phosphorylation and translocation during priming and activation. J Leukoc Biol 2005;78:1025.

27. Segal AW. How neutrophils kill microbes. Annu Rev Immunol 2005;23:197.

28. Soehnlein O. Direct and alternative antimicrobial mechanisms of neutrophil-derived granule proteins. J Mol Med (Berl) 2009;87:1157.
29. Brinkmann V, Reichard U, Goosmann C, et al. Neutrophil extracellular traps kill bacteria. Science 2004;303:1532.
30. Chuammitri P, Ostojic J, Andreasen CB, et al. Chicken heterophil extracellular traps (HETs): Novel defense mechanism of chicken heterophils. Vet Immunol Immunopathol 2009;129:126.
31. Lippolis JD, Reinhardt TA, Goff JP, et al. Neutrophil extracellular trap formation by bovine neutrophils is not inhibited by milk. Vet Immunol Immunopathol 2006;113:248.
32. Palic D, Ostojic J, Andreasen CB, et al. Fish cast NETs: Neutrophil extracellular traps are released from fish neutrophils. Dev Comp Immunol 2007;31:805.
33. Buchanan JT, Simpson AJ, Aziz RK, et al. DNase expression allows the pathogen group A Streptococcus to escape killing in neutrophil extracellular traps. Curr Biol 2006;16:396.
34. Martinelli S, Urosevic M, Daryadel A, et al. Induction of genes mediating interferon-dependent extracellular trap formation during neutrophil differentiation. J Biol Chem 2004;279:44123.
35. Urban CF, Ermert D, Schmid M, et al. Neutrophil extracellular traps contain calprotectin, a cytosolic protein complex involved in host defense against Candida albicans. PLoS Pathog 2009;5:e1000639.
36. Fuchs TA, Abed U, Goosmann C, et al. Novel cell death program leads to neutrophil extracellular traps. J Cell Biol 2007;176:231.
37. Urban CF, Reichard U, Brinkmann V, et al. Neutrophil extracellular traps capture and kill Candida albicans yeast and hyphal forms. Cell Microbiol 2006;8:668.
38. Beiter K, Wartha F, Albiger B, et al. An endonuclease allows Streptococcus pneumoniae to escape from neutrophil extracellular traps. Curr Biol 2006;16:401.
39. Wartha F, Beiter K, Albiger B, et al. Capsule and D-alanylated lipoteichoic acids protect Streptococcus pneumoniae against neutrophil extracellular traps. Cell Microbiol 2007;9:1162.
40. Soehnlein O, Lindbom L. Neutrophil-derived azurocidin alarms the immune system. J Leukoc Biol 2009;85:344.
41. Deban L, Russo RC, Sironi M, et al. Regulation of leukocyte recruitment by the long pentraxin PTX3. Nat Immunol 2010;11:328.
42. Inforzato A, Jaillon S, Moalli F, et al. The long pentraxin PTX3 at the crossroads between innate immunity and tissue remodelling. Tissue Antigens 2011;77:271.
43. McEver RP. Rolling back neutrophil adhesion. Nat Immunol 2010;11:282.
44. Cassatella MA. Neutrophil-derived proteins: selling cytokines by the pound. In: Frank JD, editor. Adv Immunol 1999;73:369.
45. Massberg S, Grahl L, von Bruehl ML, et al. Reciprocal coupling of coagulation and innate immunity via neutrophil serine proteases. Nat Med 2010;16:887.
46. Kehrli ME Jr, Schmalstieg FC, Anderson DC, et al. Molecular definition of the bovine granulocytopathy syndrome: identification of deficiency of the Mac-1 (CD11b/CD18) glycoprotein. Am J Vet Res 1990;51:1826.
47. Mathew EC, Shaw JM, Bonilla FA, et al. A novel point mutation in CD18 causing the expression of dysfunctional CD11/CD18 leucocyte integrins in a patient with leucocyte adhesion deficiency (LAD). Clin Exp Immunol 2000;121:133.
48. Sipes KM, Edens HA, Kehrli ME Jr, et al. Analysis of surface antigen expression and host defense function in leukocytes from calves heterozygous or homozygous for bovine leukocyte adhesion deficiency. Am J Vet Res 1999;60:1255.

49. Ackermann MR, Kehrli ME, Laufer JA, et al. Alimentary and respiratory tract lesions in eight medically fragile Holstein cattle with bovine leukocyte adhesion deficiency (BLAD). Vet Pathol Online 1996;33:273.

50. Nagahata H. Bovine leukocyte adhesion deficiency (BLAD): a review. J Vet Med Sci 2004;66:1475.

51. Giger U, Boxer L, Simpson P, et al. Deficiency of leukocyte surface glycoproteins Mo1, LFA-1, and Leu M5 in a dog with recurrent bacterial infections: an animal model. Blood 1987;69:1622.

52. Trowald-Wigh G, Håkansson L, Johannisson A, et al. Leucocyte adhesion protein deficiency in Irish setter dogs. Vet Immunol Immunopathol 1992;32:261.

53. Kijas JMH, Bauer TR, Gäfvert S, et al. A missense mutation in the β-2 integrin gene (ITGB2) causes canine leukocyte adhesion deficiency. Genomics 1999;61:101.

54. Cauvin A, Connolly D. Immunodeficiency syndrome in Irish setters. Vet Rec 1997; 141:556.

55. Trowald-Wigh G, Ekman S, Hansson K, et al. Clinical, radiological and pathological features of 12 Irish setters with canine leucocyte adhesion deficiency. J Small Anim Pract 2000;41:211.

56. Prieur DJ, Collier LL. Neutropenia in cats with the Chediak-Higashi syndrome. Can J Vet Res 1987;51:407.

57. Kramer JW, Davis WC, Prieur DJ. The Chediak-Higashi syndrome of cats. Lab Invest 1977;36:554.

58. Kramer JW, Davis WC, Prieur DJ, et al. An inherited disorder of Persian cats with intracytoplasmic inclusions in neutrophils. J Am Vet Med Assoc 1975;166:1103.

59. Meyers KM, Seachord CL, Holmsen H, et al. Evaluation of the platelet storage pool deficiency in the feline counterpart of the Chediak-Higashi syndrome. Am J Hematol 1981;11:241.

60. Colgan SP, Gasper PW, Thrall MA, et al. Neutrophil function in normal and Chediak-Higashi syndrome cats following administration of recombinant canine granulocyte colony-stimulating factor. Exp Hematol 1992;20:1229.

61. Padgett GA. Neutrophilic function in animals with the Chediak-Higashi syndrome. Blood 1967;29:906.

62. Ayers JR, Leipold HW, Padgett GA. Lesions in Brangus cattle with Chediak-Higashi syndrome. Vet Pathol 1988;25:432.

63. Renshaw HW, Davis WC, Fudenberg HH, et al. Leukocyte dysfunction in the bovine homologue of the Chediak-Higashi syndrome of humans. Infect Immun 1974;10:928.

64. Shiraishi M, Ogawa H, Ikeda M, et al. Platelet dysfunction in Chediak-Higashi syndrome-affected cattle. J Vet Med Sci 2002;64:751.

65. Hirsch VM, Cunningham TA. Hereditary anomaly of neutrophil granulation in Birman cats. Am J Vet Res 1984;45:2170.

66. Cheville NF. The gray Collie syndrome. J Am Vet Med Assoc 1968;152:620.

67. Lund JE, Padgett GA, Ott RL. Cyclic neutropenia in grey collie dogs. Blood 1967;29: 452.

68. Lothrop CD Jr, Warren DJ, Souza LM, et al. Correction of canine cyclic hematopoiesis with recombinant human granulocyte colony-stimulating factor. Blood 1988;72:1324.

69. Dale DC, Alling DW, Wolff SM. Cyclic hematopoiesis: the mechanism of cyclic neutropenia in grey collie dogs. J Clin Invest 1972;51:2197.

70. Adamson JW, Dale DC, Elin RJ. Hematopoiesis in the grey collie dog: studies of the regulation of erythropoiesis. J Clin Invest 1974;54:965.

71. Dunn CD, Jones JB, Jolly JD, et al. Progenitor cells in canine cyclic hematopoiesis. Blood 1977;50:1111.

72. Patt HM, Lund JE, Maloney MA. Cyclic hematopoiesis in grey collie dogs: a stem-cell problem. Blood 1973;42:873.
73. Horwitz M, Benson KF, Person RE, et al. Mutations in ELA2, encoding neutrophil elastase, define a 21-day biological clock in cyclic haematopoiesis. Nat Genet 1999;23:433.
74. Horwitz MS, Duan Z, Korkmaz B, et al. Neutrophil elastase in cyclic and severe congenital neutropenia. Blood 2007;109:1817.
75. Pacheco JM, Traulsen A, Antal T, et al. Cyclic neutropenia in mammals. Am J Hematol 2008;83:920.
76. Benson KF, Li FQ, Person RE, et al. Mutations associated with neutropenia in dogs and humans disrupt intracellular transport of neutrophil elastase. Nat Genet 2003;35:90.
77. Dell'Angelica EC, Shotelersuk V, Aguilar RC, et al. Altered trafficking of lysosomal proteins in Hermansky-Pudlak syndrome due to mutations in the beta 3A subunit of the AP-3 adaptor. Mol Cell 1999;3:11.
78. Meng R, Bridgman R, Toivio-Kinnucan M, et al. Neutrophil elastase-processing defect in cyclic hematopoietic dogs. Exp Hematol 2010;38:104.
79. Bowles CA, Alsaker RD, Wolfle TL. Studies of the Pelger-Huet anomaly in foxhounds. Am J Pathol 1979;96:237.
80. Gill AF, Gaunt S, Sirninger J. Congenital Pelger-Huet anomaly in a horse. Vet Clin Pathol 2006;35:460.
81. Grondin TM, DeWitt SF, Keeton KS. Pelger-Huet anomaly in an Arabian horse. Vet Clin Pathol 2007;36:306.
82. Latimer KS, Rakich PM, Thompson DF. Pelger-Huet anomaly in cats. Vet Pathol 1985;22:370.
83. Nachtsheim H. The Pelger-anomaly in man and rabbit; a mendelian character of the nuclei of the leucocytes. J Hered 1950;41:131.
84. Hoffmann K, Dreger CK, Ollns AL, et al. Mutations in the gene encoding the lamin B receptor produce an altered nuclear morphology in granulocytes (Pelger-Huet anomaly). Nat Genet 2002;31:410.
85. Latimer KS, Rowland GN, Mahaffey MB. Homozygous Pelger-Huet anomaly and chondrodysplasia in a stillborn kitten. Vet Pathol 1988;25:325.
86. Cohen TV, Klarmann KD, Sakchaisri K, et al. The lamin B receptor under transcriptional control of C/EBPepsilon is required for morphological but not functional maturation of neutrophils. Hum Mol Genet 2008;17:2921.
87. Latimer KS, Kircher IM, Lindl PA, et al. Leukocyte function in Pelger-Huet anomaly of dogs. J Leukoc Biol 1989;45:301.
88. Aroch I, Ofri R, Aizenberg I. Haematological, ocular and skeletal abnormalities in a samoyed family. J Small Anim Pract 1996;37:333.
89. Degousee N, Ghomashchi F, Stefanski E, et al. Groups IV, V, and X phospholipases A2s in human neutrophils: role in eicosanoid production and gram-negative bacterial phospholipid hydrolysis. J Biol Chem 2002;277:5061.
90. Kaushansky K, Williams WJ. Williams hematology. 8th edition. New York: McGraw-Hill Medical; 2010.

Evaluation and Clinical Application of Platelet Function Testing in Small Animal Practice

Pete W. Christopherson, DVM, PhD*,
Elizabeth A. Spangler, DVM, PhD,
Mary K. Boudreaux, DVM, PhD

KEYWORDS

- Primary hemostasis • Platelet adhesion • Platelet aggregation
- Platelet granule secretion • Clot retraction

Platelets are the first line of defense at sites of vascular injury and are often referred to as agents of primary hemostasis. Platelets adhere to exposed subendothelial surfaces, form aggregates, and release granule contents that serve a variety of functions including recruitment of additional platelets, providing a localized source of coagulation and fibrinolytic proteins, and providing proteins chemotactic for fibroblasts and other cells necessary for tissue repair. Platelets also serve as a scaffold for the assembly of coagulation proteins necessary for the efficient formation of fibrin, also known as secondary hemostasis. Additionally, platelets provide the muscle needed to retract and stabilize the clot, an important event for preventing premature clot dissolution. Disruption of platelet function at virtually any level can lead to abnormal hemorrhage. Platelet-type bleeding is usually characterized by mucosal bleeding and/or petechial to ecchymotic hemorrhages that may appear on the skin or mucosal surfaces. Often platelet-type hemorrhages are insidious (microscopic gastrointestinal and urinary tract bleeding as examples) and with time can result in iron-deficiency anemia. Platelet function assays can assist the clinician in determining the level at which platelet function has been compromised (**Fig. 1**). Examples of assays to consider are presented next. Availability in veterinary medicine is variable, and many of these methods are only offered at centers focused on evaluation of platelet function.

The authors have nothing to disclose.
Department of Pathobiology, Auburn University College of Veterinary Medicine, 166 Greene Hall, Auburn, AL 36849, USA
* Corresponding author.
E-mail address: chrispw@auburn.edu

Vet Clin Small Anim 42 (2012) 173–188
doi:10.1016/j.cvsm.2011.09.013
0195-5616/12/$ – see front matter © 2012 Elsevier Inc. All rights reserved.

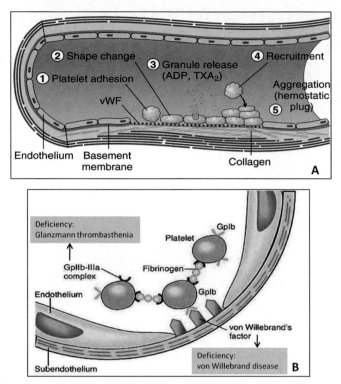

Fig. 1. (*A*) Illustration of the major platelet processes involved in primary hemostasis. With vessel injury, platelet adherence to the subendothelium is mediated primarily by von Willebrand factor (vWF). Platelets concurrently undergo shape change and release granule contents, which recruit more platelets to the site of vascular damage. Platelet aggregation occurs by activated platelets binding fibrinogen and leads to the formation of a primary hemostatic plug. (*B*) Illustration of platelet interactions during adhesion and aggregation. Adhesion occurs primarily through the binding of glycoprotein Ib (GpIb) on platelet surfaces to von Willebrand factor bound to subendothelial collagen. Aggregation is mediated through platelet glycoprotein IIb-IIIa complexes (GpIIb-IIIa) binding to fibrinogen. Quantitative or qualitative deficiencies in von Willebrand factor or glycoprotein IIb-IIIa result in von Willebrand disease or Glanzmann thrombasthenia, respectively. (*Adapted from* Mitchell RN, Cotran RS. Hemodynamic disorders, thrombosis, and shock. In: Cotran RS, Kumar V, Collins T, editors. Pathologic basis of disease. 6th edition. Philadelphia: W.B. Saunders Company; 1999. p. 113–38; with permission.)

WHOLE BLOOD ASSAYS OF PLATELET FUNCTION
Buccal Mucosal Bleeding Time

The buccal mucosal bleeding time (BMBT) is a screening test for disorders of primary hemostasis that is readily available in veterinary practice. The bleeding time is performed on the buccal mucosa using a spring-loaded cassette that delivers two incisions of a precise depth and length.[1] The buccal mucosa is everted and held gently in place with a gauze strip during performance of the test. The incisions are observed until bleeding stops, primarily due to platelet adhesion and aggregation, using care not to disturb the incisions during the procedure. The technique may require that the animal be anesthetized, particularly if the animal is fractious, shakes its head, or licks at the incisions. Use of the bleeding time to evaluate primary hemostasis should be reserved for those patients in which the platelet count is normal and platelet function is questioned. The technique is especially useful in dogs with suspected von Willebrand disease (VWD) prior to surgery. A normal BMBT should be 2 to 3 minutes. The BMBT can be prolonged with thrombocytopenia, acquired platelet function defects, VWD, or intrinsic platelet function disorders. The BMBT is not useful for the detection of coagulopathies, including hemophilia.[2]

Aperture Closure Instruments

The Platelet Function Analyzer–100 (PFA-100, Siemens Healthcare Diagnostics, Deerfield, IL, USA) is an example of an aperture closure instrument that can be used to document global platelet adhesion and aggregation that occurs under high shear.[3] The instrument aspirates citrated whole blood through a capillary tube and a compartment containing test cartridge membranes. The test cartridge membranes have a small centrally located aperture and are coated with collagen and either adenosine diphosphate (ADP) or epinephrine. As blood flows under high shear across the membrane and through the aperture, platelets become activated and begin to adhere and aggregate, resulting in closure of the aperture within 1 to 3 minutes. The instrument measures the decrease in flow rate with time until flow completely stops. The final closure time (CT) and volume of blood flow are recorded by the instrument. The CT is affected by many variables in addition to platelet function including platelet count, hematocrit, von Willebrand factor (vWF) levels, and improper sample handling including errors in anticoagulant to blood ratio. The PFA-100 has shown value when used in combination with the vWF antigen and collagen binding assays to characterize canine VWD.[4] Dogs with acquired type 2 VWD secondary to high shear associated with heart valve disorders have prolonged CT,[5,6] and a study using the PFA-100 also identified platelet dysfunction in a group of dachshunds with mild to moderate myxomatous mitral valve disease.[7]

Viscoelastic Coagulation Analyzers

Thrombelastography (TEG; Haemoscope Corporation, Niles, IL, USA) and Rotational Thromboelastometry (ROTEM; Pentapharm GmbH, Munich, Germany) are similar methods that detect viscoelastic changes in whole blood during polymerization of fibrin under low shear conditions and provide a dynamic view of hemostasis.[8,9] The Sonoclot Analyzer (Sienco Inc, Arvada, CO, USA) also detects viscoelastic changes during clot formation, but few reports describe the use of this instrument in veterinary medicine,[10,11] and it is not described in detail in this report. A comparative description of each method is provided in a recent review.[12] Readouts from TEG/ROTEM provide a graphic view of clot formation and clot lysis over time (**Fig. 2**). In the clinical laboratory setting citrated whole blood samples are usually evaluated and clot formation is initiated by recalcification of the sample at a defined time after blood collection. Activators of coagulation such as kaolin or tissue factor can be used to decrease the time required to generate a tracing and may decrease analytical variation.[13,14] Standardization within the laboratory, including the time period between sample collection and performance of the assay, is critical for the interpretation of results.[15] Values measured by the instruments reflect the time to initial fibrin formation, rate of clot development, maximum clot strength, and rate of fibrinolysis (**Table 1**). Platelet number and function are major determinants of clot strength, but fibrinogen concentration and efficiency of fibrin production also contribute. The sensitivity of TEG/ROTEM to specific defects in platelet function is variable. For example, maximum clot strength is substantially decreased in animals with

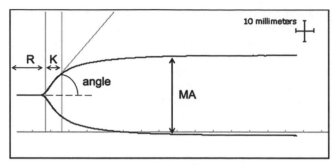

Fig. 2. TEG tracing from a normal dog. R (minutes) is the time for initial fibrin formation, and is measured from the start of the reaction until the tracing reaches an amplitude of 2 mm. K (minutes) reflects the rate of clot accumulation, and is the time required to reach a defined clot strength, with a tracing amplitude of 20 mm. The α-angle (degrees) also reflects the rate of clot accumulation and is determined by a line drawn tangential to the tracing from 2 to 20 mm amplitude. MA (millimeters) is the maximum width of the tracing and is an indication of maximum clot strength.

Glanzmann thrombasthenia, in which a quantitative or qualitative decrease in the platelet glycoprotein IIb-IIIa (GPIIb-IIIa) complex impairs platelet aggregation and clot retraction (E. A. Spangler, unpublished observation).[16] Because these methods are performed under low shear conditions, they are not sensitive to defects in platelet adhesion or vWF deficiency. The platelet contribution to clot strength has been specifically evaluated through modification of TEG/ROTEM by addition of cytochalasin D, which inhibits actin polymerization and thus impairs platelet function by preventing events that require the actin cytoskeleton.[17,18] Conventional TEG/ROTEM are not sensitive methods for evaluating the effects of platelet function inhibitors that target specific pathways of platelet activation, such as clopidogrel, because thrombin produced during coagulation results in strong platelet activation. A modified strategy for TEG (PlateletMapping) uses blood collected with heparin to eliminate thrombin activity. Reptilase and factor XIII are used to generate a cross-linked fibrin clot, and

Table 1
Comparison of values routinely measured by thrombelastography (TEG) and rotational thromboelastometry (ROTEM)

Variable	TEG	ROTEM	Units
Time to initial fibrin formation (0–2 mm amplitude)	R	CT	minutes
Time to standard clot strength (2–20 mm amplitude)	K	CFT	minutes
Slope of the tracing between 2 and 20 mm amplitude	α angle	α angle	degrees
Maximum clot strength	MA	MCF	millimeters
Maximum clot strength	G	. . .	dynes/cm²
Clot lysis	LY30, LY60	CL30, CL60	%

TEG measurements: R, reaction time; MA, maximum amplitude; LY30, % lysis at 30 minutes; LY60, % lysis at 60 minutes. K and α-angle indicate the rate of clot formation. G is calculated from MA (G = 5000 × MA/(100 − MA). ROTEM measurements: CT, clot time; CFT, clot formation time; MCF, maximum clot firmness; CL30, % clot lysis at 30 minutes; CL60, % clot lysis at 60 minutes. CFT and α-angle indicate the rate of clot formation.

platelet activation is initiated by the addition of agonists such as ADP or arachidonic acid. Maximum hemostatic activity of the blood sample is measured in citrated blood activated with kaolin, and the combined results of these tests are used to calculate platelet function.[19,20] This approach has been used in dogs to assess the effects of clopidogrel,[21] but clinical application of this method may be limited by cost. In addition, because canine platelets have a variable response to arachidonic acid, evaluation of platelet responses to arachidonic acid–induced platelet activation should be done with caution in dogs.[22]

VerifyNow

The sample analyzed with the VerifyNow (Accumetrics, San Diego, CA, USA) is citrated or heparinized whole blood. The assay uses fibrinogen-coated beads that are bound by activated platelets. The change in light transmission that occurs with platelet aggregation/agglutination is recorded and compared to a control sample. Agonists used include ADP (to check for effectiveness of ADP antagonists such as clopidogrel), arachidonic acid (to check for aspirin effectiveness), and thrombin receptor activation peptide (TRAP; to check for GPIIb-IIIa antagonist effectiveness). As mentioned previously, canine platelets have a variable response to arachidonic acid.[22] Additionally, TRAPs are not effective in activating canine platelets.[23] Therefore, the assays assessing aspirin effectiveness or inhibition of GPIIb-IIIa are not recommended for use in dogs.

PlateletWorks

The PlateletWorks assay (Helena Laboratories UK, Ltd, Sunderland, England) compares platelet counts obtained prior to and after the addition of a platelet activating agent such as ADP or collagen. One sample is collected into EDTA; other samples are collected into tubes containing 3.2% citrate and either ADP, arachidonic acid, or collagen for platelet activation. Platelet counts are performed on the EDTA-anticoagulated sample and on the activated samples within 10 minutes of collection using an impedance counter. Percentage aggregation is calculated by the following equation: Percent (%) Aggregation = (Baseline Platelet Count − Agonist Platelet Count) ÷ Baseline Platelet Count × 100. Percent Inhibition can be calculated using the following equation: Percent Inhibition = Agonist Platelet Count ÷ Baseline Platelet Count × 100. While the technique is simple and rapid and requires a fairly small volume of blood, it is highly operator-dependent and lack of correlation with other methods of evaluating platelet function has been reported.[24] The method appeared to be useful in the evaluation of clopidogrel effects on feline platelets.[25]

Multiplate

The Multiplate analyzer or Multiplate electrical impedance aggregometry (MEA) (Dynabyte, Munich, Germany) is also known as Multiplate impedance platelet aggregometry (IPA). The sample for this instrument is whole blood collected in either heparin or hirudin, a direct thrombin inhibitor. The manufacturers of the system recommend using thrombin inhibitors as anticoagulants, instead of calcium chelators such as citrate, in an effort to maintain near physiologic concentrations of calcium. However, samples are diluted 1:1 with 0.9% NaCl before analysis,[26] and as a result, calcium concentrations are still reduced. The instrument uses two silver-coated copper wires to detect platelet adhesion/aggregation after agonist addition by measuring the increase in electrical resistance between the two wires. An aggregation tracing is generated, which allows the user to assess the quality and quantity of platelet activation. Results are expressed in aggregation units and plotted against time over 6 minutes. The extent of aggregation can be measured at the maximal height of the tracing and the rate of the reaction can be determined by measuring the slope of the tracing. Platelet activity is quantified and reported as area under the curve (AUC) and is affected by the height and slope of the aggregation tracing. Several agonists are marketed by the manufacturer including ADP (with and without PGE[1]), collagen, arachidonic acid, ristocetin, and TRAP-6. Ristocetin is marketed as an agonist for detection of VWD; however, the usefulness of this assay in dogs is not clear. TRAPs are ineffective and arachidonic acid is inconsistent for activation of canine platelets.[22,23]

Impact-R

The Impact Cone and Plate(let) analyzer (Matis Medical, Beersel, Belgium) is marketed as a research instrument under the name Impact-R (Image analysis, Monitoring, Platelet, Adhesion, Cone & Plate Technology). Citrated whole blood is subjected to uniform shear by the spinning of a cone in a cup. The system mimics platelet adhesion and aggregation in response to addition of an agonist under physiologic conditions. Platelet adhesion and aggregation are evaluated using image analysis software after automated staining of adhered platelets in the cup. Agonist (ADP, collagen) addition allows determination of the effectiveness of antiplatelet medications such as clopidogrel or aspirin.[27,28] The authors are not aware of any studies using this instrument in domestic animals.

ADHESION ASSAYS
Collagen Binding

The collagen-binding activity assay (CBA) is a method of evaluating the function of vWF and is useful for the identification of dogs with acquired or inherited Type 2 VWD.[29] CBA ELISA assays use collagen-coated microtiter plates to assess for vWF binding capacity. The ratio of vWF-antigen to vWF-CBA can be used to distinguish Type 2 VWD from Types 1 and 3. Dogs with Type 2 VWD will have vWF antigen assay results that are discordant with their CBA results due to the reduced presence of the more functional high molecular weight multimers of vWF. Ratios of vWF-antigen to vWF-CBA greater than 2 are consistent with the diagnosis of Type 2 VWD. Distinguishing acquired and inherited forms of Type 2 VWD requires treatment of potential underlying causes of acquired VWD and subsequent reevaluation of the vWF-antigen to vWF-CBA ratio.

vWF Antigen

The vWF antigen ELISA is a useful quantitative method for the diagnosis of Type 1 and Type 3 VWD.[30] Type 1 VWD is the most common form of VWD in dogs, although several breeds have been identified with Type 3 VWD.[30,31] Inherited Type 2 VWD is rare and has only been identified in German shorthair pointers and German wirehair pointers.[32,33] Dogs with Type 1 VWD generally have vWF antigen levels that are less than 15%, while dogs with Type 3 VWD have no detectable vWF. The quantitative nature of these assays makes them unsuitable as stand-alone assays for the diagnosis of Type 2 VWD.

vWF Function

Functional assays for diagnosis of VWD include the ristocetin and botrocetin (venom coagglutinin) assays.[34,35] These agents bind to distinct sites on vWF, resulting in a change in the conformation of the vWF A1 domain and subsequent vWF binding to platelet GPIb-IX-V receptors.[36] The resulting platelet agglutination is proportional to the amount of vWF present in the sample. These assays are performed at very few research laboratories.

PLATELET AGGREGATION ASSAYS
Platelet Aggregometry

Platelet aggregation testing is the gold standard for evaluation of platelet function. Platelet aggregometers assess the ability of platelets to form aggregates using light transmission (platelet-rich-plasma) or impedance (whole blood, see section on MultiPlate) as monitoring methods. Light transmission methods are more sensitive to subtle changes in platelet function than impedance methods. Platelet-rich plasma is isolated from citrated blood samples and exposed to platelet agonists such as gamma thrombin, collagen, ADP, and platelet activating factor. Platelet aggregation is measured by detection of increased light transmission (**Fig. 3**). By using a variety of agonists at varying concentrations, specific pathways of platelet signaling can often be dissected using this technique. This can greatly facilitate the characterization of inherited disorders at the biochemical and molecular levels.[37] Patients with Glanzmann thrombasthenia (Great Pyrenees, Otterhounds, and horses) have a reduced or absent platelet aggregation response to all agonists[37–40] (**Fig. 4**), while animals with platelet signal transduction disorders (Basset Hound, Eskimo Spitz, Landseer-ECT, and bovine CalDAG-GEFI disorders) have a reduced to absent platelet aggregation response to most agonists and an impaired response to thrombin.[37,41–44]

Platelet aggregation testing can also be useful for monitoring the effectiveness of anti-platelet medications. Drug dosages can be tailored specifically to patients based on their degree of platelet inhibition. In some prothrombotic conditions, medication dosages may have to be increased to maintain platelet inhibition, and in others, platelet inhibition may not be possible using certain medications, including COX inhibitors.[45,46] Platelet aggregation methods require specialized equipment and expertise in the methods of platelet isolation (for light transmission methods) and evaluation of results. Because optical aggregometry assays must be completed within 4 hours of blood collection, the patient usually must be on or near the premises of the testing facility.

Clot Retraction

Clot retraction is a test of platelet function that can be performed in a clinical setting. As with the bleeding time, this technique should be reserved for animals that are known to have normal platelet numbers but questionable platelet function. The clot retraction test should also not be performed in animals known to be on medication that will inhibit platelet function. The clot retraction test is a test of platelet function that relies on the normal interaction between thrombin, platelet receptors, and fibrinogen. Because the assay specifically documents the ability of platelets to respond to thrombin, not all animals with a platelet function defect will have an abnormal clot retraction test. Basset Hounds and Eskimo Spitz dogs with CalDAG-GEFI thrombopathia have platelets that will interact with thrombin and express fibrinogen receptors; therefore, the clot retraction test in these patients is normal.[41,47] Otterhounds, Great Pyrenees, and horses with Glanzmann thrombasthenia have platelets that either lack or have reduced amounts of the receptor needed for normal interaction with fibrinogen.[38–40] These patients have abnormal clot retraction (**Fig. 5**). Patients with VWD have normal clot retraction.

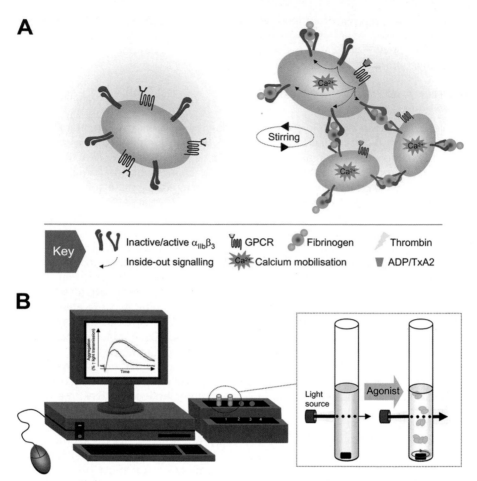

Fig. 3. Traditional model of platelet aggregation. (*A*) Three important blood and platelet elements are important for platelet aggregation testing: an activating stimulus (typically a soluble agonist), fibrinogen, and platelet surface fibrinogen receptors (GPIIb-IIIa complexes). Activation of the GPIIb-IIIa complexes is essential for fibrinogen binding and subsequent platelet aggregation. (*B*) Platelet aggregometry is a technique that involves stirring a suspension of platelets (platelet-rich-plasma or PRP) in the presence of a platelet agonist and detecting changes in light transmission. Light transmission increases with platelet aggregation and is recorded digitally or on a strip chart recorder. (*From* Jackson SP. The growing complexity of platelet aggregation. Blood 2007;109:5087–95; with permission.)

FLOW CYTOMETRY
Membrane Glycoproteins

Monoclonal antibodies recognizing glycoproteins IIb and IIIa (alpha IIb and beta 3 integrin subunits) or polyclonal antibodies recognizing the entire GPIIb-IIIa complex are available commercially and can be used to diagnose or rule out Glanzmann thrombasthenia in dogs and horses (**Fig. 6**).[38,48] This methodology is relatively quick and definitive for identifying affected animals but does not reliably identify heterozygous animals. Monoclonal antibodies recognizing other platelet integrins or proteins

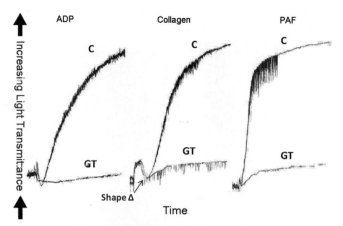

Fig. 4. Aggregometry tracings demonstrating markedly reduced platelet aggregation responses to ADP, collagen, and platelet activating factor (PAF) in a horse with Glanzmann thrombasthenia (reduced light transmittance) compared with a normal control horse. Similar responses were observed to all concentrations of agonists. Traces from the control horse are labeled C; traces from the affected horse are labeled GT. The shape change response, which is present in both horses for all agonists, is indicated in the collagen aggregation tracing. (*Adapted from* Livesey L, Christopherson P, Hammond A, et al. Platelet dysfunction (Glanzmann's thrombasthenia) in horses. J Vet Intern Med 2005;19:917–9; with permission.)

such as the collagen receptor or vWF receptor are not readily available for dogs, cats, or horses.

FLOW CYTOMETRY: ACTIVATION-SPECIFIC CHANGES

Antibodies that bind specifically to activated platelets and minimally to nonactivated platelets are considered activation-specific antibodies.[49] These antibodies can be used to evaluate platelet dysfunction, detect in vivo platelet activation, and monitor efficacy of medications. Although these antibodies have primarily been developed against human platelets, some do cross-react with platelets from other species. Studies assessing the detection of activated platelets in dogs[50] and in horses[51] have been published. Activation-specific changes on platelets that can be detected using antibodies and flow cytometric techniques include the following categories:

Receptor-Induced Binding Sites (RIBS)

Antibodies that bind preferentially to surface bound rather than soluble ligand due to the presence of antigens on the ligand that become expressed as a result of binding a receptor are termed RIBS antibodies. CAP-1 is a monoclonal antibody that recognizes an RIBS epitope on canine fibrinogen.[52] This antibody binds minimally to soluble fibrinogen but binds avidly to fibrinogen that has become bound to the GPIIb-IIIa complex and thus can be used to evaluate the functionality of the GPIIb-IIIa receptor in response to various agonists. Recently the antibody was found to be useful in evaluating platelet function in samples that had been collected 24 hours earlier using CPDA-1 as the anticoagulant. This allowed evaluation of platelets in samples from dogs that were not on the premises of the testing facility and in one instance led to the identification of a previously undocumented intrinsic platelet disorder.[53]

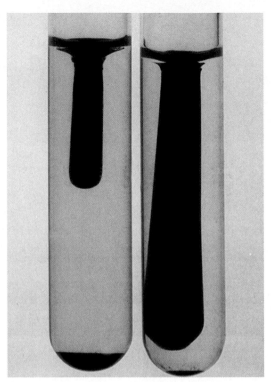

Fig. 5. Photograph depicting dilute whole-blood clot retraction for samples obtained from an unaffected Otterhound (*left tube*) and an otterhound with Glanzmann thrombasthenia (*right tube*). Samples were stimulated with 0.2 U of bovine thrombin and allowed to incubate undisturbed for 4 hours at 37°C. Notice the failure (score of 1+, reference range, 3 to 4+) of the platelets of the affected otterhound to effect retraction of the clot. (*From* Boudreaux MK, Catalfamo JL. Molecular and genetic basis for thrombasthenic thrombopathia in Otterhounds. Am J Vet Res 2001;62:1797–804; with permission.)

Ligand-Induced Binding Sites (LIBS)

Antibodies that recognize epitopes on GPIIb-IIIa that become expressed when an RGD-containing ligand binds to the receptor are called LIBS antibodies.[54] Several LIBS antibodies, most of which recognize epitopes on GPIIIa, have been developed for use in people.[54] Many of these antibodies show promise of being useful in other species since the epitopes they recognize are highly conserved across species.[55] D3 has been shown to recognize LIBS on canine, rabbit, and porcine platelets,[56] while LIBS1 has been shown to recognize LIBS on rabbit platelets.[57] These antibodies have been shown to recognize activated platelets in vivo and in vitro. More recently, LIBS antibodies coupled to microparticles of iron oxide have been used to visualize areas of platelet accumulation in arteries using magnetic resonance imaging techniques.[58,59]

Granule Membrane Proteins

Antibodies that recognize granule lining membrane proteins that become exteriorized following platelet granule release fall into this category. The most well-known

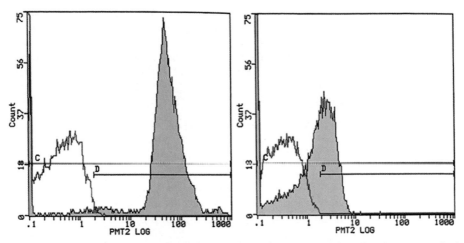

Fig. 6. Flow cytometric analysis of the binding of anti–CD41/CD61 (GPIIb-IIIa complex) antibody to platelets from a control horse and from a horse with Glanzmann thrombasthenia. The unshaded peaks (to the left of gate D) represent nonspecific binding of secondary FITC-labeled antibody only. The shaded peaks (within gate D) represent binding of antibody to control horse platelets (*left*) and affected horse platelets (*right*) incubated with primary and secondary antibody. Binding of antibody to platelets of the Glanzmann horse was markedly reduced when compared with binding of antibody to normal horse platelets. (*Adapted from* Livesey L, Christopherson P, Hammond A, et al. Platelet dysfunction (Glanzmann's thrombasthenia) in horses. J Vet Intern Med 2005;19:917–9; with permission.)

granule membrane protein that is used for evaluation of platelet activation is P-selectin. A monoclonal antibody that recognizes P-selectin on dog platelets has been developed.[60]

Granule Secreted Proteins

Antibodies that recognize soluble proteins unique to platelets that have been secreted during the platelet release reaction fall into this category. Monoclonal antibodies recognizing beta-thromboglobulin are used extensively for the evaluation of human platelet activation.[61] Unfortunately, commercial antibodies that recognize dog, cat, or horse beta-thromboglobulin are not available.

Activated GPIIb-IIIa

Monoclonal antibodies recognizing activated GPIIb-IIIa complexes can be used to help distinguish disorders in which the complex is present but not functional. PAC-1, which does not cross-react with canine platelets, is the most well-recognized antibody of this type for evaluating human platelet activation.[62] Unfortunately, antibodies that cross-react with activated GPIIb-IIIa receptors on dog, cat, or horse platelets are not commercially available.

Annexin V Binding

Activated platelets provide a negatively charged surface for the assembly of coagulation protein complexes. This procoagulant surface results primarily from exteriorization of phosphatidylserine (PS).[63] Annexin V is a protein that preferentially binds to negatively charged phospholipids such as PS, and FITC-labeled annexin V detected via flow cytometry can be used as a marker for the expression of PS on the surface of activated platelets.[64] The inability of platelets to express a procoagulant surface has been described in humans and is called Scott syndrome.[65] A similar disorder has been characterized in a family of German shepherd dogs.[66] Because thrombin generation and subsequent clot formation are severely impaired in this disorder, clinical signs resemble those seen with a coagulopathy rather than those typically seen with a thrombopathia.

GRANULE DISORDERS/FUNCTIONAL AND QUANTITATIVE ASSAYS
Electron Microscopy

Platelets have three main types of granules: alpha, dense, and lysosomal. Granules can be evaluated both quantitatively (amount of granules—are they absent or reduced?) and qualitatively (content of granules—are these absent or reduced?) at the electron microscopic level. Dense granules can be evaluated using Uranaffin-stained platelets. Granules can be counted and then categorized based on quantity and quality of their contents.

Serotonin Uptake and Release

^{14}C-serotonin can be used to monitor the ability of platelets to take up and release serotonin simultaneous with evaluation of platelet aggregation. The technique is very useful for evaluation of platelet disorders caused by primary granule defects (storage pool deficiency) or signal transduction defects that result in the inability of platelets to undergo normal granule release.[42,67]

ATP Release

ATP release can be monitored concurrent with evaluation of platelet aggregation using luciferin-luciferase–based methodology. The technique does not require the use of radioactive materials. ATP release defects can be seen with primary granule disorders as well as with signal transduction disorders.

SUMMARY

Tests that evaluate many aspects of platelet function have been applied in both human and veterinary medicine for the monitoring of treatment with platelet function inhibitors and for detection of platelet function abnormalities (inherited or acquired). Interspecies variation in the response to various platelet agonists is an important consideration when methods that have been developed for people are applied in other species. At the present time, many of these assays are not readily available in standard veterinary practice. Advanced platelet function testing for veterinary patients is offered at select academic institutions. Discussion with a specialist is recommended when considering the use of these tests, and the relative strengths and limitations of each assay should be considered in the interpretation of test results.

REFERENCES

1. Jergens AE, Turrentine MA, Kraus KH, et al. Buccal mucosa bleeding times of healthy dogs and of dogs in various pathologic states, including thrombocytopenia, uremia, and von Willebrand's disease. Am J Vet Res 1987;48:1337–42.
2. Brooks M, Catalfamo J. Buccal mucosa bleeding time is prolonged in canine models of primary hemostatic disorders. Thromb Haemost 1993;70:777–80.
3. Harrison P. The role of PFA-100 testing in the investigation and management of haemostatic defects in children and adults. Br J Haematol 2005;130:3–10.

4. Burgess HJ, Woods JP, Abrams-Ogg ACG, et al. Evaluation of laboratory methods to improve characterization of dogs with von Willebrand disease. Can J Vet Res 2009;73:252–9.
5. Tarnow I, Kristensen AT, Texel H, et al. Decreased platelet function in Cavalier King Charles Spaniels with mitral valve regurgitation. J Vet Intern Med 2003;17:680–6.
6. Tarnow I, Kristensen AT, Olsen LH, et al. Dogs with heart diseases causing turbulent high-velocity blood flow have changes in platelet function and von Willebrand factor multimer distribution. J Vet Intern Med 2005;19:515–22.
7. Moesgaard SG, Sørensen TM, Sterup A, et al. Changes in platelet function in Dachshunds with early stages of myxomatous mitral valve disease. Res Vet Sci 2009;86:320–4
8. Kol A, Borjesson DL. Application of thrombelastography/thromboelastometry to veterinary medicine. Vet Clin Pathol 2010;39:405–16.
9. Brooks MB, Stokol T, Catalfamo JL. Comparative hemostasis: animal models and new hemostasis tests. Clin Lab Med 2011;31:139–59.
10. Dallap Schaer BL, Wilkins PA, Boston R, et al. Preliminary evaluation of hemostasis in neonatal foals using a viscoelastic coagulation and platelet function analyzer. J Vet Emerg Crit Care (San Antonio) 2009;19:81–7.
11. Dallap Schaer BL, Bentz AI, Boston RC, et al. Comparison of viscoelastic coagulation analysis and standard coagulation profiles in critically ill neonatal foals to outcome. J Vet Emerg Crit Care (San Antonio) 2009;19:88–95.
12. McMichael MA, Smith SA. Viscoelastic coagulation testing: technology, applications, and limitations. Vet Clin Pathol 2011;40:140–53.
13. Johansson PI, Bochsen L, Andersen S, et al. Investigation of the effect of kaolin and tissue-factor-activated citrated whole blood, on clot-forming variables, as evaluated by thromboelastography. Transfusion 2008;48(11):2377–83.
14. Wiinberg B, Kristensen AT. Thromboelastography in veterinary medicine. Semin Thromb Hemost 2010;36:747–56.
15. Wiinberg B, Jensen AL, Rojkjaer R, et al. Validation of human recombinant tissue factor-activated thromboelastography on citrated whole blood from clinically healthy dogs. Vet Clin Pathol 2005;34:389–93.
16. Macieira S, Rivard GE, Champagne J, et al. Glanzmann thrombasthenia in an Oldenbourg filly. Vet Clin Pathol 2007;36:204–8.
17. Nielsen VG, Geary BT, Baird MS. Evaluation of the contribution of platelets to clot strength by thromboelastography in rabbits: the role of tissue factor and cytochalasin D. Anesth Analg 2000;91:35–9.
18. Theusinger OM, Nurnberg J, Asmis LM, et al. Rotation thromboelastometry (ROTEM) stability and reproducibility over time. Eur J Cardiothorac Surg 2010;37:677–83.
19. Craft RM, Chavez JJ, Bresee SJ, et al. A novel modification of the Thrombelastograph assay, isolating platelet function, correlates with optical platelet aggregation. J Lab Clin Med 2004;143:301–9.
20. Bochsen L, Wiinberg B, Kjelgaard-Hansen M, et al. Evaluation of the TEG platelet mapping assay in blood donors. Thromb J 2007;5:3.
21. Brainard BM, Kleine SA, Papich MG, et al. Pharmacodynamic and pharmacokinetic evaluation of clopidogrel and the carboxylic acid metabolite SR 26334 in healthy dogs. Am J Vet Res 2010;71:822–30.
22. Johnson GJ, Leis LA, Rao GH, et al. Arachidonate-induced platelet aggregation in the dog. Thromb Res 1979;14:147–54.
23. Catalfamo J, Andersen TT, Fenton JW II. Thrombin receptor-activating peptides unlike thrombin are insufficient for platelet activation in most species [abstract]. Thromb Haemost 1993;69:1195.

24. van Werkum JW, Kleibeuker M, Postma S, et al. A comparison between the Platelet-works-assay and light transmittance aggregometry for monitoring the inhibitory effects of clopidogrel. Int J Cardiol 2010;140:123–6.

25. Hamel-Jolette A, Dunn M, Bedard C. Plateletworks: a screening assay for clopidogrel therapy monitoring in healthy cats. Can J Vet Res 2009;73:73–6.

26. Can MM, Tanboga IH, Turkyilmaz E, et al. The risk of false results in the assessment of platelet function in the absence of antiplatelet medication: comparison of the PFA-100, multiplate electrical impedance aggregometry and verify now assays. Thromb Res 2010;125:e132–7.

27. Michelson AD, Frelinger AL 3rd, Furman MI. Current options in platelet function testing. Am J Cardiol 2006;98:4N–10N.

28. Shenkman B, Savion N, Dardik R, et al. Testing of platelet deposition on polystyrene surface under flow conditions by the cone and plate(let) analyzer: role of platelet activation, fibrinogen and von Willebrand factor. Thromb Res 2000;99:353–61.

29. Sabino EP, Erb HN, Catalfamo JL. Development of a collagen-binding activity assay as a screening test for type II von Willebrand disease in dogs. Am J Vet Res 2006;67:242–9.

30. Brooks M, Dodds WJ, Raymond SL. Epidemiologic features of von Willebrand's disease in Doberman pinschers, Scottish terriers, and Shetland sheepdogs: 260 cases (1984–1988). J Am Vet Med Assoc 1992;200:1123–7.

31. Raymond SL, Jones DW, Brooks MB, et al. Clinical and laboratory features of a severe form of von Willebrand disease in Shetland sheepdogs. J Am Vet Med Assoc 1990;197:1342–6.

32. Johnson GS TM, Dodds WJ. Type II von Willebrand's disease in German shorthair pointers [abstract]. Vet Clin Pathol 1987;16:7.

33. Brooks M, Raymond S, Catalfamo J. Severe, recessive von Willebrand's disease in German Wirehaired Pointers. J Am Vet Med Assoc 1996;209:926–9.

34. Johnson GS, Turrentine MA, Tomlinson JL. Detection of von Willebrand's disease in dogs with a rapid qualitative test, based on venom-coagglutinin-induced platelet agglutination. Vet Clin Pathol 1985;14:11–8.

35. Read MS, Smith SV, Lamb MA, et al. Role of botrocetin in platelet agglutination: formation of an activated complex of botrocetin and von Willebrand factor. Blood 1989;74:1031–5.

36. De Luca M, Facey DA, Favaloro EJ, et al. Structure and function of the von Willebrand factor A1 domain: analysis with monoclonal antibodies reveals distinct binding sites involved in recognition of the platelet membrane glycoprotein Ib-IX-V complex and ristocetin-dependent activation. Blood 2000;95:164–72.

37. Boudreaux MK. Characteristics, diagnosis, and treatment of inherited platelet disorders in mammals. J Am Vet Med Assoc 2008;233:1251–9.

38. Boudreaux MK, Kvam K, Dillon AR, et al. Type I Glanzmann's thrombasthenia in a Great Pyrenees dog. Vet Pathol 1996;33:503–11.

39. Livesey L, Christopherson P, Hammond A, et al. Platelet dysfunction (Glanzmann's thrombasthenia) in horses. J Vet Intern Med 2005;19:917–9.

40. Boudreaux MK, Catalfamo JL. Molecular and genetic basis for thrombasthenic thrombopathia in otterhounds. Am J Vet Res 2001;62(11):1797–804.

41. Boudreaux MK, Crager C, Dillon AR, et al. Identification of an intrinsic platelet function defect in Spitz dogs. J Vet Intern Med 1994;8:93–8.

42. Catalfamo JL, Raymond SL, White JG, et al. Defective platelet-fibrinogen interaction in hereditary canine thrombopathia. Blood 1986;67:1568–77.

43. Gentry PA, Cheryk LA, Shanks RD, et al. An inherited platelet function defect in a Simmental crossbred herd. Can J Vet Res 1997;61:128–33.

44. Johnstone IB, Lotz F. An inherited platelet function defect in Basset hounds. Can Vet J 1979;20:211–5.
45. Boudreaux MK, Dillon AR, Ravis WR, et al. Effects of treatment with aspirin or aspirin/dipyridamole combination in heartworm-negative, heartworm-infected, and embolized heartworm-infected dogs. Am J Vet Res 1991;52(12):1992–9.
46. Boudreaux MK, Dillon AR, Sartin EA, et al. Effects of treatment with ticlopidine in heartworm-negative, heartworm-infected, and embolized heartworm-infected dogs. Am J Vet Res 1991;52:2000–6.
47. Johnstone IB, Lotz F. An inherited platelet function defect in Basset hounds. Can Vet J 1979;20:211–5.
48. Christophorcon PW, Insalaco TA, van Santen VL, et al. Characterization of the cDNA encoding alphaIIb and beta3 in normal horses and two horses with Glanzmann thrombasthenia. Vet Pathol 2006;43:78–82.
49. Abrams C, Shattil SJ. Immunological detection of activated platelets in clinical disorders. Thromb Haemost 1991;65:467–73.
50. Wills TB, Wardrop KJ, Meyers KM. Detection of activated platelets in canine blood by use of flow cytometry. Am J Vet Res 2006;67:56–63.
51. Segura D, Monreal L, Perez-Pujol S, et al. Assessment of platelet function in horses: ultrastructure, flow cytometry, and perfusion techniques. J Vet Intern Med 2006;20: 581–8.
52. Boudreaux MK, Panangala VS, Bourne C. A platelet activation-specific monoclonal antibody that recognizes a receptor-induced binding site on canine fibrinogen. Vet Pathol 1996;33:419–27.
53. Boudreaux MK, Martin M. P2Y12 receptor gene mutation associated with postoperative hemorrhage in a Greater Swiss Mountain dog. Vet Clin Pathol 2011;40:202–6.
54. Frelinger AL, 3rd, Cohen I, Plow EF, et al. Selective inhibition of integrin function by antibodies specific for ligand-occupied receptor conformers. J Biol Chem 1990;265: 6346–52.
55. Honda S, Tomiyama Y, Pelletier AJ, et al. Topography of ligand-induced binding sites, including a novel cation-sensitive epitope (AP5) at the amino terminus, of the human integrin beta 3 subunit. J Biol Chem 1995;270:11947–54.
56. Jennings LK, White MM, Mandrell TD. Interspecies comparison of platelet aggregation, LIBS expression and clot retraction: observed differences in GPIIb-IIIa functional activity. Thromb Haemost 1995;74:1551–6.
57. Santoro ML, Sano-Martins IS. Platelet dysfunction during Bothrops jararaca snake envenomation in rabbits. Thromb Haemost 2004;92:369–83.
58. von Zur Muhlen C, von Elverfeldt D, Choudhury RP, et al. Functionalized magnetic resonance contrast agent selectively binds to glycoprotein IIb/IIIa on activated human platelets under flow conditions and is detectable at clinically relevant field strengths. Mol Imaging 2008;7:59–67.
59. von zur Muhlen C, Peter K, Ali ZA, et al. Visualization of activated platelets by targeted magnetic resonance imaging utilizing conformation-specific antibodies against glycoprotein IIb/IIIa. J Vasc Res 2009;46:6–14.
60. Doré M, Hawkins HK, Entman ML, et al. Production of a monoclonal antibody against canine GMP-140 (P-selectin) and studies of its vascular distribution in canine tissues. Vet Pathol 1993;30:213–22.
61. Gurney D, Lip GY, Blann AD. A reliable plasma marker of platelet activation: does it exist? Am J Hematol 2002;70:139–44.
62. Shattil SJ, Hoxie JA, Cunningham M, et al. Changes in the platelet membrane glycoprotein IIb.IIIa complex during platelet activation. J Biol Chem 1985;260: 11107–14.

63. Tzima E, Walker JH. Platelet annexin V: the ins and outs. Platelets 2000;11:245–51.
64. Dachary-Prigent J, Pasquet JM, Freyssinet JM, et al. Calcium involvement in amino-phospholipid exposure and microparticle formation during platelet activation: a study using Ca2+-ATPase inhibitors. Biochemistry 1995;34:11625–34.
65. Zwaal RF, Comfurius P, Bevers EM. Scott syndrome, a bleeding disorder caused by defective scrambling of membrane phospholipids. Biochim Biophys Acta 2004;1636: 119–28.
66. Brooks MB, Catalfamo JL, Brown HA, et al. A hereditary bleeding disorder of dogs caused by a lack of platelet procoagulant activity. Blood 2002;99:2434–41.
67. Callan MB, Bennett JS, Phillips DK, et al. Inherited platelet delta-storage pool disease in dogs causing severe bleeding: an animal model for a specific ADP deficiency. Thromb Haemost 1995;74:949–53.

Laboratory Diagnosis of Disseminated Intravascular Coagulation in Dogs and Cats: The Past, the Present, and the Future

Tracy Stokol, BVSc, PhD

KEYWORDS

- Hemostasis • Thromboelastography • Laboratory tests
- Disseminated intravascular coagulation • Diagnosis
- Review

The hemostatic system is an intricate co-operative network of proteins and cells that produces then dissolves fibrin clots. Disruptions in the balance between stimulatory and inhibitory forces that drive clotting and fibrinolysis cause hemorrhagic or thrombotic disorders, the most severe of which is disseminated intravascular coagulation (DIC). DIC is a secondary complication of infections, inflammation and neoplasia. It contributes to morbidity and mortality through systemic microvascular thrombosis. Since clinical signs and imaging techniques are insensitive to thrombosis, laboratory testing is essential for DIC detection. Early diagnosis and mitigation can potentially improve survival and decrease hospitalization costs of affected animals.

PATHOPHYSIOLOGY OF DIC

Our view of physiologic hemostasis has evolved from the concept of a series of sequential cascading "waterfall" enzymatic reactions to more complex interrelated reactions that are grounded on cell surfaces, primarily provided by activated platelets. For a more in-depth appreciation of this "cell-based model" of hemostasis, the reader is referred to a recent review.[1] DIC essentially represents this normal hemostatic process gone viral—instead of being localized to a site of vessel injury and to platelet surfaces, hemostasis becomes unrestricted, uncontrolled, and systemic in DIC. Bacterial sepsis is one of the main causes of DIC in humans and animals.[2,3] As such,

The author has nothing to disclose.
Department of Population Medicine and Diagnostic Sciences, S1-058 Schurman Hall, College of Veterinary Medicine, Upper Tower Road, Cornell University, Ithaca, NY 14853, USA
E-mail address: ts23@cornell.edu

animal models of sepsis have provided substantial insight into how hemostasis becomes sufficiently perturbed to manifest in DIC.[4–6] There is some redundancy in the ways in which the hemostatic system responds to triggering stimuli; however, it is unlikely that "one rule fits all." The type of stimulus and the resulting interplay between the different cellular and enzymatic hemostatic components and between hemostasis and inflammation likely dictate the mechanisms by which DIC is initiated and progresses in different disorders and the interventions required to limit or halt this process.[7–9] Below is a summary of current concepts on the pathophysiology of DIC.

Two central themes of DIC are that thrombin generation is excessive and uncontrolled and that thrombin generation occurs and is amplified and disseminated on cell surfaces.[2,10] This indicates that the coagulation cascade must be excessively activated in DIC and that cell surfaces must be available to propagate and disseminate thrombin generation. Tissue factor (coagulation factor III, tissue thromboplastin) has been designated the main culprit in activation of coagulation in DIC.[2,10,11] Exposure of large amounts of tissue factor in the extravascular space or intravascular expression of tissue factor on circulating cells or cell membrane–derived microparticles begins the process of DIC (**Fig. 1**). Tissue factor activates the coagulation cascade (in health and in DIC) by binding to and activating its circulating enzymatic partner, coagulation factor VII (FVII), in the extrinsic pathway of coagulation. When complexed with tissue factor, activated FVII efficiently activates surface-bound factor X (FX) and factor IX. Once the extrinsic pathway generates thrombin via activated FX, thrombin amplifies its own production by activating other coagulation factor enzymes (factor XI) and cofactors (factors VIII and V) of the intrinsic and common pathways. This eventually terminates in fibrin production (and thrombus formation).[1,2] When tissue factor is exposed intravascularly or in large amounts, the normal spatial restriction of coagulation is lost and inhibitory mechanisms are disrupted, leading to excessive thrombin generation. Although tissue factor is important in initiation of DIC, there are other ways in which the coagulation cascade can be activated in disease states. For example, snake venom components and cancer proteases can directly activate other coagulation factors, including FX, inducing a DIC-like syndrome.[12,13]

Tissue factor fuels the fire of DIC, but alone is insufficient to result in dissemination of coagulation. Rather, thrombin generation is facilitated and propagated systemically through phospholipid-containing microparticles, lack of appropriate inhibition and a feedback cycle that is initiated (at least in inflammatory causes of DIC) between coagulation and inflammation.[2,10] Microparticles are small (<1 μm) vesicles that are shed from the surface membrane of many different cell types (platelets, monocytes, granulocytes, erythrocytes, and endothelial cells), particularly after activation.[14] Membrane-derived microparticles are enriched in phosphatidylserine, a negatively charged phospholipid that is normally found on the inner leaflet of cell membranes, but is flipped to the outer membrane when cells become activated. Phosphatidylserine is the binding site for Gla-domain–containing coagulation factors and enables the assembly of the tenase (FX activating) and prothrombinase (thrombin activating) complexes on cell surfaces. The formation of coagulation factor complexes on phosphatidylserine-bearing surfaces produces high local factor concentrations, protects factors from inhibition, and amplifies their activity over 1000-fold.[14,15] Due to their small size, microparticles are not restricted to an injured site and persist in the circulation, thus providing a large functional surface area on which coagulation can propagate systemically.[14] Under physiologic conditions, activated platelets are the main source of phosphatidylserine membranes (both the intact cell and shed microparticles); however, in DIC, additional procoagulant membranes are provided by

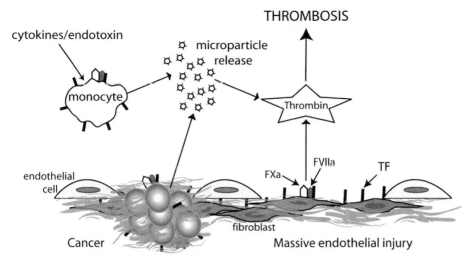

Fig. 1. Sources of tissue factor in DIC. Tissue factor is constitutively expressed on subendo-thelial fibroblasts and smooth muscle cells, where it is sequestered from its plasma ligand, FVII. Under physiologic conditions, this localizes activation of coagulation to a site of blood vessel injury. With massive endothelial or tissue injury, large amounts of this extravascular tissue factor are exposed to FVII, which subsequently binds to tissue factor and becomes activated (FVIIa). The tissue factor–FVIIa complex then binds to and activates factor IX (not shown) and factor X (FXa), the latter of which cleaves prothrombin to thrombin, initiating coagulation. In inflammatory states or sepsis, tissue factor expression is induced in circulating monocytes by endotoxin or inflammatory cytokines (interleukin-1β and tumor necrosis factor-α), which also shed tissue factor–bearing microparticles from their membranes.[16,63] This mechanism is also likely operative in other inflammatory states that initiate DIC, such as pancreatitis and heatstroke. Cancer cells can constitutively express high concentrations of tissue factor and also release tissue factor–enriched microparticles.[12,42,64] Release of large amounts of tissue factor generates excessive thrombin, which overwhelms inhibitory mech-anisms and disseminates, resulting in widespread thrombosis. Although it is possible that other cells (granulocytes, platelets, and endothelial cells) can express tissue factor in disease states, it is now thought that these cells derive tissue factor from fusion of monocyte-derived microparticles versus synthesizing this protein de novo.[63]

other cell types, notably tissue factor–expressing monocytes, cancer cells, and apoptotic cells.[6,14,16,17] Thus, the driving force for coagulation—tissue factor—and the membrane support—phosphatidylserine—are colocalized to a greater degree in DIC than under physiologic conditions. Studies in humans demonstrate that oxidized lipoproteins can also provide phospholipid membrane support for coagulation and may have a role in dissemination of coagulation in DIC associated with sepsis[18]; however, the extent to which this occurs in domestic species is unknown.

Concurrent with thrombin generation is activation of fibrinolysis, resulting in the release of fibrin split products. However, fibrinolysis may be inhibited to some degree in DIC, particularly in later stages of sepsis and trauma. Inhibition is mediated through thrombin itself, high concentrations of which result in the production of thick strands of lysis-resistant fibrin and activation of a carboxypeptidase that inhibits fibrinolysis (thrombin-activatable thrombolysis inhibitor).[1,19] The concomitant release of polyphosphates from activated platelets[20] and tissue plasminogen activator inhibitors from the endothelium contributes to inhibition of fibrinolysis, particularly in sepsis.[2]

Inhibition of fibrinolysis would favor the development of thrombi, which is characteristic of DIC. However, since increased concentrations of fibrin split products are a characteristic and early laboratory finding in DIC with tests for these products having high negative predictive values,[21,22] fibrinolysis is always occurring in DIC to some degree.

Thrombin generation is normally balanced by inhibitors, specifically antithrombin (AT), activated protein C, and tissue factor pathway inhibitor.[1] Inhibitory function can be defective in DIC, either as a direct consequence of this process or secondary to the underlying disease. During DIC, inhibitors (AT, activated protein C) are consumed as they complex with their activated targets and are cleared from the circulation. In inflammation-induced DIC, inflammatory cytokines can downregulate production of inhibitors or their cofactors or receptors, resulting in decreased inhibitor activity. Inhibitors or their cofactors can also be degraded by neutrophil proteases.[2,10,23,24] Thus, inhibitors no longer constrain coagulation, which is excessive to begin with, resulting in the progression and dissemination of DIC.

It is now well accepted that coagulation and inflammation are intertwined.[2,24] Inflammation is one of the most common instigators of DIC, with inflammatory cytokines and complement components upregulating tissue factor, downregulating inhibitors, and activating various cells inducing vesiculation and phosphatidylserine exposure.[24,25] Conversely, activated coagulation factors (notably thrombin, FX, and the tissue factor–FVII complex) can potentiate the inflammatory response by binding to and activating protease-activated receptors (PARs) on platelets, leukocytes, and endothelial cells.[24,26] Activated PAR induce G protein–coupled cell signaling in these cells, resulting in upregulation of adhesion molecules (eg, intracellular adhesion molecule-1) and secretion of inflammatory mediators (eg, interleukin-6 and interleukin-8). Coagulation-induced inflammation is potentiated by the loss of hemostasis inhibitors, which can elicit anti-inflammatory and cell-protective responses, particularly activated protein C.[24,27] The extent to which this positive feedback loop is initiated in DIC may depend on the underlying cause of DIC and the precise balance between coagulation activating and opposing forces. The recognition of these intimate links between inflammation and coagulation has advanced the use of activated protein C concentrates for treating DIC,[28] with the intent on capitalizing on the inflammatory versus the anticoagulant properties of this inhibitor.

This summary of the pathophysiology of DIC has focused on the coagulation cascade, cell surfaces, and inhibitors, with little emphasis being placed on platelets. Yet platelets are important in perpetuating and disseminating coagulation and their contribution cannot be underestimated. Whether platelets are activated directly by the primary disease or as a consequence of generation of activated coagulation factor proteases, activated platelets are still likely the main structural scaffold on which DIC proceeds and are a rich source of phosphatidylserine-expressing microparticles, platelet and inflammatory agonists, and coagulation factors. However, it is unlikely that platelet activation or phosphatidylserine exposure alone will result in DIC without concurrent direct activation of the coagulation cascade.

THE DIC CONTINUUM

In 2001, a Scientific Subcommittee of the International Society on Thrombosis and Haemostasis (ISTH) on DIC produced a series of recommendations aimed at standardizing diagnostic criteria for DIC to improve clinical outcomes.[29] This subcommittee defined DIC as "an acquired syndrome characterized by intravascular activation of coagulation with loss of localization arising from different causes. It can originate from and cause damage to the microvasculature, which if sufficiently severe,

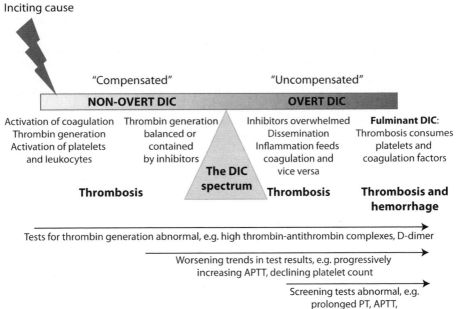

Fig. 2. The DIC continuum. A primary disease (inflammation, neoplasia, infection, trauma) activates the coagulation cascade, resulting in generation of thrombin, which subsequently amplifies its own production. Simultaneously, platelets and leukocytes are activated (by the underlying disease or activated coagulation factors) and release microparticles and exteriorize phosphatidylserine, providing a supportive enhancing framework for thrombin production. Thrombin generation is initially restrained by several inhibitors in the "compensated" or nonovert phase of DIC. Some degree of thrombosis is likely occurring and abnormalities in tests that detect thrombin generation, such as thrombin-antithrombin complexes and D-dimer, may be observed. As the inciting stimulus continues to activate coagulation, inhibitors become overwhelmed and inflammation is exacerbated by the hyperactive coagulation system. An "uncompensated" phase or overt DIC then ensues, in which thrombin generation becomes uncontrolled and systemic. This results in widespread thrombosis with abnormal hemostatic test results that are typical of DIC. Platelets and coagulation factors eventually become deficient manifesting as hemorrhage. Deficiencies have been mostly attributed to consumption with thrombosis; however, other mechanisms are likely operative (such as enhanced hepatic clearance of platelets[65] and cleavage of coagulation factors by proteases). Serial monitoring of hemostatic test results may detect progressive disruption of hemostasis as it becomes more and more unrestrained in non-overt DIC, eventually transforming into overt DIC. Note that these phases of DIC do not always naturally segue into one another. For instance, massive head trauma may immediately result in overt DIC from release of tissue factor in the brain, whereas low-grade inflammation may incite a more slow-burning controlled process (nonovert DIC) that may not progress.

can produce organ dysfunction." The subcommittee advanced the concept that DIC is an evolving process that can be separated into different stages: nonovert DIC, "controlled" overt DIC, and "uncontrolled" overt DIC (**Fig. 2**). In nonovert DIC, coagulation has been activated (usually through tissue factor exposure); however, thrombin generation is constrained by inhibitors and there is minimal incitement of inflammation. The subcommittee also refers to this stage as "a stressed but compensated" hemostatic system, and this stage likely encompasses what has been previously referred to as "low-grade or chronic DIC."[30] Although not clearly stated, it is likely that microvascular thrombosis is occurring to some extent in this nonovert stage of DIC. This stage of DIC is difficult to diagnose because it is characterized primarily by thrombin generation, which cannot be reliably detected by routine coagulation screening assays, such as the prothrombin time (PT) and activated partial thromboplastin time (APTT).[21] Overt DIC reflects an activated and uncompensated hemostatic system, where inhibitors are overwhelmed, thrombin generation proceeds unopposed, the inflammation-hemostasis feedback loop is operative, and thrombosis is causing organ dysfunction. The subcommittee defines "controlled" overt DIC as a temporary condition, which can be ceased by intervention (eg, ruptured placenta), whereas "uncontrolled" overt DIC cannot be reversed by sole removal of the underlying cause. As thrombosis proceeds in overt DIC, platelets and coagulation factors are consumed, cleared, or cleaved, resulting in abnormalities in screening hemostasis assays, which are designed to pick up deficiencies in these cells and proteins. With time, these deficiencies may dominate the clinical syndrome, resulting in hemorrhage, which is more clinically discernable than thrombosis. This is the most severe manifestation of DIC and has been referred to as "fulminant" or "end-stage" DIC. Since this is the most clinically apparent and readily diagnosed stage of DIC, the moniker "death is coming" was coined for this hemostatic disorder. Although there is some evidence that nonovert DIC can progress to overt DIC in some patients,[31] this progression is not inevitable and likely depends on many factors, including the nature of the underlying disease, inherent differences in susceptibility to DIC, and disease- or DIC-related variables that influence activation or containment of coagulation.

LABORATORY TESTING OF DIC IN DOGS AND CATS
The Past

In veterinary medicine, DIC has been traditionally diagnosed on a combination of clinical and laboratory criteria (**Box 1**). To diagnose DIC, animals must fulfill both clinical criteria (a primary disease and clinical symptoms) and have two or more abnormal laboratory tests, reflecting abnormalities in all pathways of hemostasis.[3,32–36] The rationale for using a combination of test results for DIC diagnosis is sound, because none of these tests alone are specific for DIC. Although detection of fibrin thrombi in the microvasculature on histopathologic examination is considered the "gold standard" for diagnosis of DIC, it is a poor standard because fibrin thrombi can lyse rapidly after death[37]; thus, DIC is essentially an antemortem clinical and laboratory diagnosis. Nevertheless, this traditional method for diagnosing DIC has major shortcomings. Hemorrhage manifests late in the course of DIC and may not be evident at all in cats with this syndrome.[35,36,38] Unfortunately, thrombosis is far more difficult to recognize in affected patients and yet is the more important abnormality, being the major factor responsible for the high morbidity and mortality associated with DIC. Thus, clinical signs of hemorrhage or thrombosis cannot be relied upon to facilitate the diagnosis of DIC and these symptoms are not included in currently recommended DIC scoring systems in human medicine.[29] Since we rely heavily on clinical assessment (which depends on the index of suspicion harbored by the attending clinician), this means that the presence of DIC is likely frequently missed in animals, removing a potential opportunity for altering patient outcome. There is no standardization regarding the tests (type, number, or cut-offs) used to diagnose DIC, which makes it difficult to compare across published studies. Coagulation screening assays (PT, APTT, thrombin clot time, and fibrinogen concentration) are optimized for detection of factor deficiencies and are thus geared toward detection of the most

---

Box 1
Traditional criteria for diagnosis of disseminated intravascular coagulation

Clinical findings

Presence of a primary disease initiating DIC

Excessive hemorrhage or thrombosis

Laboratory tests

Consumption of platelets

  Thrombocytopenia

Consumption of coagulation factors

  Prolonged PT

  Prolonged APTT

  Prolonged thrombin clot time

  Hypofibrinogenemia

Consumption of inhibitors

  Low AT

Evidence of fibrinolysis

  Increased fibrin(ogen) degration products

  Increased D-dimer

Evidence of a microangiopathy

  Red blood cell fragments in a blood smear (schistocytes, keratocytes, acanthocytes)

---

advanced stages of DIC. These tests are insensitive to an activated but contained hemostatic system (nonovert DIC) or earlier stages of overt DIC where coagulation activation dominates over consumption.[21,39,40] Furthermore, test sensitivity to DIC differs between species and criteria used in dogs are not necessarily applicable to cats. DIC is an infrequent diagnosis in cats, likely because cats rarely demonstrate clinical signs of excessive hemorrhage and routine hemostatic assays are insensitive to DIC in this species. Reduced AT activity and high fibrin(ogen) degradation product (FDP) or D-dimer concentrations are two of the more sensitive tests for diagnosis of DIC in dogs,[32,33,41] but low AT activity is uncommon and FDP or D-dimer concentrations are not as reliably increased in cats with DIC (personal observations, 2011).[35,38] It is difficult to diagnose overt DIC in the face of a normal platelet count in dogs, yet cats with DIC may not be thrombocytopenic.[38] As indicated earlier, none of the laboratory tests are specific for DIC (even when used in combination) and some of the tests are so nonspecific (such as red blood cell fragments in cats), that they are not useful for DIC diagnosis.

The Present

To overcome the inherent limitations of traditional criteria, the diagnostic emphasis in humans has shifted toward the application of scoring systems for diagnosis of nonovert and overt DIC and new tools for detection of thrombin activation or hypercoagulability.[21,40] Although several assays for thrombin activation (eg, thrombin–AT complexes, fibrinopeptides, prothrombin fragments) and microparticle detection have been evaluated in human patients,[21,40,42] little information exists on these assays in veterinary medicine and none have been tested in animals with DIC. Rather there is enormous interest in viscoelastographic-based coagulation testing for the detection of hypercoagulability (including that due to DIC) in animals. Thus, this section will focus on scoring systems and viscoelastographic testing.

In order to standardize DIC diagnosis for clinical use and outcome assessment, the DIC Scientific Subcommittee of the ISTH proposed a scoring system for nonovert and overt DIC.[29] The scheme was deliberately based on widely available standard diagnostic assays in human medicine, such as the PT and platelet count, without the need for specialized tests, such as AT or protein C activity, fibrinopeptides, or thrombin–AT complexes. For overt DIC, the scoring system can only be applied to patients that have a predisposing disorder and no points are given for the underlying disease. Since overt DIC was defined as an excessively activated and uncontrolled hemostatic system that is characterized by widespread and ongoing thrombosis, results of routine assays that detect platelet and coagulation factor depletion and release of fibrinolytic products should be abnormal in this stage of DIC. Therefore, the overt DIC score was based a moderate thrombocytopenia, a prolonged PT, low fibrinogen, increased fibrinolytic products (FDP, D-dimer), or soluble fibrin monomer (which is produced from the action of thrombin on fibrinogen). In essence, the overt DIC score represents a standardized format for traditional DIC testing (without a requirement for relevant clinical signs). In contrast, laboratory detection of nonovert DIC is far more difficult because this stage is characterized by an activated but contained hemostatic system (i.e., thrombin generation) and most of the routine screening assays of coagulation are insensitive to thrombin generation.[39] Thus, for the nonovert score, points were given for the underlying disease (i.e., the patient is at risk of DIC) and trends in data from routine assays (PT, platelet count, fibrinolytic products, or soluble fibrin monomer) were included in order to detect a progressively activated hemostatic system with deteriorating inhibitory control. Specialized tests that reflect thrombin activation (thrombin–AT complexes, low activity of inhibitors) could be done and were included in the scheme but were not necessary for attaining a score consistent with nonovert DIC. The recommended testing interval for evaluating dynamic trends was 24 to 48 hours. Weaknesses in the ISTH scoring system were a relatively low platelet cut-off ($<100 \times 10^6$/L) and no defined test or cut-offs for fibrinolytic products or soluble fibrin monomer (which could be used interchangeably with FDP or D-dimer). Other scoring systems for overt DIC have been used for several years in Japan.[21] Prospective validation of the ISTH scoring system, particularly that for overt DIC, has been accomplished and the scheme has been subjected to a 5-year review.[21] The performed studies support the continued use of the ISTH scoring system for overt DIC because patients classified with overt DIC have higher mortality rates and incidence of organ dysfunction than those not in overt DIC in most studies. Clinical treatment trials also show that the overt DIC score is useful in evaluating beneficial responses to therapy with regard to standardized patient outcomes.[28,43] The studies also illustrated that the overt DIC score is largely dependent on the PT and platelet count, that fibrinogen could be eliminated from the scoring scheme, and that fibrinolytic products or soluble fibrin monomer do not contribute substantially to the score due to their high sensitivity. There is still uncertainty over which test and test cut-off for fibrin generation or lysis should be used for ISTH scoring and there is a substantial lack of concordance between the ISTH and Japanese schemes (the Japanese scoring systems, particularly that from the Japanese Association for Acute Medicine, appear to perform better overall, perhaps due to regional differences in disease demographics or because they ascribe points for the primary disorder). Less validation of nonovert DIC has been done; however, one study demonstrated that patients in nonovert DIC have higher mortality rates than patients without DIC and some progress to overt DIC.[31] The latter study also showed that serial monitoring of screening assays (PT, platelet count, fibrinolytic products, or soluble fibrin monomer) were useful for the diagnosis of nonovert DIC, with inhibitor assays for AT and activated protein C activity not contributing substantially to the score.

There has been one preliminary study on application of a modified ISTH scoring system for diagnosis of nonovert DIC in dogs.[44] In this study, the authors used total hospitalization days and 28-day mortality rates as outcome measures in 24 dogs with diseases associated with DIC. They combined selected nonovert and overt DIC criteria (points were given for underlying disease, a prolonged PT, thrombocytopenia, high D-dimer, and low AT activity) for diagnosing DIC and compared it to traditional assessment (three or more abnormal tests including thrombocytopenia and pro-longed coagulation times) on daily blood samples, selecting the highest values for comparison. They found that more dogs were diagnosed in DIC with traditional criteria but mortality rates were higher in the dogs that were classified in DIC by modified ISTH criteria. Total days of hospitalization were no different between groups. This study suggests that ISTH criteria are potentially applicable to dogs. However, the tests and cutoffs selected for the canine ISTH scoring scheme may not have been optimized for the dog, resulting in the reduced sensitivity of the scheme compared to traditional assessment (which has since been corroborated by subsequent studies by these authors in larger numbers of dogs[45]). For example, the APTT is more sensitive than the PT as an indicator of DIC in dogs.[32,33]

The same authors have recently published a diagnostic scoring algorithm for DIC based on multiple logistic regression analysis of hemostatic assays. To develop the model, dogs admitted to a single academic veterinary hospital were tested daily for various hemostatic test results (PT, APTT, D-dimer, platelet count, fibrinogen, AT, and protein C) and results were scored per ISTH overt DIC criteria. Using data from the day of the highest ISTH DIC score, a diagnosis of DIC was made by a simple majority opinion of three experts based on traditional DIC criteria (abnormal test results reflecting coagulation factor and platelet consumption, inhibitor depletion, and fibrinolytic activity). The final model was based on results from the PT, APTT, fibrinogen, and dichotomized D-dimer (>0.5 mg/L for a latex agglutination-based card assay) from 63 dogs (37% of which had DIC per expert opinion). A logistic value of $P>.40$ was designated as the optimal diagnostic cut-off for the model. The model was tested on a different population of dogs from another academic institution, with the assays presumably being performed at the first institution. Dogs with P values greater than the cut-off had a higher relative risk of death (the latter was not defined). This same study also revealed that the sensitivity of ISTH overt criteria for diagnosis of DIC in dogs was lower than expert opinion. This proposed model may be a promising way to standardize diagnosis of DIC in later stages of overt disease (although is no better than expert opinion), but the model still awaits verification from additional independent studies, particularly using different methods and reagents since these assay variables may markedly influence usefulness of the model.[46] For instance, the latex agglutination D-dimer assay used in the model is not commercially available in the United States and a previous study has shown a lack of concordance between diagnostic assays for this marker.[47]

Viscoelastographic testing is a source of tremendous interest in veterinary medi-cine, yielding a plethora of recent publications, particularly with respect to the use of these assays for diagnosing hypercoagulability in animals, such as nonovert DIC. Viscoelastograph-based testing is referred to as a "global" hemostatic assay because it is performed in whole blood, thus assessing all soluble factors and cellular constituents involved in hemostasis, with the exception of the endothelium and tissue-derived proteins. Interestingly, these assays are used to dictate or assess response to transfusion therapy in humans undergoing surgery and are not generally used for diagnosis of specific hemostatic disorders.[10,48] There have been several recent substantive reviews on the use of viscoelastographic coagulation testing in veterinary medicine[49,50]; hence, only a few points will be emphasized here. Important factors that influence coagulation results from these analyzers are the type and concentration of the activator (if one is used), the timing of analysis, and hematocrit.[49–53] Tissue factor and kaolin are two commonly used activators, with tissue factor activation being analogous to a whole blood PT and kaolin activation with a whole blood APTT. In support of this, tissue factor-activated thromboelastographic (TEG, performed with the TEG 5000 analyzer from Haemoscope Corporation) results display no abnormalities (similar to the PT) in blood from dogs with hemophilia A (M. Brooks, personal communication, 2011). There is a trend toward hypercoagulable tracings with storage of blood and lower hematocrits (which may be an artifact of the technique, since it is unlikely all anemic dogs are truly hypercoagulable).[49,50] Thus, studies using different viscoelastic techniques, activators, and time of analysis cannot be directly compared and hematocrit is clearly a confounding variable that must be taken into consideration. Furthermore, there is no consensus on the definition of hypercoagulability, with some authors using the G or global clot strength[54,55] and others using one or more abnormal TEG results, including mathematical formulae that combines most of the major tests, the coagulation index, or total thrombin generation (area under the TEG curve).[56–60]

Only one viscoelastographic study has been performed in dogs with DIC.[55] In this study, tissue factor–activated TEG was performed 30 minutes after blood was collected from 50 dogs admitted to the intensive care unit of two university hospitals. Similar to that done previously by these authors,[45] the diagnosis of DIC was based on expert opinion. Overall coagulation state (hyper-, normo-, and hypocoagulability) from the TEG was defined on global clot strength or G, a direct mathematical derivation of the maximum amplitude (MA) of clot formation, using data from the highest ISTH overt DIC score. Outcome was based on 28-day mortality rates. The authors found that hypercoagulability was the most common coagulation state in dogs with DIC but that hypocoagulable dogs had a higher risk of mortality than dogs with normal or hypercoagulable status. The influence of hematocrit on test results was not evaluated. This study and others by the same and other authors[22,54,59] also illustrated the dependence of the G (or MA) on the platelet count and fibrinogen concentration, with blood from dogs with platelet counts less than 30×10^6/L being hypocoagulable and high fibrinogen being associated with hypercoagulability. These data suggest that TEG results defined by G (or MA) may provide no information on overall coagulation status in severely thrombocytopenic dogs or dogs with hyperfibrinogenemia. Indeed, hyperfibrinogenemia may be an independent risk factor for thrombosis[61] and measuring fibrinogen in dogs may yield similar information on hypercoagulability than in vogue viscoelastographic techniques.

The Future

It is likely that we will continue to use traditional criteria to diagnose DIC in animals, with DIC remaining a rare diagnosis in cats. Time and additional studies will tell whether viscoelastographic coagulation testing will live up to the hoped for promise for detecting earlier nonovert or thrombotic phases of overt DIC. However, a recent study suggests TEG is not a good screening tool for detection of early hemostatic abnormalities in experimental endotoxemia in dogs.[22] It is also unlikely that a single sensitive and specific diagnostic assay for DIC will be discovered in the next few years, although new prognostic tests may become available.[21,62] The search for molecular markers of thrombin activation will no doubt continue and potentially become more targeted as our understanding of the complex hemostatic system evolves. In the interim, we will continue to rely upon clinical acumen and a battery of affordable and readily available imaging and laboratory assays to diagnose DIC and detect thrombosis. Although costly, daily or alternate-day testing to monitor for trends in hemostatic test results (such as a normal but declining platelet count, progressively increasing D-dimer concentrations, or decreasing AT activity) may prove the best means to identify dogs in early or thrombotic phases of DIC.[21,40] To effectively evaluate risk factors and new diagnostic tests and treatment strategies, it is imperative that we reach consensus and standardize, to the best of our ability, the definition of DIC, the best tests and test cut offs used to diagnose DIC, and outcome assessment for clinical trials or research studies in dogs and cats. The multiple logistic regression model proposed by Wiinberg and colleagues[45] may be a good starting point to reach this consensus, once it has been independently verified and applied across clot detection methods and reagents.

REFERENCES

1. Smith S. Overview of hemostasis. In: Weiss DJ, Wardrop KJ, editors. Schalm's veterinary hematology. 6th edition. Ames (IA): Blackwell Publishing; 2010. p. 635–53.
2. Levi M, Schultz M, van der Poll T. Disseminated intravascular coagulation in infectious disease. Semin Thromb Hemost 2010;36:367–77.
3. de Laforcade AM, Freeman LM, Shaw SP, et al. Hemostatic changes in dogs with naturally occurring sepsis. J Vet Intern Med 2003;17:674–9.
4. Taylor FB Jr, Chang A, Ruf W, et al. Lethal E. coli septic shock is prevented by blocking tissue factor with monoclonal antibody. Circ Shock 1991;33:127–34.
5. Warr TA, Rao LV, Rapaport SI. Disseminated intravascular coagulation in rabbits induced by administration of endotoxin or tissue factor: effect of anti-tissue factor antibodies and measurement of plasma extrinsic pathway inhibitor activity. Blood 1990;75:1481–9.
6. Pawlinski R, Wang JG, Owens AP 3rd, et al. Hematopoietic and non-hematopoietic cell tissue factor activates the coagulation cascade in endotoxemic mice. Blood 2010;116:806–14.
7. Asakura H, Suga Y, Yoshida T, et al. Pathophysiology of disseminated intravascular coagulation (DIC) progresses at a different rate in tissue factor-induced and lipopolysaccharide-induced DIC models in rats. Blood Coagul Fibrinolysis 2003;14:221–8.
8. Ontachi Y, Asakura H, Takahashi Y, et al. No interplay between the pathways mediating coagulation and inflammation in tissue factor-induced disseminated intravascular coagulation in rats. Crit Care Med 2006;34:2646–50.
9. Patel KN, Soubra SH, Lam FW, et al. Polymicrobial sepsis and endotoxemia promote microvascular thrombosis via distinct mechanisms. J Thromb Haemost 2010;8:1403–9.
10. Toh CH, Downey C. Back to the future: testing in disseminated intravascular coagulation. Blood Coagul Fibrinolysis 2005;16:535–42.
11. Berthelsen LO, Kristensen AT, Tranholm M. Purified thromboplastin causes haemostatic abnormalities but not overt DIC in an experimental rabbit model. Thromb Res 2010;126:337–44.
12. Zwicker JI, Furie BC, Furie B. Cancer-associated thrombosis. Crit Rev Oncol Hematol 2007;62:126–36.

13. Isbister GK. Snakebite doesn't cause disseminated intravascular coagulation: coagulopathy and thrombotic microangiopathy in snake envenoming. Semin Thromb Hemost 2010;36:444–51.

14. Freyssinet JM. Cellular microparticles: what are they bad or good for? J Thromb Haemost 2003;1:1655–62.

15. Sinauridze EI, Kireev DA, Popenko NY, et al. Platelet microparticle membranes have 50- to 100-fold higher specific procoagulant activity than activated platelets. Thromb Haemost 2007;97:425–34.

16. Satta N, Toti F, Feugeas O, et al. Monocyte vesiculation is a possible mechanism for dissemination of membrane-associated procoagulant activities and adhesion molecules after stimulation by lipopolysaccharide. J Immunol 1994;153:3245–55.

17. Wang JG, Manly D, Kirchhofer D, et al. Levels of microparticle tissue factor activity correlate with coagulation activation in endotoxemic mice. J Thromb Haemost 2009;7:1092–8.

18. Dennis MW, Downey C, Brufatto N, et al. Prothrombinase enhancement through quantitative and qualitative changes affecting very low density lipoprotein in complex with C-reactive protein. Thromb Haemost 2004;91:522–30.

19. Weisel JW. Structure of fibrin: impact on clot stability. J Thromb Haemost 2007; 5(Suppl 1):116–24.

20. Smith SA, Morrissey JH. Polyphosphate enhances fibrin clot structure. Blood 2008; 112:2810–6.

21. Favaloro EJ. Laboratory testing in disseminated intravascular coagulation. Semin Thromb Hemost 2010;36:458–67.

22. Eralp O, Yilmaz Z, Failing K, et al. Effect of experimental endotoxemia on thrombelastography parameters, secondary and tertiary hemostasis in dogs. J Vet Intern Med 2011;25:524–31.

23. Massberg S, Grahl L, von Bruehl ML, et al. Reciprocal coupling of coagulation and innate immunity via neutrophil serine proteases. Nat Med 2010;16:887–96.

24. van der Poll T, Boer JD, Levi M. The effect of inflammation on coagulation and vice versa. Curr Opin Infect Dis 2011;24:273–8.

25. Laudes IJ, Chu JC, Sikranth S, et al. Anti-c5a ameliorates coagulation/fibrinolytic protein changes in a rat model of sepsis. Am J Pathol 2002;160:1867–75.

26. Coughlin SR. Thrombin signalling and protease-activated receptors. Nature 2000; 407(6801):258–64.

27. Danese S, Vetrano S, Zhang L, et al. The protein C pathway in tissue inflammation and injury: pathogenic role and therapeutic implications. Blood 2010;115:112111–30.

28. Dhainaut JF, Yan SB, Joyce DE, et al. Treatment effects of drotrecogin alfa (activated) in patients with severe sepsis with or without overt disseminated intravascular coagulation. J Thromb Haemost 2004;2:1924–33.

29. Taylor FB Jr, Toh CH, Hoots WK, et al. Towards definition, clinical and laboratory criteria, and a scoring system for disseminated intravascular coagulation. Thromb Haemost 2001;86:1327–30.

30. Bick RL. Disseminated intravascular coagulation: a review of etiology, pathophysiology, diagnosis, and management: guidelines for care. Clin Appl Thromb Hemost 2002;8:1–31.

31. Toh CH, Downey C. Performance and prognostic importance of a new clinical and laboratory scoring system for identifying non-overt disseminated intravascular coagulation. Blood Coagul Fibrinolysis 2005;16:69–74.

32. Feldman BF, Madewell BR, O'Neill S. Disseminated intravascular coagulation: antithrombin, plasminogen, and coagulation abnormalities in 41 dogs. J Am Vet Med Assoc 1981;179:151–4.

33. Stokol T, Brooks M, Erb H, et al. Evaluation of kits for the detection of fibrin(ogen) degradation products in dogs. J Vet Intern Med 1999;13:478–84.

34. Bateman SW, Mathews KA, Abrams-Ogg ACG, et al. Diagnosis of disseminated intravascular coagulation in dogs admitted to an intensive care unit. J Am Vet Med Assoc 1999;215:798–804.

35. Peterson JL, Couto CG, Wellman ML. Hemostatic disorders in cats: a retrospective study and review of the literature. J Vet Intern Med 1995;9:298–303.

36. Thomas JS, Green RA. Clotting times and antithrombin III activity in cats with naturally developing diseases: 85 cases (1984–1994). J Am Vet Med Assoc 1998;213:1290–5.

37. Moser KM, Guisan M, Bartimmo EE, et al. In vivo and post mortem dissolution rates of pulmonary emboli and venous thrombi in the dog. Circulation 1973;48:170–8.

38. Estrin MA, Wehausen CE, Jessen CR, et al. Disseminated intravascular coagulation in cats. J Vet Intern Med 2006;20:1334–9.

39. Taylor FB Jr, Wada H, Kinasewitz G. Description of compensated and uncompensated disseminated intravascular coagulation (DIC) responses (non-overt and overt DIC) in baboon models of intravenous and intraperitoneal Escherichia coli sepsis and in the human model of endotoxemia: toward a better definition of DIC. Crit Care Med 2000;28(9 Suppl):S12–9.

40. Levi M, Meijers JC. DIC: which laboratory tests are most useful. Blood Rev 2011;25:33–7.

41. Stokol T, Brooks MB, Erb HN, et al. D-dimer concentrations in healthy dogs and dogs with disseminated intravascular coagulation. Am J Vet Res 2000;61:393–8.

42. Langer F, Spath B, Haubold K, et al. Tissue factor procoagulant activity of plasma microparticles in patients with cancer-associated disseminated intravascular coagulation. Ann Hematol 2008;87:451–7.

43. Kienast J, Juers M, Wiedermann CJ, et al. Treatment effects of high-dose antithrombin without concomitant heparin in patients with severe sepsis with or without disseminated intravascular coagulation. J Thromb Haemost 2006;4:90–7.

44. Wiinberg B, Jensen AL, Rojkjaer R, et al. Prospective pilot study on performance and prognostic value of a new human, ISTH-based scoring system for identifying non-overt disseminated intravascular coagulation in dogs [abstract]. J Vet Intern Med 2006;20:765.

45. Wiinberg B, Jensen AL, Johansson PI, et al. Development of a model based scoring system for diagnosis of canine disseminated intravascular coagulation with independent assessment of sensitivity and specificity. Vet J 2010;185:292–8.

46. Stokol T, Brooks MB, Erb HN. Effect of citrate concentration on coagulation test results in dogs. J Am Vet Med Assoc 2000;217:1672–7.

47. Stokol T, Erb HN, De Wilde L, et al. Evaluation of latex agglutination kits for detection of fibrin(ogen) degradation products and D-dimer in healthy horses and horses with severe colic. Vet Clin Pathol 2005;34:375–82.

48. Luddington RJ. Thrombelastography/thromboelastometry. Clin Lab Haematol 2005;27:81–90.

49. McMichael MA, Smith SA. Viscoelastic coagulation testing: technology, applications, and limitations. Vet Clin Pathol 2011;40:140–53.

50. Kol A, Borjesson DL. Application of thrombelastography/thromboelastometry to veterinary medicine. Vet Clin Pathol 2010;39:405–16.

51. Wiinberg B, Jensen AL, Rojkjaer R, et al. Validation of human recombinant tissue factor-activated thromboelastography on citrated whole blood from clinically healthy dogs. Vet Clin Pathol 2005;34:389–93.

52. Marschner CB, Bjornvad CR, Kristensen AT, et al. Thromboelastography results on citrated whole blood from clinically healthy cats depend on modes of activation. Acta Vet Scand 2010;52:38.
53. Smith SA, McMichael M, Galligan A, et al. Clot formation in canine whole blood as measured by rotational thromboelastometry is influenced by sample handling and coagulation activator. Blood Coagul Fibrinolysis 2010;21:692–702.
54. Wiinberg B, Jensen AL, Rozanski E, et al. Tissue factor activated thromboelastography correlates to clinical signs of bleeding in dogs. Vet J 2009;179:121–9.
55. Wiinberg B, Jensen AL, Johansson PI, et al. Thromboelastographic evaluation of hemostatic function in dogs with disseminated intravascular coagulation. J Vet Intern Med 2008;22:357–65.
56. Sinnott VB, Otto CM. Use of thromboelastography in dogs with immune-mediated hemolytic anemia: 39 cases (2000–2008). J Vet Emerg Crit Care (San Antonio 2009;19:484–8.
57. Fenty RK, Delaforcade AM, Shaw SE, et al. Identification of hypercoagulability in dogs with primary immune-mediated hemolytic anemia by means of thromboelastography. J Am Vet Med Assoc 2011;238:463–7.
58. Donahue SM, Otto CM. Thromboelastography: a tool for measuring hypercoagulability, hypocoagulability, and fibrinolysis. J Vet Emerg Crit Care 2005;15:9–16.
59. Wagg CR, Boysen SR, Bedard C. Thrombelastography in dogs admitted to an intensive care unit. Vet Clin Pathol 2009;38:453–61.
60. Vilar Saavedra P, Lara Garcia A, Zaldivar Lopez S, et al. Hemostatic abnormalities in dogs with carcinoma: a thromboelastographic characterization of hypercoagulability. Vet J 2011.
61. Machlus KR, Cardenas JC, Church FC, et al. Causal relationship between hyperfibrinogenemia, thrombosis, and resistance to thrombolysis in mice. Blood 2011;117:4953–63.
62. Hwang SM, Kim JE, Han KS, et al. Thrombomodulin phenotype of a distinct monocyte subtype is an independent prognostic marker for disseminated intravascular coagulation. Crit Care 2011;15:R113.
63. Pawlinski R, Mackman N. Cellular sources of tissue factor in endotoxemia and sepsis. Thromb Res 2010;125(Suppl 1):S70–3.
64. Stokol T, Daddona J, Mubayed L, et al. Tissue factor expression in canine tumor cell lines. Am J Vet Res 2011;72:1097–106.
65. Grozovsky R, Hoffmeister KM, Falet H. Novel clearance mechanisms of platelets. Curr Opin Hematol 2010;17:585–9.

Index

Note: Page numbers of article titles are in **boldface** type.

Vet Clin Small Anim 42 (2012) 203–217
doi:10.1016/S0195-5616(11)00213-0
0195-5616/12/$ – see front matter © 2012 Elsevier Inc. All rights reserved.

vetsmall.theclinics.com

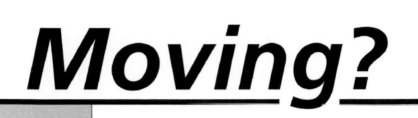

Moving?

Make sure your subscription moves with you!

To notify us of your new address, find your **Clinics Account Number** (located on your mailing label above your name), and contact customer service at:

Email: journalscustomerservice-usa@elsevier.com

800-654-2452 (subscribers in the U.S. & Canada)
314-447-8871 (subscribers outside of the U.S. & Canada)

Fax number: 314-447-8029

Elsevier Health Sciences Division
Subscription Customer Service
3251 Riverport Lane
Maryland Heights, MO 63043

*To ensure uninterrupted delivery of your subscription,
please notify us at least 4 weeks in advance of move.